Case History and
Data Interpretation
in Medical Practice

Case History and Data Interpretation in Medical Practice

Concerned mainly with Case Histories, Data Interpretation,
Cardiac Catheter, Pedigree, Spirometry,
Pictures of Multiple Diseases and a Brief Short Notes

Third Edition

ABM Abdullah MRCP (UK) FRCP (Edin)
Dean
Faculty of Medicine
and
Professor of Medicine
Bangabandhu Sheikh Mujib Medical University
Dhaka, Bangladesh

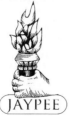

JAYPEE *The Health Sciences Publishers*

New Delhi | London | Philadelphia | Panama

Jaypee Brothers Medical Publishers (P) Ltd

Headquarters

Jaypee Brothers Medical Publishers (P) Ltd
4838/24, Ansari Road, Daryaganj
New Delhi 110 002, India
Phone: +91-11-43574357
Fax: +91-11-43574314
Email: jaypee@jaypeebrothers.com

Overseas Offices

J.P. Medical Ltd
83 Victoria Street, London
SW1H 0HW (UK)
Phone: +44 20 3170 8910
Fax: +44 (0)20 3008 6180
Email: info@jpmedpub.com

Jaypee Medical Inc
The Bourse
111 South Independence Mall East
Suite 835, Philadelphia, PA 19106, USA
Phone: +1 267-519-9789
Email: jpmed.us@gmail.com

Jaypee Brothers Medical Publishers (P) Ltd

Bhotahity, Kathmandu, Nepal
Phone: +977-9741283608
Email: kathmandu@jaypeebrothers.com

Jaypee-Highlights Medical Publishers Inc
City of Knowledge, Bld. 237, Clayton
Panama City, Panama
Phone: +1 507-301-0496
Fax: +1 507-301-0499
Email: cservice@jphmedical.com

Jaypee Brothers Medical Publishers (P) Ltd
17/1-B Babar Road, Block-B, Shaymali
Mohammadpur, Dhaka-1207
Bangladesh
Mobile: +08801912003485
Email: jaypeedhaka@gmail.com

Website: www.jaypeebrothers.com
Website: www.jaypeedigital.com

Case History and Data Interpretation in Medical Practice
First Edition: 2006
Second Edition: 2010
Third Edition: **2015**
ISBN 978-93-5152-375-8
Printed at : Samrat Offset Pvt. Ltd.

"Some patients, though conscious that their condition is perilous, recover their health simply through their contentment with the goodness of the physician."

— Hippocrates, 400 BC

Dedicated to

Professor AKM Rafique Uddin
Ex-Professor and Head, Department of Medicine
Dhaka Medical College and Hospital
Dhaka, Bangladesh

Preface to the Third Edition

Wide acceptability by the students, many doctors and senior teachers encouraged me to prepare the third edition of this book. Medicine is an enormously expanding subject with no leaps and bounds. This new edition is designed with presentation of many common and uncommon medical scenarios that I have faced in my day-to-day practice. With advancement of knowledge and new invention, I have also added new cases, new data, and latest information as far as possible. Also, I have added many new photographs.

In the answer part, a detail description of the disease is provided, so that the reader can gain basic information of the specific disease, even without going through a voluminous textbook. The skills needed to be competent clinician can only be mastered by thinking and exercising the brain, which are the essential part applied in this book.

My special thanks to Shri Jitendar P Vij (Group Chairman), Mr Ankit Vij (Group President), Mr Tarun Duneja (Director–Publishing), Ms Samina Khan, Mr Rajesh Sharma, Mr Prasun Kumar, Mr Kulwant Singh, Mr Sumit Kumar, and other staff of M/s Jaypee Brothers Medical Publishers (P) Ltd, New Delhi, India, for their untiring endeavor and hard work, which made it possible for the timely publication of this book.

Last but not least, I do not know how to express my gratitude to my wife and children for their untiring support, sacrifice, tolerance and understanding during preparation of such a book.

I would like to invite constructive criticism and suggestions regarding this book from my readers, students, colleagues and doctors that would help me improve it further.

ABM Abdullah

Preface to the First Edition

Case history and data interpretation are becoming a very important tool in clinical medicine. These are designed and formulated in such a way that maximum time may be used by the candidate in thinking and minimum in writing, the best way of brain exercise. I think, this will increase a doctor's competence, confidence, efficiency and skill, in diagnosing a particular disease, formulating specific investigations and proper management. In addition, it is the best tool to be a good clinician and physician.

One must remember that specific answer is required, and if there are multiple possibilities, the best one should be mentioned. Answer must be precise and specific, vague one should be avoided. In this book, I have prepared many long and short questions with proper investigations, largely based on the real cases. Answers are given with brief short notes of the specific problems, so that the candidate may get some idea without going through a big textbook.

Questions are fun to do and answers are instructive. I hope, postgraduate students and other equivalent doctors will find this book a very useful one and will enjoy the questions. I do not claim that this book is adequate for the complete clinical medicine and one must consult standard textbook.

I would invite and appreciate the constructive criticism and good suggestions from the valued readers. I must apologize for the printing mistakes, which, in spite of my best effort, have shown their ugly face.

I gratefully acknowledge the publications and books, from where much information have been taken and included. I am always grateful and thankful to all my students who were repeatedly demanding and encouraged me for writing such a book. I am grateful to Kh Atikur Rahman (Shamim), Md Oliullah and Mr Biswanath Bhattacharjee (Kazal) for their great help in computer composing and graphic designing that made the book a beautiful and attractive one. My special thanks to Mr Saiful Islam Khan, proprietor and other staffs of "Asian Color Printing" whose hard work and cooperation have made almost "painless delivery" of this book.

Last but not least, I would like to express my gratitude to my wife and children for their untiring support, sacrifice and encouragement in preparing such a book of its kind.

ABM Abdullah

Acknowledgments

I had the opportunity to work with many skilled and perspicacious clinicians, from whom I have learned much of clinical medicine and still learning. I pay my gratitude and heartiest respect to them. I am also grateful to those patients whose clinical history and investigations are mentioned in this book. I would like to express my humble respect and gratefulness to Prof Pran Gopal Datta, Vice-Chancellor, Bangabandhu Sheikh Mujib Medical University, Dhaka, Bangladesh, whose valuable suggestions, continuous encouragement and support helped me to prepare this book. I am also highly grateful to Dr Ahmed-Al-Muntasir-Niloy and Dr Mohammad Abul Kalam Azad, who have worked hard, checking the whole manuscript and making necessary corrections and modifications.

I also acknowledge the contributions of my teachers, colleagues, doctors and students, who helped me by providing pictures, advice, corrections and many new clinical problems:

❖ Prof MA Zaman, MRCP (UK), FRCP (Glasgow), FRCP (London)
❖ Prof MU Kabir Chowdhury, FRCP (Glasgow)
❖ Prof Md Gofranul Hoque, FCPS
❖ Prof AKM Khorshed Alam, FCPS
❖ Prof Md Abdul Mannan MD (EM), MCPS (Medicine), PhD (Endocrine)
❖ Prof Md Farid Uddin DEM, MD (EM)
❖ Prof Akhtarun Naher M Phil (Microbiology), WHO (Fellow)
❖ Dr Moral Nazrul Islam, MBBS (Dhaka), DD (Singapore), FDCS, FICD, DHRS (USA), Fellow, University of Miami School of Medicine, Florida, USA
❖ Dr Tahmida Hassan, MBBS, DDV, MD
❖ Dr Tazin Afrose Shah, FCPS (Medicine)
❖ Dr Shahnoor Sharmin, MCPS, FCPS, MD (Cardiology)
❖ Dr Mohammad Abul Kalam Azad, MBBS, FCPS (Medicine)
❖ Dr Md Razibul Alam, MBBS, MD, BSMMU
❖ Dr Samprity Islam, MBBS, BSMMU
❖ Dr Sadi Abdullah, MBBS, DTCD (DU)
❖ Dr Imtiaz Ahmed, MBBS
❖ Dr Faiza Mukarrama, MBBS
❖ Dr Sadia Sabah, MBBS
❖ Dr Shakawat Hossain (Rokon), MBBS.

Acknowledgments

Contents

Case History and Data Interpretation

(For answers: See page 315-445)

"It is impossible for anyone to find the correct function of any part unless he is perfectly acquainted with the action of the whole instrument."

— Galen

"It is much more important to know what sort of patient has a disease than what sort of disease a patient has,"

— Sir William Osler

CASE NO. 001

A man of 63 years presented with the complaints of weakness, dizziness, lethargy, palpitation, breathlessness on mild exertion and weight loss for 6 months.

On examination, appearance—pigmented, anemia—moderate, jaundice—nil, edema—mild, pitting. BP—90/60 mm Hg, pulse—110/min. No other physical findings.

Investigations

❖ Urine	- Protein (+).
❖ Full blood count	- Hb – 7.2 g/dL, WBC – 4,000/cmm, Poly – 55%, lympho – 45%, Platelets – 1,90,000/cmm, ESR – 52 mm in 1st h.
❖ Peripheral blood film (PBF)	- Microcytic, hypochromic, Few normocytic and normochromic.
❖ Reticulocyte count	- 0.8% (normal 0.2 to 2%).
❖ Bilirubin	- 28 µmol/L (normal 2 to 17).
❖ Serum glutamic-pyruvic transaminase (SGPT)	- 39 IU/L (normal 10 to 40).
❖ Alkaline phosphatase	- 110 IU/L (normal 25 to 100).
❖ Serum creatinine	- 1.3 mg/dL (normal 0.5 to 1.13).
❖ Serum iron	- 45 µmol/L (normal 4 to 30).
❖ Total iron-binding capacity (TIBC)	- 88 µmol/L (normal 45 to 72).
❖ Serum ferritin	- 550 µg/L (normal 20 to 300).

QUESTIONS

a. What is the likely diagnosis?
b. Mention one investigation to confirm your diagnosis.
c. Suggest one single therapeutic advice to the patient.

CASE NO. 002

A 27-year-old female with 8 months pregnancy is referred for jaundice. She is admitted in the hospital with suspected pre-eclampsia. No significant past medical history.

On examination, the patient is ill looking, anemia—moderate, jaundice—moderate, and edema—mild and pitting. BP—150/105 mm Hg. Examination of other systems—no abnormality.

Investigations

❖ Urine	- Protein (++).
❖ Full blood count	- Hb – 8.2 g/dL, WBC – 15,000/cmm, poly – 75%, lympho – 25%, platelets – 90,000/cmm, ESR – 62 mm in 1st h.
❖ Bilirubin	- 118 µmol/L (normal 2 to 17).

❖ Serum glutamic-
pyruvic transaminase
(SGPT)   - 99 IU/L (normal 5 to 40).
❖ Alkaline phosphatase - 290 IU/L (normal 20 to 100).
❖ Serum creatinine   - 1.3 mg/dL (normal 0.5 to 1.13).
❖ Serum electrolytes   - Sodium—138 mmol/L. Chloride—100 mmol/L. Potassium—
4.6 mmol/L. Bicarbonate—23 mmol/L.

QUESTIONS

a. What is your diagnosis?
b. What two further investigations would you suggest?
c. What treatment would you give?

CASE NO. 003

A 49-year-old lady, non-diabetic and non-hypertensive, presented with frequent attacks of dizziness, vertigo, palpitation, weakness and sweating for 10 months. Initially, these symptoms were present in the morning after waking from sleep and relieved by breakfast. For the last 6 months, these symptoms are more frequent any time of the day and relieved by taking food. Recently, the patient has gained weight of about 12 kg.

On examination, the patient looks obese, multiple linear striae are present. BP—130/80 mm Hg, pulse—84/min.
Examinations of other systems reveal no abnormality.

QUESTIONS

a. What is your diagnosis?
b. Suggest one alternative diagnosis.
c. Suggest two other causes of such case.
d. Suggest three investigations.

CASE NO. 004

A 16-year-old school student has been suffering from weakness, polyuria, nocturia and cramps in legs for 3 years. No history of diarrhea or vomiting. No significant past medical history.

On examination, the patient looks emaciated, moderately anemic. BP—110/75 mm Hg, pulse—76/min. Muscle power and tone–diminished. All reflexes–diminished. Other systems reveal no abnormality.

Investigations

❖ Full blood count   - Hb – 10.2 g/dL, WBC – 10,000/cmm, poly – 65%, lympho – 35%,
platelets – 2,70,000/cmm, ESR – 42 mm in 1st h.
❖ RBS   - 6.1 mmol/L.
❖ Urine   - Protein (+).
❖ Serum creatinine   - 1.1 mg/dL.

* Serum electrolytes - Sodium 141 mmol/L. Chloride 100 mmol/L.
                        Potassium 2.6 mmol/L. Bicarbonate 32 mmol/L.
* USG of abdomen   - Normal.
* Chest X-ray   - Normal.

QUESTIONS

a. What is your diagnosis?
b. Suggest three further investigations.
c. Suggest two differential diagnoses.

CASE NO. 005

A 35-year-old receptionist is admitted in the surgical unit with severe abdominal pain, frequent vomiting and constipation for 9 days. On inquiry, it was found that she had similar attack many times since 10 years and she was admitted four times in the hospital. Five years back, appendicectomy was done, but her symptoms did not improve. For the last 6 months, she is complaining of insomnia, anxiety and confusion.

On examination, BP—160/115 mm Hg, pulse—124/min, abdomen—diffuse tenderness. No other physical findings.

Investigations

* Full blood count   - Hb – 12.2 g/dL, WBC – 13,900/cmm, poly – 62%, lympho – 35%,
                        eosinophil – 3%, platelets – 2,90,000/cmm, ESR – 42 mm in 1st hr.
* Random blood
  sugar (RBS)   - 7.1 mmol/L.
* Urine R/E   - Normal.
* Serum creatinine   - 1.2 mg/dL.
* Serum electrolytes - Sodium 131 mmol/L. Chloride 98 mmol/L.
                        Potassium 4.6 mmol/L. Bicarbonate 26 mmol/L.
* Serum bilirubin   - 55 µmol/L (normal 2 to 17).
* SGPT   - 96 IU/L (normal 10 to 40).
* USG of abdomen   - Normal.
* X-ray chest   - Normal.
* Barium meal   - Normal.
* Follow through
  Barium enema   - Normal.

QUESTIONS

a. What is your diagnosis?
b. List three investigations for your diagnosis.

CASE NO. 006

A 30-year-old housewife, living in a slum area, is complaining of severe pain in lower abdomen, high grade, continuous fever, burning micturition and purulent vaginal discharge for 2 days.

She was given oral antibiotic and pain-killer (indomethacin) as suppository. After 3 days, she is hospitalized, because of severe pain in right hypochondrium, which radiates to the right shoulder, associated with vomiting and dry cough.

On examination, looks ill, dehydrated. BP—90/60 mm Hg, pulse—120/min, temperature—38.9°C.

Liver—enlarged, 2 cm, tender. Hepatic rub—present. Stony dull in right lower chest with absent breath sound.

QUESTIONS

a. What is your diagnosis?
b. Suggest two differential diagnoses.
c. Suggest four investigations.

CASE NO. 007

A 39-year-old school teacher presented with low grade continuous fever, pain in multiple joints, weight loss and dry cough for 6 months. For the last 3 months, she is also complaining of swelling of both parotid gland and few red lesions in the leg.

On examination, the patient is ill looking and emaciated, BP—95/60 mm Hg, pulse—106/min.

Temperature—37.8°C. Both parotid glands are enlarged. One right supraclavicular lymph node is palpable and non-tender. Spleen—just palpable. No hepatomegaly .

QUESTIONS

a. Suggest four differential diagnoses.
b. What is the likely diagnosis?
c. Suggest five investigations.

CASE NO. 008

A 20-year-old student presented with gross hematuria, 3 days after sore throat, fever and headache. There is no significant past medical history.

On examination, no abnormality in general examination. Throat—congested with enlarged tonsils. BP—110/70 mm Hg, pulse—80/min, temperature—38.2°C. Examination of other systems reveals no abnormality.

Investigations

❖ Full blood count	-	Hb – 14.3 g/dL, WBC – 10,900/cmm, poly – 62%, lympho – 38%, platelets – 3,95,000/cmm, ESR – 55 mm in 1st hour.
❖ Urine microscopy	-	Red cell casts (+++) and granular casts (+++).
❖ Urinary protein	-	0.16 g/24 hours
❖ Urea	-	3.6 mmol/L.
❖ Creatinine	-	1.2 mg/dL.
❖ Serum electrolytes	-	Sodium 138 mmol/L. Potassium 4.2 mmol/L. Bicarbonate 26 mmol/L. Chloride 101 mmol/L.
❖ Creatinine clearance	-	68 mL/min (normal 98 to 168).

❖ Throat swab   - No growth.
❖ Chest X-ray   - Normal.
❖ USG of abdomen   - Cortex and medulla of both kidneys are irregular.

QUESTIONS

a. What is the most likely diagnosis?
b. Suggest three diagnostically helpful investigations.
c. Mention one alternative diagnosis.

CASE NO. 009

A 31-year-old housewife has been suffering from occasional loose motions, weight loss, weakness, palpitation and insomnia for 6 months. She was hospitalized. Three days before admission, she has been suffering from high grade, continuous fever, cough with yellow sputum, right-sided chest pain, nausea and vomiting. On the 3rd day, she feels drowsiness, dizziness, followed by confusion, incoherent talk and delirium.

On examination, the patient looks very anxious and emaciated. Anemia—mild, few submandibular lymph nodes palpable, small smooth goiter is present, temperature—40°C, BP—160/70 mm Hg, pulse—140/min, irregularly irregular.
Heart—systolic murmur in pulmonary area.

Investigations

❖ Full blood count   - Hb – 10.5 g/dL, WBC – 23,540/cmm, poly – 88%, lympho – 12%, platelets – 1,80,000/cmm, ESR – 49 mm in 1st h.
❖ Chest X-ray   - Homognous opacity in the left upper zone.
❖ ECG   - Atrial fibrillation.
❖ RBS   - 12.1 mmol/L.
❖ Serum electrolytes - Sodium 128 mmol/L. Potassium 4.1 mmol/L. Bicarbonate 21.8 mmol/L. Chloride 105 mmol/L.
❖ Urea   - 45 mg/dL.
❖ Creatinine   - 1.2 mg/dL.

QUESTIONS

a. What is the likely diagnosis?
b. What investigation should be done to confirm your diagnosis?

CASE NO. 010

A 70-year-old lady is suffering from fever, frequency of micturition and feeling unwell for 10 days. She is hospitalized, because of confusion, drowsiness, followed by unconsciousness. There was no history of diabetes mellitus, hypertension or any drug intake.

On examination, the patient is semiconscious, response to painful stimulus, tongue—dry, skin turgor—reduced, BP—90/60 mm Hg, pulse—110/min, low volume. Temperature—39.2°C. Neck rigidity—slightly present. Plantar—extensor on both sides. Lower abdomen—very tender.

Investigations

- Full blood count   - Hb – 11.2 g/dL, WBC – 17,000/cmm, poly – 85%, lympho – 15%, platelets 2,10,000/cmm, ESR – 12 mm in 1st hr.
- Serum electrolytes   - Sodium 158 mmol/L. Chloride 110 mmol/L. Potassium 4.6 mmol/L. Bicarbonate 19 mmol/L.
- Bilirubin   - 18 µmol/L (Normal 2 to17).
- SGPT   - 29 IU/L (Normal 10 to 40).
- Alkaline phosphatase - 90 IU/L (Normal 20 to100).
- Serum creatinine   - 1.4 mg/ dL (Norma 0.8 to1.2).
- Serum urea   - 38 mg/dL (Normal 20 to 40).
- Urine   - Plenty of pus cells, albumin (++), glucose (+++).
- Chest X-ray   - Normal.
- CT scan of brain   - Diffuse age-related cerebral atrophy.

QUESTIONS

a. What is the likely diagnosis?
b. Suggest four investigations.
c. What immediate therapeutic measures would you start?

CASE NO. 011

A 59-year-old man, smoker, diabetic had an attack of acute myocardial infarction. During recovery, on the 3rd day of illness, he developed sudden blindness.

There is no significant finding on general examination. BP—100/60 mm Hg, pulse—82/min, irregular. Heart—pansystolic murmur in mitral area. Lungs and abdomen – no abnormality. Pupil—normal in size and shape, equally reactive to light and accommodation. No other neurological finding. Fundoscopy—normal.

QUESTIONS

a. Where is the site of lesion of blindness?
b. What is the likely cause?
c. Suggest one investigation to confirm your diagnosis.
d. What is the prognosis?
e. Mention two causes of murmur.

CASE NO. 012

A 29-year-old clerk is hospitalized with the complaints of high grade, continuous fever, polyarthritis involving all the joints, generalized bodyache, right-sided chest pain, abdominal pain, nausea and occasional vomiting for 8 weeks. She also lost weight about 3 kg within this period. There is no history of cough or hemoptysis.

On examination, the patients—looks unwell, anemia—moderate, cervical and inguinal lymphadenopathy, which are soft, discrete and non-tender. Liver—enlarged, 2 cm, non-tender. Spleen—just palpable. Pleural rub—present on right lower chest. Abdomen—diffusely tender and slightly rigid. Both knee joints—swollen and tender. Cervical spine—painful restricted movement. Left shoulder and both wrist joints are tender.

Investigations

- ❖ Full blood count - Hb – 8.5 g/dL, WBC – 33, 540/cmm, poly – 81%, lympho – 19%, platelets–1,88,000/cmm, ESR – 138 mm in 1st hour.
- ❖ Chest X-ray - Small consolidation in right lower zone with small pleural effusion on left.
- ❖ RBS - 8.1 mmol/L.
- ❖ Blood and urine C/S - No growth.
- ❖ RA test and ANA - Negative.
- ❖ CRP - 54 g/L (normal <10).
- ❖ ASO titer - 400 IU/L.
- ❖ Urea - 45 mg/dL.
- ❖ Creatinine - 1.2 mg/dL.
- ❖ USG of abdomen - Hepatosplenomegaly, mild ascites and para-aortic lymphadenopathy.

QUESTIONS

a. What further history will you take from the patient?
b. What diagnosis would you consider first?
c. Suggest two differential diagnoses.
d. Suggest three investigations.

CASE NO. 013

An 18-year-old girl presented with the complaints of irregular menstruation and hirsutism. The problem is present for 4 years, but becoming worse for the last 1 year, for which she was always depressed.

Investigations	Result	Normal value
1. TSH	1.8 mIU/L	< 5.5 mIU/L
2. Prolactin	295 u/L	< 400 u/L
3. LH	19.3 u/L	1 to 13 u/L
4. FSH	21.1 u/L	4 to 13 u/L
5. Testosterone	34.9 u/L	1 to 12 u/L
6. 17-hydroxyprogesterone and 30 minutes after synacthen injection	13 nmol/L 272 nmol/L	1 to 12 nmol/L

QUESTIONS

a. What is the diagnosis?
b. Suggest one alternative diagnosis.
c. What test should be done to differentiate between these two?
d. What is the treatment?
e. Suggest two investigations for your diagnosis.

CASE NO. 014

A young patient is hospitalized with the complaints of high fever, severe headache, repeated vomiting and exhaustion for 6 days. One day before admission, he noticed some red spots in different parts of the body.

On examination, the patient looks toxic, anemia—mild, jaundice—nil. Temperature—104°F, BP—90/60 mm Hg. pulse—110/min. Few petechial rash in trunk and some red spots in different parts of the body. Neck rigidity—slight. Kernig's sign—absent. Fundoscopy—normal. No other physical findings.

Investigations

- ❖ Full blood count - Hb – 11.9 g/dL, WBC – 26,000/cmm, poly – 87%, lympho – 13%, ESR – 40 mm in 1st hr, platelets – 80,000/cmm.
- ❖ Urine - Few pus cells, protein (+).
- ❖ Chest X-ray - Normal.
- ❖ Serum electrolytes - Sodium 140 mmol/L. Chloride 100 mmol/L. Potassium 3.9 mmol/L. Bicarbonate 22 mmol/L.
- ❖ Blood glucose - 3.2 mmol/L.
- ❖ ECG - Sinus tachycardia.

QUESTIONS

a. What is the likely diagnosis?
b. Suggest one alternative diagnosis.
c. Suggest three investigations.
d. Mention one confirmatory test for your diagnosis.
e. Suggest one further investigation.

CASE NO. 015

A 59-year-old, retired male was suffering from chronic liver disease with hepatitis B infection for 3 years. For the last one month, he has been suffering from weakness, anorexia, abdominal distension and jaundice. He was on diuretics and vitamins. For the last 9 days, he was hospitalized because of increasing abdominal distension, diffuse abdominal pain, scanty urine and continuous fever.

On examination, the patient is pale, anemia—moderate, jaundice—mild, BP—105/60 mm Hg, pulse—70/min. Ascites—huge, spleen—just palpable, abdomen—mild diffuse tenderness present.

Investigations

- ❖ Full blood count - Hb –8.5 g/dL, WBC –13,540/cmm, poly – 84%, lympho – 13%, eosinophil-3%, platelets – 88,000/cmm, ESR – 88 mm in 1st hour.
- ❖ Chest X-ray - Bilateral mild pleural effusion.
- ❖ ECG - Normal.
- ❖ RBS - 8.1 mmol/L.
- ❖ Urine - A few pus cells.
- ❖ Urea - 25 mg/dL.
- ❖ Creatinine - 1.2 mg/dL.
- ❖ USG of abdomen - Liver—small with high, coarse echogenicity, splenomegaly and huge ascites.

QUESTIONS

a. What is the likely diagnosis?
b. What single investigation would you suggest?
c. Mention one specific treatment may be required in such case.

CASE NO. 016

A 26-year-old lady developed nausea, vomiting and severe abdominal pain for one week. She is also complaining of pain in both hip joints for the same duration. There is no history of trauma. She has been suffering from SLE for 5 years, well controlled with steroid and chloroquine.

On examination, she looks—pale, anemia—moderate, jaundice—absent. Liver—just palpable, non-tender, spleen—enlarged 1 cm. Abdomen—diffusely tender.

Investigations

❖ Full blood count   - Hb – 8.2 g/dL, WBC – 10,100/cmm, poly – 76%, lympho – 24%
                          ESR – 90 mm in 1st hour.
❖ Urine   - Plenty of pus cells, albumin (++), glucose (+).
❖ Serum creatinine   - 1.1 mg/dL.
❖ Serum urea   - 38 mg/dL.
❖ Chest X-ray   - Normal.
❖ Plain X-ray abdomen - Subacute intestinal obstruction.
❖ Electrolytes   - Sodium 129 mmol/L. Chloride 98 mmol/L. Potassium 4.6 mmol/L.
                          Bicarbonate 23 mmol/L.
❖ Bilirubin   - 17 µmol/L (Normal 2 to17).
❖ SGPT   - 35 IU/L (Normal 20 to 40).
❖ Alkaline phosphatase - 93 IU/L (Normal 40 to 100).

QUESTIONS

a. What is the diagnosis?
b. What is the cause of her hip pain?
c. Suggest one definite investigation for her hip pain.

CASE NO. 017

A lady of 62 years was admitted in the hospital with the history of confusion, incoherent talk, difficulty in breathing and incontinence of urine for 2 days. Six hours after admission, she became unconscious. Five days before this, there was a history of fall with fracture of neck of right femur. No significant past medical history.

On examination, the patient looks unwell, responds to painful stimuli, BP—105/65 mm Hg, pulse—58/min, neck rigidity—absent, plantar—extensor on both sides. Examination of other systems reveal no abnormality.

Investigations

- ❖ Full blood count   - Hb—12.7 g/dL, WBC—5,200/cmm, poly—62%, lympho—38%, ESR—30 mm in 1st hour, platelets—1,80,000/cmm.
- ❖ Blood sugar   - 5.1 mmol/L.
- ❖ Serum electrolytes - Sodium 142 mmol/L. Chloride 102 mmol/L. Potassium 4 mmol/L. Bicarbonate 23 mmol/L.

QUESTIONS

a. What is the likely diagnosis?
b. Suggest two investigations.

CASE NO. 018

A lady aged 32 years is referred from obstetric department for an urgent medical opinion. Two days after delivery, the patient developed cough with profuse frothy sputum, respiratory distress with difficulty on lying flat, compression in the chest and sweating. She was otherwise well before delivery. She is the mother of two children. No significant past medical history.

On examination, the patient looks exhausted, sweaty and dyspneic. Cyanosis—mild and central. Anemia—moderate, edema—present and pitting. BP—95/55 mm Hg, pulse—120/min, irregular. Respiratory rate—26/min. JVP—raised, pulsatile. Liver—enlarged, 3 cm and tender. Heart—apex shifted to the left, pansystolic murmur in mitral area. Bilateral basal crepitations—present.

Investigations

- ❖ Full blood count   - Hb – 8.7 gm/dl, WBC – 13,640/cmm, poly – 80%, lympho – 20%, platelets – 2,88,000/cmm, ESR – 78 mm in 1st hr.
- ❖ Chest X-ray   - Cardiomegaly, upper lobe diversion and small bilateral pleural effusion.
- ❖ RBS   - 7.1 mmol/L.
- ❖ Urea   - 35 mg/dL.
- ❖ Creatinine   - 1.6 mg/dL.
- ❖ USG of abdomen   - Hepatomegaly and bulky uterus.
- ❖ ECG   - Low voltage and atrial fibrillation.

QUESTIONS

a. What is the likely diagnosis?
b. What two investigations would you suggest?

CASE NO. 019

A 52-year-old woman presented with frequency of micturition, extreme weakness, loss of appetite, constipation, abdominal pain and weight loss for 7 months. On examination, anemia—mild, tongue—dry, BP—140/100 mm Hg, pulse—86/min. Tenderness in epigastric region, no organomegaly.

Investigations

❖ Full blood count	-	Hb – 10.6 g/dL, WBC – 8,900/cmm
❖		poly – 55%, lympho – 43%, mono – 2%, ESR – 90 mm in 1st hr,
❖ Plain X-ray KUB	-	Nephrocalcinosis.
❖ USG of abdomen	-	Calcification in both kidneys.
❖ Urine	-	Protein (+), few pus cells.
❖ RBS	-	6.9 mmol/L.
❖ Urea	-	8.2 mmol/L.
❖ Creatinine	-	1.4 mg/dL.
❖ Serum electrolytes	-	Sodium 139 mmol/L. Chloride 110 mmol/L. Potassium 3.6 mmol/L. Bicarbonate 22 mmol/L.

QUESTIONS

a. What is the likely diagnosis?
b. Suggest five investigations to confirm your diagnosis.
c. What single treatment should be given immediately?

CASE NO. 020

A 23-year-old lady is admitted in the psychiatry department with the complains of violent behavior, refusal of food intake, excitability, no speech or no response to any command and insomnia for the last one month. Her mother told that she was suffering from occasional low grade fever, arthralgia, pain in both eyes with redness, frequency of micturition and weight loss for the last 10 months.

On examination, face—puffy, anemia—severe, edema—pitting and mild. BP—125/75 mmHg, pulse—90/min, spleen—enlarged, 2 cm. Higher psychic functions—no response and uncooperative. Reflexes—all exaggerated. Plantar—equivocal, cranial nerves—apparently normal. Fundoscopy—soft exudate in both eyes.

Investigations

❖ Full blood count	-	Hb – 6.1 g/dL, WBC – 5,600/cmm, poly – 61%, lympho – 36%, eosinophil – 3%, platelets – 87,000/cmm, ESR – 130 mm in 1st hour.
❖ PBF	-	Macrocytosis and polychromasia.
❖ Reticulocyte	-	5.2% (normal 0.2 to 2%).
❖ Coomb's test	-	Positive.
❖ Urine	-	Protein (++).
❖ Chest X-ray	-	Cardiomegaly with small bilateral pleural effusion.
❖ RBS	-	7.1 mmol/L.
❖ Urea	-	35 mg/dL.
❖ Creatinine	-	2.6 mg/dL (normal 0.57 to 1.36).
❖ USG of abdomen	-	Splenomegaly with mild ascites.
❖ CT scan of brain	-	Widening of the cortical sulci with small infarction in the parietal region on left side.

QUESTIONS

a. What is the likely diagnosis?
b. Suggest four investigations.

CASE NO. 021

A 20-year-old student is complaining of sore throat, pain in the right ear with discharge, which developed three days after a trauma in the head during playing. He was always in good health. No fracture in skull, no obvious head injury. After 3 days, he developed high fever, headache, transient loss of consciousness lasted for few seconds, blurring of vision, followed by convulsion. On examination:

* Neck rigidity—present.
* Weakness on the left side of body.
* Musle tone—increase on the left side. All reflexes on the left side—exaggerated.
* Plantar—extensor on both sides.
* Homonymous hemianopia—left side. Ataxia—left side.
* Two-point discrimination—present.
* No sensory change.
* Fundoscopy—normal.

Lumbar puncture and CSF study show:

* Pressure	-	30 cm of H_2O (normal 50 to 180).
* Cells	-	4/cmm, all lymphocytes (normal 0 to 4).
* Protein	-	15 mg/dL (normal 15 to 40).
* Glucose	-	41 mg/dL (normal 28 to 45).

QUESTIONS

a. What is your diagnosis?
b. Suggest three investigations which will help in your diagnosis.

CASE NO. 022

A 27-year-old lady is referred from psychiatry department for an urgent medical opinion. This lady was suffering from psychiatric disorder for 3 years, feeling better with antipsychotic drugs. For the last 3 weeks, she has been suffering from high grade continuous fever, associated with chill and rigor, subsides with high dose paracetamol. She is also complaining of anorexia, loss of weight, difficulty in deglutition, stiffness of muscles, palpitation and syncopal attack. Five years back, she was suffering from pulmonary tuberculosis, completed full course of anti-TB drugs.

On examination, she is emaciated, mildly anemic, BP—90/65 mm Hg, pulse—120/min, Temperature—105.2ºF.

Heart and lungs—Normal. No organomegaly.

Neck rigidity—present. Higher psychic functions—the patient is uncooperative. No or little response to command. Muscle tone—increased in both upper and lower limbs. Musle power—dimnished in both upper and lower limbs. Reflexes—difficult to elicit. Plantar—equivocal on both sides.

Investigations

❖ Full blood count	- Hb—11.1 g/dL, WBC – 15,600/cmm, poly—87%, lympho—13%, platelets—1,87,000/cmm, ESR—60 mm in 1st hour.
❖ Urine	- Pus cells – few and protein (++).
❖ Blood and urine culture	- Negative.
❖ Chest X-ray	- Normal.
❖ RBS	- 7.1 mmol/L.
❖ Urea	- 35 mg/dL.
❖ Creatinine	- 1.2 mg/dL.
❖ Serum electrolytes	- Sodium 138 mmol/L. Potassium 4.2 mmol/L. Bicarbonate 22.8 mmol/L. Chloride 105 mmol/L.
❖ MT	- 12 mm.
❖ USG of abdomen	- Normal.
❖ CT scan of brain	- Normal.

QUESTIONS

a. What is the likely diagnosis?
b. Suggest three investigations.
c. Suggest one investigation helpful to confirm your diagnosis.

CASE NO. 023

A lady aged 70 years presented with the complaints of breathlessness even on mild exertion, occasional dry cough and marked loss of weight for 2 years.

Lung Function Test Shows

❖ Vital capacity	- 2.3 liters/sec (predicted 3.28 to 4.43 L).
❖ FEV$_1$	- 0.7 liters/sec (predicted 2.44 to 3.33 L).
❖ Residual volume	- 5.11 liters/sec (predicted 1.35 to 1.83 L).

QUESTIONS

a. What does this lung function test indicate?
b. What is the likely diagnosis?
c. Suggest two further investigations.

CASE NO. 024

A school-going girl aged 14 years is admitted in a surgical ward with severe acute abdominal pain, repeated vomiting and bloody diarrhea. On the 3rd day, she develops pain in both knee and ankle joints, multiple urticarial rash, few purpura and scanty micturition.

On examination, the patient looks pale, BP—150/100 mm Hg, pulse—100/min, anemia—mild, jaundice—absent. Abdomen—tenderness in the epigastrium and around umbilicus.

Both knee and ankle joint—swollen and tender. Examination of other systems reveals no abnormality.

Investigations

- ❖ Full blood count   - Hb – 9.8 g/dL, WBC – 6,200/cmm, poly – 74%, lympho – 26%, ESR – 57 mm in 1st hr, platelets – 1,95,000/cmm.
- ❖ MCV   - 71 fl.
- ❖ Plain X-ray abdomen - Multiple fluid level and gas shadow.
- ❖ Blood sugar   - 5.1 mmol/L.
- ❖ Serum electrolytes   - Sodium 136 mmol/L. Chloride 98 mmol/L. Potassium 4.1 mmol/L. Bicarbonate 21 mmol/L.
- ❖ Urine   - Protein (+), RBC cast (++).
- ❖ USG of abdomen   - Full of gas shadow.
- ❖ Chest X-ray   - Normal.

QUESTIONS

a. What is your diagnosis?
b. Suggest two investigations which will help in your diagnosis.
c. Suggest one investigation which will help in prognosis.

CASE NO. 025

A young student presented with weakness, anorexia, nausea and high colored urine for 2 days. He was suffering from fever, cough, pain in the throat and headache 10 days back. There is history of previous similar attack several times. No significant past medical illness.

On examination, anemia—mild, jaundice—mild, liver—just palpable, non-tender. No other physical finding.

Investigations

- ❖ Full blood count   - Hb – 10.2 g/dL, ESR – 32 mm in 1st hr, WBC – 9,900/cmm, poly – 61%, lympho – 35%, monocyte – 4%.
- ❖ Reticulocyte count   - 0.7% (normal 0.2 to 2).
- ❖ Total bilirubin   - 52 µmol/L (normal <17).
- ❖ ALT (SGPT)   - 15 IU/L (normal <20).
- ❖ AST (SGOT)   - 21 IU/L (normal <25).
- ❖ Alkaline phosphatase - 42 IU/L (normal 20 to 100).
- ❖ USG of abdomen   - Slight hepatomegaly.

QUESTIONS

a. What is the diagnosis?
b. Suggest two investigations.
c. What treatment would you give to the patient?

CASE NO. 026

A middle-aged man was hospitalized with the complaints of anorexia, nausea, vomiting and frank blood-stained urine. On the third day of illness, there is complete anuria. One day before admission, there was history of fall with multiple injuries in the body, but no fracture.

On examination, face—puffy. BP—160/110 mm Hg, pulse—97/min, anemia—mild, edema—pitting. Multiple bruise and ecchymoses—in trunk and buttock.

Investigations

❖ Full blood count — Hb—9 g/dL, WBC—13,200/cmm, poly—67%, lympho—33% ESR—70 mm in 1st hr, platelets—1,99,000/cmm.
❖ Urea — 14 mmol/L (normal 2.5 to 6.6).
❖ Creatinine — 9 mg/dL (normal 0.68 to 1.36).
❖ Blood sugar — 4.8 mmol/L.
❖ Serum electrolytes — Sodium 132 mmol/L. Chloride 92 mmol/L. Potassium 6.1 mmol/L. Bicarbonate 14 mmol/L.
❖ Urine — Mild proteinuria, no RBC or pus cell.

QUESTIONS

a. What is your diagnosis?
b. Suggest two investigations to confirm your diagnosis.
c. What immediate treatment should be given?

CASE NO. 027

A 68-year-old woman has been suffering from low grade, continuous fever, arthralgia, loss of appetite, sweating mostly at night and weight loss for 5 months. For the last 2 months, she is also complaining of severe pain in both knee joints and frequent headache, mostly on temporal and occipital region with occasional difficulty in vision. There is no history of previous illness. She was treated by local physician by multiple drug, the name of which she could not mention. But no improvement.

Investigations

❖ Full blood count — Hb—9.8 g/dL, WBC—10,500/cmm, poly—63%, lympho—25%, eosinophil—8%, monocyte—4%, platelets—3,98,000/cmm, ESR—135 mm in 1st hour.
❖ Urine — Proteinuria (++), few RBC and pus cells.
❖ Chest X-ray — Normal.
❖ USG of abdomen — Normal.
❖ MT — 07 mm.
❖ CRP — 39 mg/dL (normal <10).
❖ RA test — Negative.
❖ ANA — Negative.
❖ Blood and urine culture — No growth.
❖ CT scan of brain — Mild cerebral atrophy.

QUESTIONS

a. What is the likely diagnosis?
b. Suggest one investigation to confirm the diagnosis.
c. What drug should be started immediately and why?

■ CASE NO. 028

A man aged 40 years presented with the complaints of weight loss, anorexia, occasional loose stool and abdominal distension for 6 months. There is history of itchy vesicular rash on his buttock and around both the knees five years ago. No significant past medical history.

On examination, anemia—moderate, jaundice—absent. Tongue—smooth and shiny. No other abnormality.

Investigations

❖ Full blood count	-	Hb—8.7 g/dL, WBC—10,700/cmm, poly—70%, lympho—30%, ESR—50 mm in 1st hour.
❖ MCHC	-	31.3 g/dL.
❖ MCV	-	98 fl.
❖ USG of abdomen	-	Mild hepatomegaly.
❖ PBF	-	Macrocytosis, microcytosis, anisopoikilocytosis, few pencil cell and hypersegmented neutrophils.
❖ Stool	-	Vegetable cells plenty, no growth on culture.

■ QUESTIONS

a. What is the cause of hematological findings?
b. Suggest the likely diagnosis.
c. What two investigations would confirm the diagnosis?
d. What was the cause of rash?
e. What two additional findings may be seen in blood film?
f. What advice would you give to the patient?

■ CASE NO. 029

A 19-year-old girl is admitted in the hospital with severe abdominal pain, burning micturition, vomiting, bloody diarrhea, bodyache, multiple skin rashes and high fever for 5 days. Her menstruation is irregular, but this time it is persistent for 10 days with heavy bleeding. Tonsillectomy was done at the age of 5 and also appendicectomy at the age of 17 years.

On examination, the patient looks very ill, BP—70/50 mm Hg, pulse—120/min, lower abdomen—very tender. Temperature—39.7°C. There are multiple maculopapular, reddish skin rashes all over the body.

Investigations

❖ Full blood count	-	Hb – 11.3 g/dL, WBC – 19,570/cmm, poly – 86%, lympho – 14%, platelets – 1,00,000/cmm.
❖ Urine	-	Plenty of pus cells and RBCs.
❖ Chest X-ray	-	Normal.
❖ Urea	-	65 mg/dL.
❖ Creatinine	-	1.2 mg/dL.
❖ Serum electrolytes	-	Sodium 125 mmol/L. Potassium 3.1 mmol/L. Bicarbonate 28.8 mmol/L. Chloride 95 mmol/L.
❖ Prothrombin time	-	17.3 sec (control 11).

QUESTIONS

a. What is your diagnosis?
b. Suggest two investigations.
c. What further history would you take?
d. Mention one serious complication.

CASE NO. 030

A lady aged 27 years is admitted in the emergency department with unconsciousness in the morning. She had marital dysharmony for few years. Her husband told that she used to take sleeping tablet, but he does not know the name of the tablet.

On examination, the patient is semiconscious, less response to painful stimulus. BP—80/60 mm Hg. Pulse—140/min. Neck rigidity—present. Muscle tone—increased. All reflexes—exaggerated. Plantar—extensor on both sides. Pupil—dilated. Few spontaneous myoclonic twitching—present. Heart and lungs—normal.

Investigations

❖ Full blood count	- Hb – 12.8 g/dL, WBC – 14,500/cmm, poly – 74%, lympho – 25%, eosinophil – 1%, platelets – 3,90,000/cmm, ESR – 15 mm in 1st hour.
❖ RBS	- 9 mmol/L.
❖ Serum electrolytes	- Sodium 135 mmol/L. Potassium 4.3 mmol/L. Bicarbonate 17.8 mmol/L. Chloride 95 mmol/L.
❖ Urea	- 46 mg/dL.
❖ Creatinine	- 1.3 mg/dL.
❖ Chest X-ray	- Normal.

QUESTIONS

a. What is your diagnosis?
b. Suggest two further investigations.
c. What two therapeutic measures would you start?

CASE NO. 031

A lady aged 61 years, known hypertensive and diabetic, is feeling unwell, weakness and sleeplessness for 10 days. On the day of admission, she was found to be drowsy and hyperventilating. She was on enalapril for hypertension and metformin for diabetes mellitus. There was a past history of myocardial infarction 3 years back with good recovery.

On examination, the patient is drowsy, unable to communicate, also hyperventilating. BP—95/65 mm Hg, pulse—82/min, low volume. No neck rigidity. No focal neurological signs. No other abnormality.

Investigations

❖ Full blood count	- Hb – 13.2 g/dL, WBC – 11,000/cmm, poly – 76%, lympho – 24%, ESR – 50 mm in 1st hour.
❖ RBS	- 11.3 mmol/L.
❖ Serum urea	- 9.1 mmol/L.
❖ Serum creatinine	- 1.2 mg/dL.

❖ Serum electrolytes   - Sodium 143 mmol/L. Chloride 97 mmol/L. Potassium 5.6 mmol/L. Bicarbonate 7.9 mmol/L.

❖ Urine   - Glucose (++).

QUESTIONS

a. What is the likely diagnosis?
b. Suggest three investigations for your diagnosis.
c. What two therapeutic measures should be started?
d. Mention four differential diagnoses of such blood picture.

CASE NO. 032

A 48-year-old man has been suffering from inflammatory bowel disease for 10 years. He is on olsalazine and his disease is well controlled. For the last few weeks, he is suffering from weakness, loss of appetite and weight loss.

On examination—anemia—moderate, clubbing—present. Leukonychia—present. BP—100/60 mm Hg, pulse—74/min. Liver—enlarged, 3 cm, tender, soft in consistency, no bruit.

Investigations

❖ Full blood count   - Hb – 8.3 g/dL, WBC – 6,500/cmm, poly – 66%, lympho – 24%, mono – 3%, eosinophil – 7%, platelets – 2,90,000/cmm, ESR – 20 mm in 1st hour.
❖ MCV   - 69 fl (normal 76 to 96).
❖ Serum bilirubin   - 20 µmol/L (normal 2 to 17).
❖ SGPT   - 117 IU/L (normal 10 to 40).
❖ Alkaline phosphatase - 390 IU/L (normal 25 to 100).
❖ γGT   - 290 IU/L (normal 5 to 30 IU/L).
❖ HBsAg and anti-HCV - Negative.
❖ Total protein   - 59 g/L (normal 62 to 80).
❖ Serum albumin   - 26 g/L (normal 35 to 50).
❖ Prothrombin time   - 12.6 sec (control 11.8).

QUESTIONS

a. What is your diagnosis?
b. Suggest two investigations to confirm your diagnosis.
c. What is the specific treatment?

CASE NO. 033

A 21-year-old student has been suffering from low grade continuous fever, diffuse abdominal pain, nausea, weight loss and constipation for 2 months. For the last 3 weeks, he noticed gradual abdominal distension with increasing pain and vomiting.

On examination, the patitent is emaciated, anemia—moderate, no jaundice. No lymphadenopathy. JVP—raised, BP—100/55 mm Hg, pulse—120/min. Liver—just palpable, ascites—moderate. Heart and lungs—Normal.

Investigations

- ❖ Full blood count — Hb – 8.0 g/dL, WBC – 9,000/cmm, poly – 62%, lympho – 35%, eosinophil – 3%, platelets – 3,10,000/cmm, ESR – 95 mm in 1st hour.
- ❖ RBS — 4.1 mmol/L.
- ❖ Serum electrolytes — Sodium 134 mmol/L. Potassium 3.4 mmol/L. Bicarbonate 28.1 mmol/L. Chloride 97 mmol/L.
- ❖ Urea — 36 mg/dL (normal 9 to 11).
- ❖ Creatinine — 1.1 mg/dL (normal 0.68 to 1.36).
- ❖ Serum bilirubin — 20 μmol/L (normal 2 to 17).
- ❖ SGPT — 37 IU/L (normal 5 to 40).
- ❖ Alkaline phosphatase — 100 IU/L (normal 20 to 100).
- ❖ Total protein — 61 g/L (normal 62 to 80).
- ❖ Serum albumin — 32 g/L (normal 35 to 50).
- ❖ Prothrombin time — 12.3 sec (control 11.8).
- ❖ USG of abdomen — Huge ascites.
- ❖ Endoscopy — Normal.

QUESTIONS

a. What is your diagnosis?
b. Suggest five investigations.
c. Mention two differential diagnoses.

CASE NO. 034

A middle-aged housewife presented with weakness, tiredness, breathlessness on exertion, loss of weight and anorexia for 6 months. She was always in good health.

On examination, she is pale and ill looking, anemia—severe, jaundice—mild, edema—mild, pitting. Few vitiligos—present in trunk and back. Heart—systolic murmur in pulmonary area. No organomegaly.

Investigations

- ❖ Full blood count — Hb – 6.0 g/dL, WBC – 3,500/cmm, poly – 58%, lympo – 42%, platelets – 1,00,000/cmm.
- ❖ MCV — 112 fl (normal 76 to 95).
- ❖ MCHC — 34 g/dL (normal 32 to 36).
- ❖ Reticulocyte — 1% (normal 0.2 to 2%).
- ❖ PBF — Macrocytosis, hypochromia and few fragmented red cells.
- ❖ Bilirubin — 25 μmol/L (normal 2 to 17).
- ❖ AST (SGOT) — 20 IU/L (normal 7 to 40).
- ❖ ALT (SGPT) — 11 IU/L (normal 5 to 40).
- ❖ Alkaline phosphatase — 55 IU/L (normal 20 to 100).

QUESTIONS

a. What hematological abnormality is seen?
b. Suggest four causes of this hematological abnormality.
c. What is the likely diagnosis?
d. Name four further tests necessary to confirm your diagnosis.
e. Why is mean corpuscular volume (MCV) high?

CASE NO. 035

A 43-year-old man, smoker and alcoholic, is admitted in the hospital with the complaints of drowsiness, confusion, incoherent talk and disorientation. He has been suffering from peptic ulcer for 10 years. For the last 5 months, he had frequent vomiting. Sometimes, there is history of induced vomiting.

On examination, BP – 90/60 mm Hg, pulse – 110/min, low volume, dehydration – present. Liver – enlarged, 3 cm, non-tender, firm in consistency.

No neck rigidity. Eye movement – right lateral rectus palsy. Nystagmus – both horizontal and vertical. Ataxia – present. Musle tone – increased, muscle power–diminished.
Reflex – exaggerated both in upper and lower limbs. Plantar–extensor on both sides.

Investigations

❖ Full blood count	-	Hb – 12.3 gm/dl, WBC – 11,000/cmm, poly – 70%, lympho – 29%, eosinophil – 1%, platelets – 3,65,000/cmm, ESR – 15 mm in 1st hour.
❖ RBS	-	8.1 mmol/L.
❖ Serum electrolytes	-	Sodium 131 mmol/L. Potassium 3.3 mmol/L. Bicarbonate 27.8 mmol/L. Chloride 95 mmol/L.
❖ Urea	-	86 mg/dL.
❖ Creatinine	-	1.3 mg/dL.
❖ Serum bilirubin	-	24 µmol/L.
❖ SGPT	-	37 IU/L.
❖ Alkaline phosphatase	-	100 IU/L (normal 25 to 100).
❖ GGT	-	39 IU/L (normal 5 to 30 IU/L).
❖ Total protein	-	60 g/L.
❖ Serum albumin	-	30 g/L.

QUESTIONS

a. What is your diagnosis?
b. What treatment should be given?
c. Suggest four investigations.

CASE NO. 036

A 62-year-old man presented with difficulty in walking and standing from sitting, tingling and numbness of upper limb, vertigo, weakness, weight loss, backache and skin rash in different parts of the body for 2 months. She also complains of occasional dry cough and weight loss for the same duration.

On examination, anemia—moderate, BP—100/60 mm Hg, pulse—98/min. Clubbing—present in fingers and toes.

Erythematous skin rashes are present in trunk and buttock.

In the upper limbs—hypertonia in right, normal in left. Reflex—exaggerated in right, diminished in left.

In the lower limbs—hypertonia, power—diminished, reflex—exaggerated, plantar—equivocal on both sides. Sensory—no abnormality. Gait—ataxia, waddling type. Right eye—Partial ptosis, pupil—meiosis, reactive to light.

QUESTIONS

a. What is your diagnosis?
b. Suggest five investigations.
c. What treatment should be given?

CASE NO. 037

A 41-year-old man presented with frequent headache, dizziness, lack of concentration, pruritus and heaviness in the left upper abdomen for 3 months. Previously, he was always in good health.

On examination, BP—140/100 mm Hg, pulse—78/min, spleen—just palpable, no hepatomegaly. Examination of other systems reveals no abnormalities.

Investigations

❖ Full blood count   - Hb – 17.6 g/dL, WBC – 21,000/cmm, poly – 83%, lympo – 15%, eosino – 2%, RBC – 8.2 million/cmm, platelets – 8,50,000/cmm, ESR – 1 mm in 1st hour.
❖ PCV   - 65%.
❖ RBS   - 7.2 mmol/L.
❖ Chest X-ray   - Normal.
❖ X-ray PNS   - Maxillary sinusitis.

QUESTIONS

a. What is your diagnosis?
b. Suggest one investigation.
c. Suggest one treatment.

CASE NO. 038

A 31-year-old young man has been suffering from severe low backache, pain in the neck, both hands and eye for 2 years. There is severe morning stiffness, improved after exercise. For the last 10 years, he has been suffering from multiple skin rashes.

He was suffering from occasional loose motions and frequency of micturition 6 months back.

On examination, BP—110/80 mm Hg, pulse—90/min. All PIP joints of right hand are swollen. There is difficulty in bending forward and backward. Tenderness over the lower part of back is present.

Investigations

❖ Full blood count   - Hb – 10.3 g/dL, WBC – 9,700/cmm, poly – 68%, lympho – 30%, eosinophil – 2%, platelets – 1,90,000/cmm, ESR – 105 mm in 1st hr.
❖ RBS   - 4.1 mmol/L.
❖ X-ray of LS spine   - Both SI joints are hazy, irregular, few syndesmophytes in lumbar vertebrae.

QUESTIONS

a. What is the likely diagnosis?
b. Suggest two investigations.
c. What single therapy would you give?

CASE NO. 039

A 53-year-old man is diagnosed as a case of chronic granulocytic leukemia. He was treated with chemotherapy and responded well. Three years later, the patient presented with the complaints of severe weakness, loss of weight, lethargy, epistaxis and pain in left upper abdomen.

On examination, anemia—severe, jaundice—mild, spleen—huge and tender. Heart and lungs—no abnormality.

Investigations

❖ Full blood count   - Hb – 7.5 g/dL, WBC – 12,800/cmm, platelets – 1,00,000/cmm, RBC – 2.8 million/cmm, ESR – 85 mm in 1st hour.
❖ Differential count   - Neutrophils-34%. Basophil-8%. Lymphocyte-6%. Myeloblast-40%. Myelocyte-10%. Metamyelocyte-2%.

QUESTIONS

a. What is the diagnosis?
b. What is the cause of abdominal pain?
c. Suggest one investigation to confirm your diagnosis.

CASE NO. 040

A 59-year-old lady has been suffering from shortness of breath on mild exertion, loss of appetite, constipation, weakness, tingling and numbness of fingers and toes for 6 months. Cholecystectomy was done 10 years back otherwise she was always in good health.

On examination, the patient is emaciated and ill, anemia—severe, tongue—smooth and shiny, angular stomatitis—present. Other systems no abnormality.

Investigations

- ❖ Full blood count   - Hb – 6.5 g/dL, WBC – 3,000/cmm, poly – 63%, lympho – 27%, mono – 4%, eosino – 6%, platelets – 1,95,000/cmm.
- ❖ MCV   - 112 fl.
- ❖ Urea   - 18 mmol/L.
- ❖ Creatinine   - 110 µmol/L (normal 55 to 125).
- ❖ Serum iron   - 25 µmol/L (normal 16 to 30).
- ❖ TIBC   - 62 µmol/L (normal 45 to 72).
- ❖ Serum B$_{12}$ - 98 ng/L (normal 200 to 800).
- ❖ Folic acid   - 11 µg/L (normal 4 to 18).

She was treated with oral B$_{12}$. Still her blood picture is the same as above.

QUESTIONS

a. Suggest three possible diagnoses of such case.
b. Suggest two investigations.
c. Suggest three other causes of such blood picture.

CASE NO. 041

A 21-year-old, pregnant female, is seen in the outpatient department for routine check-up. She was otherwise in good health.

On examination, anemia—mild, BP—100/70 mm Hg, pulse—110/min. Other systems—no abnormality.

Investigations

- ❖ Full blood count   - Hb – 10.2 g/dL, WBC – 5,000/cmm, poly – 62%, lympho – 28%, mono – 5%, eosinofils – 5%, platelets – 2,95,000/cmm, ESR – 70 mm in 1st hour.
- ❖ MCV   - 67 fl.
- ❖ Serum iron   - 16 µmol/L (normal 16 to 30).
- ❖ TIBC   - 50 µmol/L (normal 45 to 72).
- ❖ PBF   - Target cell, hypochromia and microcytosis.

QUESTIONS

a. Suggest three differential diagnoses.
b. Suggest two further investigations.

CASE NO. 042

A young lady with 4 months pregnancy presented with the complaints of palpitation, excessive sweating and intolerance to heat.

On examination, BP—150/70 mm Hg, pulse—124/min, thyroid gland—diffusely enlarged and non-tender, soft.

Investigations

* Full blood count
  - Hb – 10.5 g/dL, WBC – 9,800/cmm, poly – 66%, lympho – 30%, eosino – 4%, platelets – 2,00,000/cmm, ESR – 85 mm in 1st hour.
* Serum T_4
  - 290 nmol/L (normal 70 to 160).
* Serum T_3
  - 9 nmol/L (normal 1.32 to 3.1).
* Serum TSH
  - 4 mIU/L (normal 1.52 to 5).

QUESTIONS

a. What is your inference from the above result?
b. What further investigations should be done?
c. Mention four causes of such thyroid function abnormality.

CASE NO. 043

A 37-year-old man is presented for routine check-up. He was always in good health, but recently gaining weight about 10 kg in 3 months.

On examination, he looks obese, BP—120/80 mm Hg, pulse—80/min. No other physical findings.

Investigations

* Full blood count
  - Hb – 13.5 g/dL, WBC – 9,800/cmm, poly – 64%, lympho – 36%, platelets – 3,30,000/cmm, ESR – 15 mm in 1st hr.
* Chest X-ray
  - Normal.
* Cholesterol
  - 11.9 mmol/L (normal 3.6 to 7.8).
* Triglyceride
  - 680 mmol/L (normal < 150).
* Serum electrolytes
  - Sodium 90 mmol/L. Potassium 3.5 mmol/L. Bicarbonate 19 mmol/L.
* RBS
  - 9.3 mmol/L.

QUESTIONS

a. What is the likely biochemical diagnosis?
b. What next investigation should be done?

CASE NO. 044

A 50-year-old male, known to be hypertensive, heavy smoker, went to a wedding ceremony. One hour after heavy eating of rich food, he is suffering from nausea, repeated vomiting, breathlessness, upper abdominal pain and severe central chest pain.

On examination, the patient looks dyspneic, exhausted with profuse sweating. BP—100/60 mm Hg, pulse—110/min and low volume. ECG—sinus tachycardia.

QUESTIONS

a. What three differential diagnoses would you consider?
b. Suggest four immediate investigations.

CASE NO. 045

A 40-year-old man presented with the complaints of anorexia, weakness, abdominal pain, occasional diarrhea, dizziness, weight loss and low grade, continuous fever for 3 months. Dizziness is more on standing, with a tendency to fall sometimes.

On examination, the patient is ill-looking, emaciated, BP—90/60 mm Hg, pulse—100/min, anemia—mild. Examination of abdomen reveals slight tenderness in epigastrium. Other systems—no abnormality.

Investigations

* Full blood count   - Hb – 9.5 g/dL, WBC – 5,300/cmm, poly – 45%, lympho – 53%, mono – 2%, ESR – 81 mm in 1st hr, platelets – 2,10,000/cmm.
* MCV   - 84 fl.
* Urea   - 7.8 mmol/L.
* Serum electrolytes   - Sodium 121 mmol/L. Potassium 5.7 mmol/L. Chloride 89 mmol/L.
* RBS   - 3.1 mmol/L.
* Creatinine   - 1.2 mg/dL.
* Urine   - Plenty of pus cells and RBC—10 to 50/HPF.

QUESTIONS

a. What is the underlying diagnosis?
b. Suggest three investigations to confirm the diagnosis.
c. Mention two physical signs you should look for.

CASE NO. 046

A 14-year-old girl is hospitalized because of hematemesis, melena and huge abdominal distension for 10 days.

She had hematemesis and melena many times from the age of 7 and several units of blood transfusion were given in different occasions.

On examination—the patients looks pale, anemia—severe, spleen—enlarged, 7 cm. Ascites—huge.

Investigations

* Full blood count   - Hb – 5.5 g/dL, WBC – 2,000/cmm, poly – 70%, lympho – 20%, mono – 6%, eosino – 4%, platelets – 95,000/cmm.
* PBF   - Microcytic and hypochromic.
* Serum bilirubin   - 12 µmol/L (normal 2 to 17).
* SGPT   - 22 IU/L (normal 5 to 40).
* Alkaline phosphatase - 90 IU/L (normal 20 to 100).
* Total protein   - 55 g/L (normal 62 to 80).
* Serum albumin   - 36 g/L (normal 35 to 50).
* Prothrombin time   - 12.6 sec (control 11.8).
* USG of abdomen   - Huge splenomegaly and huge ascites.
* X-ray chest   - Normal.

❖ Urea   - 30 mg/dL.
❖ Creatinine   - 1.1 mg/dL.
❖ Anti-HCV   - Negative.
❖ HbsAg   - Negative.
❖ Endoscopy   - Esophageal varices, grade II.

QUESTIONS

a. What is the likely diagnosis?
b. Suggest three investigations to confirm your diagnosis.
c. Suggest the treatment which is most helpful in this patient.

CASE NO. 047

A 23-year-old young female, newly married, presented for routine check-up. She was well previously with normal laboratory report. This time urine examination shows glycosuria (++). She was given insulin.

During the subsequent check-up, she complains of palpitation, excessive sweating and weakness.

Investigations

❖ Full blood count   - Hb – 9.5 g/dL, WBC – 9,540/cmm, poly – 75%, lympho – 25%,
                            platelets – 2,80,000/cmm, ESR – 60/h.
❖ RBS   - 2 mmol/L.
❖ Urine   - Glucose (++).

QUESTIONS

a. What is the likely diagnosis?
b. How to explain the blood chemistry?

CASE NO. 048

A 45-year-old, obese lady, complains of increased tendency to sleep, difficulty in breathing with mild exertion, headache, vertigo, lack of concentration and weakness for 10 months.

On examination, BP—160/100 mm Hg, pulse—86/min, multiple linear striae are present in different parts of the body. Weight—96 kg.

Investigations

❖ Full blood count   - Hb – 19.5 g/dL, WBC – 5,900/cmm, poly – 65%, lympho – 33%,
                            mono – 2%, ESR – 15 mm in 1st hour, platelets – 2,30,000/cmm,
                            RBC – 8.6 million/cmm.
❖ Chest X-ray   - Normal.
❖ ECG   - Low voltage tracing with sinus bradycardia.
❖ PEFR   - 350 liters/min (predicted 400).
❖ Arterial blood gases   - PaO_2 8 kPa (60 mm Hg). $PaCO_2$ 7.5 kPa (56 mm Hg).

QUESTIONS

a. What is your diagnosis?
b. Suggest two differential diagnoses.
c. Why is there raised hemoglobin?
d. What does this blood gas show?

CASE NO. 049

A 65-year-old obese woman is hospitalized with the complaints of cough with purulent sputum, fever, chest pain and confusion for 3 days. No significant past medical illness.

On examination, anemia—mild, edema—present and non-pitting. BP—105/60 mm Hg, pulse—52/min.

Investigations

* Full blood count - Hb – 10.5 g/dL, WBC – 8,540/cmm,
                      poly – 72%, lympho – 26%, monocyte – 2%, platelets – 1,80,000/cmm.
* Chest X-ray   - Consolidation (left upper zone).
* ECG   - Low voltage tracing and sinus bradycardia.
* S. electrolytes   - Sodium 135 mmol/L. Potassium 4.1 mmol/L. Bicarbonate 21.8
                      mmol/L. Chloride 115 mmol/L.
* Urea   - 45 mg/dL.
* Creatinine   - 1.2 mg/dL.
* FT_4 - 6 pmol/L (normal 9 to 23).
* TSH   - < 0.1 mIU/L (normal 0.3 to 5).
* MRI of brain   - Normal.

QUESTIONS

a. What is the likely diagnosis of thyroid disorder?
b. What further investigation would you suggest?
c. What is the cause of ECG abnormality?

CASE NO. 050

A lady aged 35 years has been suffering from anxiety and depression for a long time. For the last 6 months, she is complaining of amenorrhea, weight loss, excessive sweating, irritability, tremor of whole body and palpitation.

On examination, the patient is anxious, BP—160/60 mm Hg, pulse—128/min. Tremor of outstretched hands—present. Thyroid—small nodular goiter is present. Systolic flow murmur is present in pulmonary area.

Investigations

* FT_3 - 4.1 pmol/L (normal 1.1 to 3.2).
* FT_4 - 293 pmol/L (normal 9 to 23).
* TSH   - 0.28 mIU/L (normal 0.3 to 5).
* Radioiodine uptake - After 2 hours, 3%. After 24 hours, 3.9%.

▌QUESTIONS

a. What is your diagnosis?
b. Suggest two investigations.

▌CASE NO. 051

A 45-year-old lady, known hypertensive, non-diabetic, gives 10 weeks history of severe headache, anorexia, nausea, vertigo and blurring of vision, which is progressively increasing. She was taking antihypertensive drug irregularly.

On examination, face—puffy, anemia—mild, edema—mild and pitting, BP—210/135 mm Hg, pulse—96/min, high volume.

Investigations

❖ Full blood count	-	Hb – 9.5 g/dL, WBC – 6,100/cmm, poly – 59%, lympho – 39%, mono – 2%, ESR – 57 mm in 1st hour, platelets – 4,90,000/cmm.
❖ Urea	-	39 mmol/L (normal 2.5 to 6.6).
❖ Creatinine	-	4.5 mg/dL (normal 0.68 to 1.36).
❖ Serum electrolytes	-	Sodium 133 mmol/L. Potassium 3.1 mmol/L. Bicarbonate–13 mmol/L.
❖ Serum cholesterol	-	450 mg/dL (normal 200 to 350).
❖ Triglyceride	-	650 mg/dL (normal 70 to 150).

▌QUESTIONS

a. What is the diagnosis?
b. What is the cause of low potassium?
c. What is the cause of this biochemical blood profile?
d. Suggest one clinical examination.
e. Mention one finding in peripheral blood film in such a case.

▌CASE NO. 052

A lady aged 63 years is admitted in the hospital with the complaints of loss of appetite, weight gain, constipation, drowsiness, confusion and extreme weakness for 2 months. She also complains of cold intolerance for the same duration. There is no significant past medical illness.

On examination, the patient looks apathetic, anemia—moderate, edema—present, non-pitting, BP—180/80 mm Hg, pulse—57/min, high volume. Other systems—no abnormality.

Investigations

❖ Full blood count	-	Hb – 7.8 g/dL, WBC – 3,540/cmm, poly – 66%, lympho – 30%, monocyte – 4%, platelets – 1,00,000/cmm.
❖ MCV	-	110 fl (normal 76 to 96).
❖ X-ray chest	-	Cardiomegaly, globular in shape.
❖ ECG	-	Low voltage.

❖ Serum electrolytes   - Sodium 125 mmol/L. Potassium 4.1 mmol/L.
                         Bicarbonate 21.8 mmol/L. Chloride 95 mmol/L.
❖ Urea   - 45 mg/dL.
❖ Creatinine   - 1.2 mg/dL.

QUESTIONS

a. What is your diagnosis?
b. What three further investigations do you suggest?
c. Mention two causes of cardiomegaly.

CASE NO. 053

A male aged 67 years developed toxic multinodular goiter. He was treated with radioiodine therapy. Two years later, hypothyroidism developed. He was on thyroxine.

After 2 years, he was seen in the thyroid clinic for routine check-up, and this time thyroid function shows the following results:
❖ FT_3 - 1.3 pmol/L (normal 1.1 to 3.2).
❖ FT_4 - 160 pmol/L (normal 9 to 23).
❖ TSH   - 15 mIU/L (normal 0.3 to 5).

QUESTIONS

a. Write three reasons for the above result.
b. What is the diagnosis?
c. What treatment is necessary now?

CASE NO. 054

A woman aged 60 years presented with fever, anorexia, weight loss, generalized muscular weakness, bodyache and polyarthritis involving the large joints for the last 4 months. She is also complaining of difficulty in deglutition and shortness of breath on mild exertion for 2 months. For the last few days, she noticed change of color of the fingers on exposure to cold.

On examination, the patient looks emaciated, anemia—moderate, BP—100/65 mm Hg, pulse—88/min. All large joints—tender. No other physical findings.

Investigations

❖ Full blood count   - Hb – 8.9 g/dL, WBC – 13,300/cmm, poly – 62%, lympho – 34%,
                        mono – 4%, ESR – 110 mm in 1st hour, platelets – 3,00,000/cmm.
❖ Serum electrolytes   Sodium 142 mmol/L. Chloride 100 mmol/L. Potassium 4.2 mmol/L.
❖ Calcium   - 9.1 mg/dL.
❖ Bilirubin   - 10 µmol/L (normal 2 to 17).
❖ AST   - 115 IU/L (normal 5 to 40).
❖ ALP   - 298 IU/L (normal 20 to 100).
❖ Serum albumin   - 30 g/L (normal 34 to 48).
❖ RA test   - Positive.

QUESTIONS

a. What is the diagnosis?
b. Mention two physical findings you would look for in this patient.
c. What three investigations should be done?

CASE NO. 055

A 53-year-old male, executive engineer, occasional smoker and alcoholic, is admitted in emergency, with the complaints of repeated hematemesis and melena, weakness and syncopal attack for 2 days. He was suffering from jaundice 7 years back with positive hepatitis B virus.

   On examination, anemia—severe, jaundice—mild, BP—60/40 mm Hg, pulse—118/min. Spleen—5 cm, liver—just palpable, non tender. Heart and lungs—normal.

Investigations

❖ Full blood count	- Hb – 4.3 g/dL, WBC – 1,19,000/cmm, poly – 57%, lympho – 06%, eosinophil - 4%, basophil – 3%, myelocyte – 15%, myeloblast – 05%, others – 6%, platelets – 2,20,000/cmm.
❖ PBF	- Anisopoikilocytosis, few nucleated RBC, WBC shift to left.
❖ Serum bilirubin	- 31 μmol/L (normal 2 to 17).
❖ SGPT	- 65 IU/L (normal 5 to 40).
❖ Alkaline phosphatase	- 115 IU/L (normal 20 to 100).
❖ Prothrombin time	- 18.8 sec (control 12.8 sec).
❖ Total protein	- 51 g/L (normal 62 to 80).
❖ Albumin	- 21 g/L (normal 34 to 48).

QUESTIONS

a. What is your diagnosis?
b. Suggest three investigations.
c. Mention two immediate treatments.

CASE NO. 056

A lady aged 65 years, who is living alone, has been suffering from weakness, polyuria, weight gain and occasional diarrhea for 2 months. She is hospitalized because of dysarthria, confusion and drowsiness for 48 hours. She was suffering from depression for long time and took varieties of drugs, the names of which she could not mention.

Investigations

❖ Full blood count	- Hb – 10.5 g/dL, WBC – 11,540/cmm, poly – 80%, lympho – 20%, platelets – 2,88,000/cmm.
❖ RBS	- 3.6 mmol/L.
❖ Serum electrolytes	- Sodium 155 mmol/L. Chloride 125 mmol/L. Potassium 6.1 mmol/L. Bicarbonate 11.8 mmol/L.
❖ Urea	- 55 mg/dL.

* Creatinine   - 1.2 mg/dL.
* TSH   - 18 mIU/L (normal 0.3 to 5 mIU/L).
* T_4 - 38 nmol/L (normal 54.05 to 173.75).
* ECG   - Low voltage, T inversion in V_1-V_6.
* Chest X-ray   - Normal.
* CT scan of brain   - Diffuse cerebral atrophy.

QUESTIONS

a. What is your diagnosis?
b. What is the likely cause of this blood picture?
c. Suggest three investigations.

CASE NO. 057

A 25-year-old man presented with anorexia, fatigue, polyuria, polydipsia, backache and generalized bodyache. He was suffering from recurrent urinary infection and chronic constipation.

Investigations

* Full blood count   - Hb – 10 g/dL, WBC – 7,300/cmm, poly – 70%, lympho – 30%, ESR – 50 mm in 1st hour, platelets – 1,80,000/cmm.
* Urea   - 8.5 mmol/L.
* Creatinine   - 1.2 mg/dL.
* S. electrolytes   - Sodium 144 mmol/L. Chloride 114 mmol/L. Potassium 2.7 mmol/l. Bicarbonate 14 mmol/l.
* Calcium   - 2.1 mmol/L (normal 2.1 to 2.62).
* Phosphate   - 1.0 mmol/L (normal 0.8 to 1.4).
* Albumin   - 42 g/L (normal 35 to 50).
* Fasting blood sugar   - 6.5 mmol/L.
* Alkaline phosphatase - 400 IU/L (normal 20 to 100).

QUESTIONS

a. What metabolic abnormality is present?
b. What is the diagnosis?
c. Suggest three investigations.
d. Why bodyache?

CASE NO. 058

A 70-year-old man, who was always in good health, presented with difficulty in walking, frequency of micturition, incontinence of urine, confusion and memory loss.

    Higher psychic functions—dementia present. Cranial nerves—normal. In the lower limb—muscle power diminished, tone increased, all reflexes—exaggerated. Plantar—extensor on both sides. No sensory loss. Ataxia—present. Other systems—normal.

QUESTIONS

a. What is the likely diagnosis?
b. Mention one alternative diagnosis.
c. Suggest two investigations.

CASE NO. 059

A 50-year-old lady, known case of rheumatoid arthritis for 15 years, was on methotrexate and sulfasalazine for years.

Recently, she presented with severe weakness, loss of appetite, breathlessness, swelling of legs, face and abdomen.

On examination, face—puffy, anemia—moderate, edema—pitting. BP—160/100 mm Hg, pulse—76/min. Liver—just palpable, spleen—mildly enlarged, ascites—mild. Others systems—normal.

Investigations

- Full blood count   - Hb – 7.5 g/dL, WBC – 2,800/cmm, poly – 60%, lympho – 30%, mono – 6%, eosinophil – 4%, platelets – 95,000/cmm.
- MCV   - 80 fl (normal 76 to 96).
- Urea   - 14 mmol/L (normal 2.5 to 6.6).
- Creatinine   - 120 μmol/L (normal 60 to 120).
- SGPT   - 220 IU/L (normal 5 to 40).
- Alkaline phosphatase - 190 IU/L normal 20 to 100).
- Total protein   - 51 g/L (normal 62 to 80).
- Serum albumin   - 26 g/L (normal 35 to 50).
- Prothrombin time   - 12.6 sec (control 12).
- Urine   - Protein (+++).
- USG of abdomen   - Splenomegaly, hepatomegaly and ascites present.
- Chest X-ray   - Small bilateral pleural effusion.

QUESTIONS

a. What is your clinical diagnosis?
b. What is the likely cause of the above picture?
c. Suggest one investigation to confirm the diagnosis.

CASE NO. 060

A 30-year-old woman has been suffering from bodyache, malaise, weakness, fever with chill and rigor for 6 months. She gives history of occasional dark color urine. In her past history, there was painful calf muscle with swelling of right leg one year back.

On examination, anemia—mild, BP—100/55 mm Hg, pulse—78/min. Other systems reveal no abnormality.

Investigations

- ❖ Full blood count — Hb – 10.2 g/dL, WBC – 3,000/cmm, poly – 32%, lympho – 58%, mono – 3%, eosinophils – 7%,ESR – 50 mm in 1st hour, platelets – 70,000/cmm.
- ❖ MCV — 104 fl.
- ❖ Reticulocytes — 8% (normal 0.2 to 2).
- ❖ Direct Coombs' test — Negative.
- ❖ Serum bilirubin — 39 µmol/L (normal 2 to 17).
- ❖ SGPT — 31 IU/L (normal 5 to 40).
- ❖ Alkaline phosphatase - 78 IU/L (normal 20 to 100).

▌QUESTIONS

a. What is the likely diagnosis?
b. Suggest two investigations.
c. What is the cause of swelling of the leg?
d. Why is mean corpuscular volume (MCV) high?

▌CASE NO. 061

A 47-year-old man presented with pain in both ankle and knee joints, swelling of right leg, fever, dry cough, shortness of breath and weight loss for 3 months. For the last 1 month, the patient also feels difficulty in hearing, more in left ear. He was treated by local doctor with multiple drugs including quinine, but his condition is deteriorated.

On examination, the patient looks emaciated, anemia—moderate BP—100/55 mm Hg, pulse—78/min. Both ankle and knee joints—swollen and tender. Heart, lung—normal. No organomegaly.

Investigations

- ❖ Full blood count — Hb – 9.3 g/dL, WBC – 10,500/cmm, poly – 60%, lympho – 28%, eosinophil – 12%, platelets – 1,95,000/cmm, ESR –105 mm in 1st hour.
- ❖ Urine — Proteinuria (++), few RBC casts, few pus cells.
- ❖ Chest X-ray — Basal consolidation on right side.
- ❖ Urea — 65 mg/dL (normal 9 to 11).
- ❖ Creatinine — 2.2 mg/dL (normal 0.68 to 1.36).

▌QUESTIONS

a. What three differential diagnoses would you consider?
b. Suggest five investigations.

▌CASE NO. 062

A 52-year-old man, presented with weakness, vertigo, loss of appetite, insomnia and occasional fainting attack for one year. He was always in good health.

On examination, the patient is emaciated and pale, BP—100/60 mm Hg, pulse—72/min, dehydration—mild.

Investigations

- ❖ Full blood count - Hb – 10.8 g/dL, WBC – 7,500/cmm, poly – 70%, lympho – 26%, eosinophil – 4%, platelets – 2,97,000/cmm, ESR – 45 mm in 1st hour.
- ❖ Chest X-ray - Normal.
- ❖ USG of abdomen - Normal.
- ❖ CT scan of brain - Normal.
- ❖ Serum electrolytes - Sodium 125 mmol/L. Potassium 4.1 mmol/L. Bicarbonate 19.8 mmol/L. Chloride 95 mmol/L.
- ❖ Urea - 45 mg/dL.
- ❖ Creatinine - 1.2 mg/dL.

QUESTIONS

a. Suggest two possible diagnoses.
b. Suggest four investigations.
c. What is the cause of the fainting attacks?

CASE NO. 063

A housewife aged 40 years, presented with frequent headache, vertigo and insomnia for 2 months. There is one miscarriage and two LUCS.

On examination, BP—210/135 mm Hg, pulse—90/min, high volume. No other physical findings. Heart, lungs and abdomen—normal.

Investigations

- ❖ Full blood count - Hb – 11.5 g/dL, WBC – 8,300/cmm, poly – 64%, lympho – 33%, mono – 3%, ESR – 48 mm in 1st hour, platelets – 2,70,000/cmm.
- ❖ Urine - Few pus cells, Glycosuria (++), proteinuria (+).
- ❖ Serum electrolytes - Sodium 145 mmol/L. Chloride 101 mmol/L. Potassium 3.1 mmol/l. Bicarbonate 30 mmol/L.
- ❖ Urea - 5.9 mmol/L.
- ❖ Creatinine - 1.3 mg/dL.
- ❖ Chest X-ray - Heart slightly enlarged.
- ❖ FBS - 8.3 mmol/L.
- ❖ Serum cholesterol - 190 mg/dL.
- ❖ Serum triglyceride - 177 mg/dL.

QUESTIONS

a. Suggest three differential diagnoses.
b. What is the likely diagnosis in this case?
c. What five physical signs will you see?
d. Mention four further investigations.

CASE NO. 064

A male aged 70 years, is admitted in the hospital with the complains of severe weakness, vertigo, loss of appetite and weight loss for one month.

On examination, the patient looks grossly chachexic. Anemia—severe, jaundice—mild, multiple purpuric spots in different parts of the body. No other physical findings.

Investigations

- ❖ Full blood count   - Hb – 4.5 g/dL, WBC – 1,540/cmm, poly – 20%, lympho – 70%, monocyte – 10%,platelets – 80,000/cmm, ESR – 70 mm in 1st hour.
- ❖ PBF   - Anisopoikilocytosis, microcytic, hypochromic and occasional macrocytic.
- ❖ Serum bilirubin   - 31 μmol/L (normal 2 to 17).
- ❖ SGPT   - 65 IU/L (normal 5 to 40).
- ❖ Alkaline phosphatase - 135 IU/L (normal 20 to 100).

QUESTIONS

a. What two differential diagnoses would you consider?
b. What single investigation would you suggest?
c. What treatment would you start immediately?

CASE NO. 065

A 55-year-old lady presented with low grade fever, lethargy, weakness, loss of appetite, weight loss and increased pigmentation for 6 months. For the last 2 months, she noticed gradually increasing abdominal distension and occasional diarrhea. Total abdominal hysterectomy (TAH) was done 3 years back.

On examination, the patient looks emaciated and there is generalized pigmentation, anemia—moderate, jaundice—mild, BP—90/65 mm Hg, pulse—90/min. Liver—enlarged, 9 cm, non-tender, firm. Spleen—enlarged, 5 cm. Few bilateral cervical lymphadenopathy, non-tender, discrete, firm in consistensy.

Investigations

- ❖ Full blood count   - Hb – 9.5 g/dL, WBC – 3,300/cmm, poly – 61%, lympho – 35%, mono – 4%, ESR – 50 mm in 1st hr, platelets – 1,00,000/cmm.
- ❖ FBS   - 8 mmol/L.
- ❖ Bilirubin   - 39 μmol/L (normal 2 to 17).
- ❖ SGPT   - 65 IU/L (normal <25).
- ❖ Alkaline phosphatase - 329 IU/L (normal 20 to 100).
- ❖ Total protein   - 85 g/L (normal 55 to 70).
- ❖ Albumin   - 32 g/L (normal 34 to 48).
- ❖ Cholesterol   - 11.2 mmol/L (normal 5.2 to 9).
- ❖ Triglyceride   - 6.10 mmol/L (normal 0.8 to 1.7).

QUESTIONS

a. What is the likely diagnosis?
b. What further single history would you like to take?
c. Mention one diagnostically useful blood test.
d. How to confirm your diagnosis?
e. What is the specific treatment of such case?

CASE NO. 066

A 35-year-old man presented with recurrent attack of headache, insomnia, sweating, and occasional palpitation for 3 months. He was well previously.

On examination, BP—160/110 mm Hg, pulse—80 /min. No other physical findings.

Investigations

- ❖ Full blood count — Hb – 13.8 g/dL, WBC – 10,500/cmm, poly – 59%, lympho – 39%, eosinophil – 2%, platelets – 3,95,000/cmm, ESR – 35 mm in 1st hour.
- ❖ Urine — Proteinuria (+), few pus cells.
- ❖ Urea — 38 mg/dL.
- ❖ Creatinine — 1.3 mg/dL.
- ❖ Chest X-ray — Heart is slightly enlarged.
- ❖ ECG — LVH.
- ❖ Urinary VMA — 99 µmol/L (normal 5 to 35 in 24 hours).

QUESTIONS

a. Suggest four causes of high VMA.
b. Suggest three investigations to confirm your diagnosis.

CASE NO. 067

A man of 60 years, smoker, presented with cough, fever, occasional headache and weakness of legs for 2 months. He is also complaining of occasional headache, insomnia and weakness for one month. He is non-diabetic, non-hypertensive. No history of past medical illnss.

On examination, anemia—mild, BP—110/70 mm Hg, pulse—70/min. No other physical findings.

CBC, blood sugar, serum electrolytes, chest X-ray, urea and creatinine are all normal.
CSF findings show:
- ❖ Pressure — 50 mm H_2O (normal 50 to 180).
- ❖ Protein — 4.75 g/L (normal 0.15 to 0.45 g/L).
- ❖ Sugar — 4.0 mmol/L (normal 2.8 to 4.5).
- ❖ Cells — Few mononuclear cells. (Normal 0 to 4).

QUESTIONS

a. Suggest four differential diagnoses.
b. Suggest three investigations.

CASE NO. 068

A young lady of 30 years has been suffering from fever, headache, bodyache, nausea and vomiting for 2 weeks.

On examination, anemia—moderate, jaundice—moderate, liver—just palpable and tender. Spleen—just palpable. Other systems—no abnormality.

Investigations

- Full blood count   - Hb – 9.9 g/dL, WBC – 4,000/cmm, poly – 49%, lympho – 51%, eosinophil – 9%, monocyte – 1%, platelets – 1,05,000/cmm.
- PBF   - Macrocytic and normochromic.
- Reticulocyte count   - 6.3% (normal 0.2 to 2).
- Chest X-ray   - Bilateral hilar lymphadenopathy.
- Bilirubin   - 100 µmol/L (normal 2 to 17).
- SGPT   - 600 IU/L (normal 5 to 40).
- SGOT   - 189 IU/L (normal 10 to 40).
- Alkaline phosphatase -   199 IU/L (normal 20 to 100).
- Urine analysis   - Urobilinogen present.

QUESTIONS

a. What is the likely diagnosis?
b. Suggest three investigations which will help in your diagnosis.

CASE NO. 069

A 42-year-old engineer presented with weakness, irritability, anorexia, dizziness, vertigo, tingling and numbness in fingers and toes for 3 months. He is also complaining of occasional loose motions and abdominal pain for 2 months.

On examination, the patient is very ill, anemia—severe, BP—90/60 mm Hg, pulse—90/min.

Investigations

- Full blood count   - Hb – 7.9 g/dL, WBC – 3,800/cmm, poly – 47%, lympho – 44%, eosinophil – 7%, monocyte – 2%, ESR – 28 mm in 1st hour.
- MCV   - 105 fl (normal 76 to 95).
- PBF   - Macrocytic, normochromic and few hypochromic.
- Reticulocyte count   - 1.3% (normal 0.2 to 2).
- Urea   - 30 mg/dL (normal 9 to 11).
- Creatinine   - 1.3 mg/dL (normal 0.68 to 1.36).
- Chest X-ray   - Heart is slightly enlarged.
- USG of abdomen   - Normal.

He was treated with vit B_{12}, folic acid and iron. After some days of treatment, his symptoms and blood pictures are not improved.

QUESTIONS

a. What is the hematological diagnosis?
b. What next investigation would you suggest?
c. Suggest three causes of this hematological picture.
d. Suggest two further investigations.

CASE NO. 070

A 35-year-old man, working in a jute industry, heavy smoker, is complaining of low grade, continuous fever with evening rise, night sweat, loss of weight, abdominal pain and dry cough for 6 months.

On examination, anemia—severe, jaundice—mild. Bilateral cervical lymphadenopathy, matted, non-tender, firm. BP—100/60 mm Hg, pulse—90/min.

Liver—enlarged, 5 cm, non-tender firm in consistency, no bruit. Spleen—enlarged, 6 cm from left anterior axillary line towards right iliac. Heart, lung—normal.

Investigations

❖ Full blood count	- Hb – 6.5 g/dL, WBC – 6,200/cmm, poly – 60%, lympho – 20%, mono – 5%, eosinophils – 15%, ESR – 110 mm in 1st hour, platelets – 1,50,000/cmm.
❖ PBF	- Macrocytic, hypochromic, polychromasia, spherocytes.
❖ Reticulocyte count	- 9% (normal 0.2 to 2).
❖ MCV	- 103 fl (normal 76 to 95).
❖ MCHC	- 33 g/dL (normal 32 to 36).
❖ Serum bilirubin	- 38 μmol/L (normal 2 to 17).
❖ SGPT	- 38 IU/L (normal 5 to 40).
❖ Alkaline phosphatase	- 400 IU/L (normal 20 to 100).
❖ Chest X-ray (CXR)	- Normal.
❖ MT	- 10 mm.

QUESTIONS

a. What is the hematological diagnosis?
b. Suggest three investigations.
c. What is the likely diagnosis?

CASE NO. 071

A young lady aged 29 years, housewife, presented with frequency of micturition, dysuria and lower abdominal pain for 10 days. For the last 3 days, she is also suffering from high grade, continuous fever with swelling and severe pain in the right knee joint. There is moderate effusion in the right knee joint. Aspiration was done.

Investigations

- ❖ Full blood count — WBC—16,400/cmm, poly—82%, lympho—18%, ESR—72 mm in 1st hour.
- ❖ Aspirated fluid shows the following:
  - ◆ Color — Turbid.
  - ◆ Cytology — Neutrophils plenty.
  - ◆ Crystals — Not found.
  - ◆ Protein — 6.1 g/dL.
  - ◆ Glucose — 1.6 mmol/L.
  - ◆ Culture — No growth.

QUESTIONS

a. Suggest two possible diagnoses.
b. List four investigations for your diagnosis.

CASE NO. 072

A patient aged 50 years, diabetic and hypertensive, has been suffering from chronic renal failure for 2 years. He is on hemodialysis. For the last 3 months, he is complaining of extreme weakness, loss of appetite and backache. For the last 2 months, he feels abnormal sensation in the leg and feet, which disturb his sleep with frequent movement of both legs.

On examination, he is pale, emaciated, pigmented, anemia—severe, edema—mild, pitting, BP—160/100 mm Hg, pulse—88/min. No other physical finding.

Investigations

- ❖ Full blood count — Hb – 5.9 g/dL, WBC – 5,200/cmm, poly – 62%, lympho – 38%, ESR – 70 mm in 1st h, platelets – 1,25,000/cmm.
- ❖ PBF — Microcytic and hypochromic.
- ❖ Random blood sugar – 4.9 mmol/L.
- ❖ Urea — 19 mmol/L (normal 2.5 to 6.6).
- ❖ Creatinine — 6.3 mg/dL (normal 0.68 to 1.36)
- ❖ Serum electrolytes — Sodium 130 mmol/L. Chloride 90 mmol/L. Potassium 6.3 mmol/L. Bicarbonate 16 mmol/L.
- ❖ USG of renal system – Both kidneys are small.

QUESTIONS

a. What is your diagnosis?
b. What treatment would you give now?

CASE NO. 073

A 60-year-old man, smoker and alcoholic, presented with continuous, low grade fever, loss of weight, anorexia and backache for 3 months. He is also complaining of dry cough, compression in the chest and frequency of micturition for one month.

On examination, the patient is emaciated, face—plethoric. Liver—enlarged, 2 cm. Right supraclavicular and cervical lymphadenopathy, non-tender, hard in consistency, some are matted, and some are discrete.

Investigations

❖ Full blood count   - Hb – 18.6 g/dL, WBC – 8,200/cmm, poly – 62%, lympho – 28%, mono – 5%, eosinophils – 5%, ESR – 90 mm in 1st hour, RBC – 7.2 million/cmm, platelets – 4,30,000/cmm.
❖ Urine   - RBC – plenty, pus cells – 10 to 25, few RBC casts, mild proteinuria.
❖ Urine culture   - No growth.
❖ Chest X-ray   - Normal.
❖ MT   - 12 mm.
❖ Blood culture   - No growth.

■ QUESTIONS

a. What is the likely diagnosis?
b. Mention one alternative diagnosis.
c. What additional history should be taken?
d. What physical findings should be seen?
e. Suggest three investigations, which will help in your diagnosis.

■ CASE NO. 074

A 29-year-old housewife was admitted in the hospital with the history of fever, weakness, headache and recurrent attacks of transient loss of consciousness for 10 days. Two days after admission, she notices epistaxis and multiple bleeding spots in different parts of the body.

On examination; she is pale, anemia—moderate, BP—180/110 mm Hg, pulse—110/min, spleen—just palpable, multiple purpura—present.

Investigations

❖ Full blood count   - Hb – 7.1 g/dL, WBC – 11,700/cmm, poly – 61%, lympho – 38%, mono – 1%, platelets – 59,000/cmm.
❖ PBF   - Microspherocytes (++), red cell fragments (++).
❖ Reticulocytes   - 3.7% (normal 0.2 to 2).
❖ Urea   - 37.8 mmol/L (normal 2.5 to 6.6)
❖ Creatinine   - 4.7 mg/dL (normal 0.68 to 1.36)
❖ Serum electrolytes   - Sodium 127 mmol/L. Chloride 93 mmol/L. Potassium 6.2 mmol/L. Bicarbonate 17 mmol/L.
❖ ANA and anti-ds DNA - Negative.

■ QUESTIONS

a. Give two possible diagnoses.
b. Suggest one investigation to confirm your diagnosis.
c. Mention one specific treatment.

CASE NO. 075

A 60-year-old male presented with fever, headache, dry cough, frequency of micturition and weakness for 10 days. Cefixime was given by a general practitioner. After 5 days, the patient complains of scanty urine, puffiness of face, swelling of legs, polyarthralgia and multiple skin rashes.

On examination, face—puffy, BP—190/110 mm Hg, pulse—106/min, edema—present, pitting. Temperature—38.3°C, multiple skin rashes—present in all over the body.

Investigations

* Full blood count — Hb – 10.9 g/dL, WBC – 11,200/cmm, poly – 64%, lympho – 28%, eosinophil – 8%, ESR – 110 mm in 1st hour, platelets – 1,75,000/cmm.
* Fasting blood sugar — 5.9 mmol/L.
* Urine — Pus cells – plenty, proteinuria (++).
* Total protein in urine — 1 g/24 hours.
* Urea — 19 mmol/L (normal 2.5 to 6.6).
* Creatinine — 833 µmol/L (normal 60 to 120).
* Serum electrolytes — Sodium 130 mmol/L. Chloride 90 mmol/L. Potassium 6.1 mmol/L. Bicarbonate 17 mmol/L.

QUESTIONS

a. What is your diagnosis?
b. Suggest two further investigations.
c. How to manage this case?
d. How to confirm the diagnosis?
e. What is the single most important treatment?

CASE NO. 076

An elderly man aged 70 years, presented with headache, dizziness, blurrring of vision, anorexia and weight loss for 5 months. He also noticed occasional bleeding from gum for 2 months.

On examination, anemia—mild, jaundice—mild. BP—100/70 mm Hg, pulse—64/min. Generalized lymphadenopathy involving the cervical, axillary and inguinal region, which are discrete, rubbery and firm in consistency.

Hepatomegaly—5 cm, firm in consistency. Non-tender, smooth surface, no bruit. Spleen—enlarged, 7 cm from left anterior axillary line towards right iliac fossa. Tenderness in the sternum. Fundoscopy—retinal hemorrhages in both eyes.

Investigations

* Full blood count — Hb – 10.3 g/dL, WBC – 3,700/cmm, poly – 35%, lympho – 55%, mono – 10%, eosinophils 5%, ESR – 115 mm in 1st hr, platelets – 1,05,000/cmm.
* Chest X-ray — Bilateral hilar lymphadenopathy.
* Urea — 32 mg/dL.
* Creatinine — 94 µmol/L.

❖ X-ray of skull   - Normal.
❖ Calcium   - 2.02 mg/dL (normal 2.1 to 2.62).
❖ Total protein   - 90 g/L (normal 62 to 80).
❖ Albumin   - 33 g/L (normal 35 to 50).
❖ Urine for Bence-Jones
  protein   - Positive.
❖ Lymph node biopsy   - Reactive hyperplasia.

QUESTIONS

a. Suggest two investigations.
b. What is your diagnosis?
c. How to treat?

CASE NO. 077

A 17-year-old girl, known case of β-thalassemia major, is admitted in the hospital with the complains of weakness, difficulty in breathing on mild exertion and swelling of both feet. Repeated blood transfusion were given every 4 to 6 months.

On examination; appearance—pigmented and emaciated. Frontal and parietal bossing—present. Anemia—severe, jaundice—mild, edema—present, pitting. JVP—engorged and pulsatile. Liver—enlarged, 4 cm, tender, soft in consistency. Spleen—enlarged, 10 cm from left anterior axillary line towards right iliac fossa.

Investigations

❖ Full blood count   - Hb – 6.1 g/dL, WBC – 7,700/cmm, poly – 63%, lympho – 34%,
                          mono – 3%, platelets – 90,000/cmm, ESR – 40 mm in 1st hr.
❖ Chest X-ray   - Heart is enlarged.
❖ Iron   - 32 μmol/L (normal 13 to 32 μmol/L).
❖ TIBC   - 84 μmol/L (normal 40 to 80 μmol/L).

QUESTIONS

a. What is the underlying diagnosis of her present symptoms?
b. Give two possible causes for her enlarged heart.
c. Suggest one single investigation.
d. What drug should be given in such case?

CASE NO. 078

A 54-year-old housewife has been suffering from recurrent attack of high grade, continuous fever, pain, redness of ear and difficulty in hearing for 5 months. She also noticed recurrent redness of both eyes with pain and nasal blockage for the last 3 months. Her deafness is progressively increasing with recent hoarseness of voice. Most of the attacks lasted for 7 to 10 days, recovered by using analgesic.

On examination, anemia—mild, BP—110/70 mm Hg, pulse—120/min. Heart—early diastolic murmur in left lower parasternal area. No organomegaly. Heart, lungs—no abnormality.

Investigations

- ❖ Full blood count   - Hb – 8.9 g/dL, WBC – 14,200/cmm, poly – 74%, lympho – 20%, eosinophil – 6%, ESR – 160 mm in 1st hr, platelets – 2,75,000/cmm.
- ❖ Blood sugar   - 5.9 mmol/L.
- ❖ Urine   - Pus cells – few, proteinuria (+).
- ❖ Blood and urine culture - No growth.
- ❖ Urea   - 7 mmol/L.
- ❖ Creatinine   - 1.3 mg/dL.
- ❖ Serum electrolytes   - Sodium 139 mmol/L. Chloride 99 mmol/L. Potassium 4.1 mmol/L. Bicarbonate 27 mmol/L.
- ❖ Chest X-ray   - Heart enlarged in TD.
- ❖ ECG   - Sinus tachycardia.
- ❖ Echocardiogram   - Aortic regurgitation, no vegetation.
- ❖ USG of abdomen   - No abnormality.

QUESTIONS

a. What is the likely diagnosis?
b. Suggest two further investigations.
c. What treatment will you give?

CASE NO. 079

A 65-year-old woman presented with pain in the epigastrium, loss of appetite, fever, generalized bodyache, night sweating, occasional headache, dizziness and weight loss for 3 months.

On examination, the patient looks pale and emaciated. Anemia—mild, jaundice—mild. No bony tenderness. Abdomen—looks distended. Spleen—massive enlargement, no hepatomegaly.

Investigations

- ❖ Full blood count   - Hb – 9.1 g/dL, WBC – 11,500/cmm, poly – 60%, lympho – 31%, myelocytes - 6%, metamyelocytes - 2%, myeloblasts - 1%, ESR – 93 mm in 1st hr, platelets – 6,65,000/cmm, Nucleated RBC – few.
- ❖ Serum bilirubin   - 28 μmol/L.
- ❖ SGPT   - 38 IU/L.
- ❖ Alkaline phosphatase - 200 IU/L.
- ❖ Chest X-ray   - Normal.

QUESTIONS

a. What is the hematological diagnosis?
b. What is the likely diagnosis?
c. What additional findings may be seen in blood film?
d. Suggest two other tests.

CASE NO. 080

A man aged 53 years had an attack of acute myocardial infarction, associated with recurrent attacks of arrhythmia, which was well controlled by antiarrhythmic drug.

During follow-up after two months, BP—95/65 mm Hg, pulse—100/min, low volume, with occasional drop beat. A multinodular goiter is present. No other physical findings.

Investigations

* Full blood count   - Hb – 12.1 g/dL, WBC – 10,700/cmm, poly – 62%, lympho – 37%, mono – 1%, platelets – 1,50,000/cmm, ESR – 50 mm in 1st hr.
* Chest X-ray   - Heart is slightly enlarged.
* ECG   - Old anterior myocardial infarction with few ventricular ectopics.
* Creatinine   - 1.2 mg/dL.
* RBS   - 7 mmol/L.
* T_4 - 312 nmol/L (normal 58 to 174).
* T_3 - 2.88 nmol/L (normal 1.23 to 3.07).
* TSH   - 0.5 mIU/L (normal 0.5 to 5).

QUESTIONS

a. Suggest a cause for the above thyroid function tests.
b. What further investigation is most useful?

CASE NO. 081

A 49-year-old housewife presented with weakness, lethargy, anorexia, dizziness, vertigo and occasional diarrhea for 3 months.

On examination, she is very pale and ill-looking, anemia—moderate, BP—110/60 mm Hg, pulse—90/min. Liver and spleen—just palpable.

Investigations

* Full blood count   - Hb – 6.9 g/dl, WBC – 5,800/cmm, poly – 69%, lympho – 30%, eosinophil – 1%, ESR – 40 mm in 1st hr.
* PBF   - Macrocytic, microcytic, normocytic and normochromic.
* Urea   - 29 mg/dL.
* Creatinine   - 1.3 mg/dL.

QUESTIONS

a. What is the hemotological diagnosis?
b. Suggest three causes of such blood picture.
c. Suggest four investigations to find out causes.

CASE NO. 082

A 47-year-old obese lady, has been suffering from frequent headache, vertigo, dizziness and insomnia for 3 months. For the last few weeks, she is also complaining of occasional difficulty in vision, double vision but no refractive error. She is a known case of bronchial asthma since her childhood, for which she was hospitalized many times with acute exacerbation. She herself took prednisolone frequently to control asthma. She used to take oral contraceptive pills for 10 years.

On examination, the patient looks obese, multiple striae—present, BP—140/95 mm Hg, pulse—70/min. Horizontal nystagmus—present in both eyes. Diplopia—present in right eye on lateral gaze. Right 6th nerve palsy—present. Other systems—normal.

Investigations

❖ Full blood count	- Hb – 13.9 g/dL, WBC – 7,800/cmm, poly – 60%, lympho – 35%, eosinophil – 3%, monocyte – 2%, ESR – 12 mm in 1st hr.
❖ RBS	- 8.1 mmol/L.
❖ Urea	- 29 mg/dL.
❖ Creatinine	- 1.2 mg/dL.
❖ Chest X-ray	- Normal.
❖ X-ray PNS	- Maxillary sinusitis.
❖ ECG	- Low voltage tracing.
❖ CT scan of brain	- Normal.
❖ MRI of brain	- Normal.

QUESTIONS

a. Mention one physical sign you will look for.
b. What is the likely cause of her headache?
c. What additional diagnosis is possible?

CASE NO. 083

A young female aged 24 years is admitted in the hospital with the complaints of anorexia, nausea and vomiting. Three weeks before, she was suffering from viral fever, associated with sore throat. 48 hours before admission, she passed dark red urine.

On examination, anemia—mild, jaundice—mild. Spleen—just palpable. Both tonsils—enlarged and congested.

Investigations

❖ Full blood count	- Hb – 9.7 g/dL, WBC – 9,500/cmm, poly – 60%, lympho – 37%, mono – 3%, platelets – 2,60,000/cmm, ESR – 30 mm in 1st hr.
❖ PBF	- Macrocytosis.
❖ Reticulocytes	- 6.3% (normal 0.2 to 2).
❖ Urine urobilinogen	- (++).
❖ Serum bilirubin	- 42 µmol/L (normal 2 to 17).
❖ SGPT	- 30 IU/L (normal 5 to 40).
❖ Alkaline phosphatase	- 84 IU/L (normal 20 to 100).
❖ Urine for bilirubin	- Negative.

QUESTIONS

a. Suggest a possible cause for this presentation.
b. What is the likely cause of discolored urine?
c. Suggest two investigations.

CASE NO. 084

A 46-year-old housewife complains of difficulty in deglutition, palpitation, weakness, headache, dizziness and breathlessness on exertion. There is no menstruation for one year.

On examination, the patient looks pale and ill looking. Anemia—moderate, BP—90/60 mm Hg, pulse—110/min. Tongue—smooth and shiny. Heart—apex beat is shifted, systolic murmur—present in apical area.

Investigations

* Full blood count - Hb – 7.1 g/dL, WBC – 5,300/cmm, poly – 57%, lympho – 41% mono – 3%, platelets – 3,25,000/cmm, ESR – 50 mm in 1st hr.
* Chest X-ray   - Heart is enlarged in transverse diameter.
* ECG   - Sinus tachycardia.
* Creatinine   - 1.2 mg/dL.
* RBS   - 7 mmol/L.
* Endoscopy   - Normal.
* USG of abdomen   - Normal.

QUESTIONS

a. What is the likely diagnosis?
b. What one physical sign will you see?
c. Suggest one simple investigation.
d. Suggest three further investigations.

CASE NO. 085

A 17-year-old girl is admitted in the hospital with the complaints of sudden weakness of all the limbs with difficulty in walking. There is history of similar attack three times in the past.

On examination, BP—110/70 mm Hg, pulse—82/min, heart and lungs—no abnormality. Neurological examination—the patient is uncooperative, no response to painful stimuli. Muscle tone—normal, muscle power—could not be tested. Reflexes—normal, plantar—flexor.

QUESTIONS

a. Suggest the most likely diagnosis.
b. Suggest one alternative diagnosis.
c. Mention one investigation.

CASE NO. 086

A young girl aged 19 years is admitted in the hospital with severe acute abdominal pain and vomiting for one day. She has been suffering from recurrent abdominal pain, palpitation, sweating, nausea and drowsiness since her childhood.

On inquiry, it was found that these symptoms usually develop after drinking fruit juice. Physical examination reveals no abnormality.

Investigations

- ❖ Full blood count - Hb – 11.9 g/dL, WBC – 10,800/cmm, poly – 63%, lympho – 37%, platelets – 1,50,000/cmm, ESR – 45 mm in 1st hr.
- ❖ RBS - 6.2 mmol/L.
- ❖ Plain X-ray abdomen - Multiple fluid level and gas shadow.
- ❖ Serum electrolytes - Sodium 132 mmol/L. Potassium 3.2 mmol/L. Bicarbonate 25.8 mmol/L. Chloride 95 mmol/L.
- ❖ USG of abdomen - Normal. Thirty minutes after drinking 150 mL of fruit juice, blood sugar is 2.3 mmol/L.

QUESTIONS

a. What is the likely underlying diagnosis?
b. Suggest one investigation which will confirm the diagnosis.
c. What advice would you give to the patient?

CASE NO. 087

A 45-year-old woman presented with swelling of both eyes with redness and gritty sensation, excess lacrimation with pain for one year.

On examination, BP—140/80 mm Hg, pulse—84/min, eye—bilateral exophthalmos, red with periorbital edema present. Thyroid—diffusely enlarged, with a small simple nodular goiter, non-tender, firm in consistency.

Investigations

- ❖ Serum FT_4 - 125 pmol/L (normal 70 to 160).
- ❖ Serum FT_3 - 2.1 pmol/L (normal 1.5 to 3.3).
- ❖ TSH - 0.90 mIU/L (normal 0.5 to 5.1).

QUESTIONS

a. What is the likely diagnosis?
b. Mention three further investigations.
c. What is the likely diagnosis of the ocular problem?

CASE NO. 088

A 13-year school going boy has been suffering from β-thalassemia major. He used to take frequent blood transfusion for anemia every 4 to 6 months. For the last few days, he is suffering from severe abdominal pain, nausea, vomiting and diarrhea.

On examination, the patient is pale and ill looking. Anemia—severe, jaundice—severe, liver—enlarged, 7 cm, tender, soft in consistency. Spleen—hugely enlarged. Abdomen—diffuse tenderness.

Investigations

* Full blood count   - Hb – 6.1 g/dL, WBC – 17,800/cmm, poly – 77%, lympho – 23%, platelets – 1,00,000/cmm, ESR – 45 mm in 1st hr.
* RBS   - 8.1 mmol/L.
* Plain X-ray abdomen - Multiple fluid level and gas shadow.
* Serum electrolytes   - Sodium 126 mmol/L. Potassium 3.1 mmol/L. Bicarbonate 29.8 mmol/L. Chloride 95 mmol/L.

After symptomatic treatment, his diarrhea is improved, but abdominal pain is still persistent.

QUESTIONS

a. Suggest three causes of abdominal pain.
b. Suggest two immediate investigations.

CASE NO. 089

A young student aged 19 years, known case of IDDM, was admitted in the hospital with extreme weakness, anorexia and polyuria for 3 days. He was hyperventilating. His diabetes was well controlled with insulin therapy. There is no significant past medical history.

On examination, the patient looks emaciated, BP—90/60 mm Hg, pulse—116/min, anemia—moderate, jaundice—absent, dehydration—present. Leukonychia—present in fingers and toes. Muscle tone and power—diminished. All the reflexes—diminished. No sensory loss.

Investigations

* Full blood count   - Hb – 10.9 g/dL, WBC – 11,200/cmm, poly – 79%, lympho – 18%, Mono – 3%, ESR – 49 mm in 1st hr.
* Serum electrolytes   - Sodium 136 mmol/L. Potassium 3.1 mmol/L. Chloride 110 mmol/L. Bicarbonate 14 mmol/L.
* Blood pH   - 7.28 (normal 7.35 to 7.45).
* Serum urea   - 40 mg/dL (normal 9 to 11).
* Serum creatinine   - 1.9 mg/dL (normal 0.68 to 1.36).
* Random blood sugar - 10.1 mmol/L.
* Lactic acid   - 3 mmol/L (normal <2).

QUESTIONS

a. What type of metabolic abnormality is present?
b. List three conditions in which this type of abnormality may be found.
c. What is the likely diagnosis in this case?
d. Why the reflexes are diminished?

CASE NO. 090

A 31-year-old young man, smoker, complains of cough with mucoid expectoration, shortness of breath, frequent hemoptysis, chest pain, weakness and vomiting for one week. No significant past medical history.

On examination, face—puffy, anemia—moderate, edema—mild and pitting. BP—150/100 mm Hg, pulse—98/min.

Investigations

❖ Full blood count	- Hb – 9.1 g/dL, WBC – 13,500/cmm, poly – 69%, lympho – 31%, ESR – 80 mm in 1st hr, platelets – 3,65,000/cmm.
❖ Serum bilirubin	- 28 µmol/L (normal 2 to 17).
❖ SGPT	- 38 IU/L (normal 5 to 40).
❖ Alkaline phosphatase	- 200 IU/L (normal 20 to 100).
❖ Urea	- 16 mmol/L (normal 2.5 to 6.6).
❖ Creatinine	- 4.7 mg/dL (normal 0.68 to 1.36).
❖ Serum electrolytes	- Sodium 132 mmol/L. Chloride 97 mmol/L. Bicarbonate 17 mmol/L. Potassium 5.7 mmol/L.
❖ Serum albumin	- 21 g/L (normal 36 to 48).
❖ Urinary total protein	- 5 g/24 hours.
❖ Urine	- Red cell casts (++), proteinuria (+++).
❖ Chest X-ray	- Multiple fluffy opacities in both lungs.

QUESTIONS

a. Give four possible diagnoses.
b. Suggest three further investigations.
c. What diagnosis would you consider first?

CASE NO. 091

A labor aged 50 years, non-diabetic, non-hypertensive, is admitted in the emergency with the complains of severe difficulty in breathing and impairment of consciousness. He is hyperventilating.

Investigations

❖ pH	- 7.52.
❖ PaO_2	- 12 kPa (normal 12 to 15).
❖ $PaCO_2$	- 8.1 kPa (normal 4.4 to 6.1).
❖ Bicarbonate	- 13 mmol/L (normal 21 to 27.5).

QUESTIONS

a. What is the diagnosis with the above result?
b. What investigations should be done?

CASE NO. 092

A 16-year-old girl presented with jaundice for 4 months. She is also complaining of weakness, loss of weight, anorexia, polyuria and depression for 2 months. Mother notices some abnormal speech.

On examination, anemia—moderate, jaundice—moderate, liver—enlarged 4 cm, tender, smooth, firm in consistency. Other systems reveal no abnormality.

Investigations

❖ Full blood count	- Hb – 8.5 g/dL, WBC – 10,700/cmm,poly – 63%, lympho – 37%, platelets – 3,00,000/cmm, ESR – 35 mm in 1st hr.
❖ Reticulocyte count	- 6% (normal 0.2 to 2).
❖ USG of abdomen	- Hepatomegaly with high echogenicity.
❖ Serum bilirubin	- 100 µmol/L (normal 2 to 17).
❖ ALT	- 200 IU/L (normal 5 to 40).
❖ AST	- 150 IU/L (normal 10 to 40).
❖ Alkaline phosphatase -	140 IU/L (normal 20 to 100).
❖ Urine	- Glycosuria (++), proteinuria (++).
❖ Viral markers	- Anti-HAV positive, other viral markers are absent.

QUESTIONS

a. What is your diagnosis?
b. Suggest two further investigations.
c. Mention one physical sign you would look for.

CASE NO. 093

A 45-year-old man has been suffering from occasional headache, heaviness in left hypochondrium and sleep disturbance for 8 months. Five days before, he had an attack of amaurosis fugax and 2 days before, one attack of transient ischemic attack (TIA). He was treated in a local clinic and referred to the hospital for further management.

On examination, liver—just palpable, spleen—enlarged 3 cm. No other physical findings.

Investigations

❖ Full blood count	- Hb – 11.4 g/dL, WBC – 15,700/cmm, poly – 85%, lympho – 10%, mono – 5%, ESR – 2 mm in 1st hour, platelets – 6,75,000/cmm, RBC – 8.2 million/cmm.
❖ PCV	- 0.55 (normal 0.40 to 0.54).
❖ MCV	- 68 fl (normal 78 to 98).
❖ MCH	- 18.5 pg (normal 27 to 32).
❖ MCHC	- 27 g/dL (normal 30 to 35).
❖ PBF	- Hypochromia (++), polychromasia (+).

QUESTIONS

a. What is the diagnosis?
b. Mention four diagnostically useful investigations.
c. What treatment is received by the patient?

CASE NO. 094

An 11-year-old school going boy presented with the history of recurrent nose bleeding from the age of six years. Bleeding used to persist few minutes to one hour, stopped by nasal pressure. There is bilateral small nasal polyp.

On examination, anemia—severe. No other physical findings.

Investigations

❖ Full blood count	-	Hb – 7.4 g/dL, WBC – 7,400/cmm, poly – 56%, lympho – 44%, platelets – 2,00,000/cmm.
❖ Bleeding time	-	15 mins 3 sec (normal up to 11 min).
❖ Prothrombin time	-	13.0 sec (control 13.0 sec).
❖ APTT	-	50 sec (control 35.0 sec).

QUESTIONS

a. What is the likely diagnosis?
b. Mention three hematological investigations to confirm your diagnosis.
c. What drug should be avoided?

CASE NO. 095

A young woman aged 32 years presented with the complains of fever, dry cough, pain in the throat, headache, bodyache, palpitation and intolerance to heat for one week.

On examination, BP—160/70 mm Hg, pulse—140/min, regular. Fine tremor of the outstretched hands.

Palm—warm and sweaty. Thyroid—diffusely enlarged, soft, non-tender, no bruit.

Investigations

❖ Full blood count	-	Hb – 11.1 g/dL, WBC – 3,500/cmm, poly – 48%, lympho – 52%, ESR – 110 mm in 1st hr, platelets – 3,65,000/cmm.
❖ Chest X-ray	-	Normal.
❖ Serum FT_3	-	8.7 pmol/L (normal 1.3 to 3.5).
❖ Serum FT_4	-	205 pmol/L (normal 70 to 160).
❖ TSH	-	0.4 mIU/L (normal 0.5 to 5.1).
❖ Radio-iodine uptake	-	After 2 hours – 7% (normal 5 to 15). After 24 hours – 5.1% (normal 15 to 30).

QUESTIONS

a. What is the likely diagnosis?
b. Suggest one investigation.
c. Mention three other causes of such thyroid functions.

CASE NO. 096

A 13-year-old girl is hospitalized with the history of tiredness, weakness, cough, hemoptysis, low grade fever and recent bruising for 3 weeks. She was suffering from measles at the age of 3 years and chicken pox at the age of 7 years.

On examination, anemia—moderate, liver and spleen—just palpable. No other physical findings.

Investigations

❖ Full blood count	- Hb – 8.3 g/dL, WBC – 6,700/cmm, poly – 30%, lympho – 51%, lymphoblast – 15%, mono – 4%, platelets – 32,000/cmm, ESR 140 mm in 1st hr.
❖ PCV	- 0.31.
❖ MCV	- 84 fl.
❖ Reticulocytes	- 0.3%.
❖ Chest X-ray	- Bilateral hilar lymphadenopathy.

QUESTIONS

a. What is the diagnosis?
b. List two essential investigations.

CASE NO. 097

A 35-year-old young man, who is otherwise healthy, presented with impotence for few years. No significant past medical illness.

On examination, looks—obese. Testes—small, pubic hair—sparse. No other physical findings.

Investigations

❖ Testosterone	- 4 mmol/L (normal 14 to 42).
❖ Prolactin	- 350 IU/L (normal <450).
❖ FT$_4$	- 18 pmol/L (normal 9 to 23).
❖ FSH	- 2 IU/L (normal 2 to 8).
❖ LH	- 3 IU/L (normal 3 to 8).

An insulin tolerance test (0.15 IU/kg) is done, which shows the following results:

Time	Glucose	Growth hormone	Cortisol
0	5	4	600
30 min	2	20	1200

QUESTIONS

a. What is the likely diagnosis?
b. Name two sites where the endocrine disturbance may have occurred.
c. Suggest one probable underlying diagnosis.
d. Suggest one investigation.

CASE NO. 098

A 46-year-old housewife was admitted in the hospital with the complaints of weight loss, abdominal pain, low back pain and night sweats for 3 months. She was treated by local doctors, but no improvement.

On examination, the patient is pale and ill-looking. Anemia—moderate. No jaundice.
No other physical findings on clinical examinations.

Investigations

❖ Full blood count	- Hb – 9.4 g/dL, WBC – 13,700/cmm, poly – 71%, lympho – 20%, platelets – 2,70,000/cmm, ESR – 65 mm in 1st hr, myelocytes – 5%, metamyelocytes – 4%, nucleated RBC – 5%.
❖ MCHC	- 30.9 g/dL (normal 30 to 35).
❖ MCV	- 90 fl (normal 78 to 98).
❖ PBF	- Normocytic and normochromic.
❖ Chest X-ray	- Normal.

QUESTIONS

a. What is the hematological diagnosis?
b. Suggest four investigations.
c. Write three causes of the above blood picture.

CASE NO. 099

A lady aged 70 years complains of tiredness, weakness, loss of appetite, cough, headache and occasional fever for 10 months. She had three attacks of pneumonia and UTI in the last 6 months.

On examination, anemia—severe, jaundice—mild. BP—90/70 mm Hg, pulse—90/min, low volume and regular.

Spleen—just palpable. No hepatomegaly. No other physical findings.

Investigations

❖ Full blood count	- Hb – 5.2 g/dL, WBC – 1,15,000/cmm, poly – 18%, lympho – 82%, ESR – 105 mm/h, platelets – 95,000/cmm.
❖ PBF	- Macrocytosis, polychromasia, anisopoikilocytosis and spherocytosis.
❖ MCV	- 106 fl (normal 78 to 98).
❖ Reticulocyte count	- 25% (normal 0.2 to 2).
❖ Serum bilirubin	- 32 μmol/L (normal 2 to 17).

❖ SGPT   - 40 IU/L (normal 5 to 40).
❖ Alkaline phosphatase - 84 IU/L (normal 20 to 100).
❖ Chest X-ray   - Bilateral hilar lymphadenopathy.

QUESTIONS

a. What are the possible diagnoses?
b. Why MCV is high?
c. Suggest two investigations.

CASE NO. 100

A housewife aged 35 years, presented with weight gain, weakness and irregular menstruation. No significant past medical illness.

On examination, looks—obese, face—plethoric, BP—150/105 mm Hg, pulse—88/min, regular. No other physical findings.

Investigations

❖ Full blood count   - Hb – 17.3 g/dL, WBC – 12,300/cmm, poly – 61%, lympho – 36%, eosinophil – 2%, mono – 1%, platelets – 3,95,000/cmm, RBC – 8.2 million/cmm, ESR – 35 mm in 1st hr.
❖ PCV   - 0.55.
❖ Chest X-ray   - Normal.
❖ Serum electrolytes - Sodium 144 mmol/L. Potassium 2.8 mmol/L. Bicarbonate 31 mmol/L. Chloride 101 mmol/L.

Oral glucose tolerance test with 75 g glucose shows the following results:

Time (min)	Glucose (mmol/L)
0	6.1
30	16.4
120	12.9

QUESTIONS

a. List four diagnostically useful investigations.
b. What is the likely diagnosis?
c. What three physical findings would you look for?
d. What further history would you like to take?

CASE NO. 101

A 29-year-old woman was admitted in the hospital with the complains of PV bleeding and high grade, continuous fever, following a self-induced abortion. She took oral contraceptive pill for 4 years.

On examination, the patient looks toxic, anemia—severe, BP—80/60 mm Hg, pulse—124/min, temperature—39.6°C. Lower abdomen—very tender. No other physical findings.

Investigations

- ❖ Full blood count   - Hb – 5.0 g/dL, WBC – 28,700/cmm, poly – 87%, lympho – 13%, platelets – 30,000/cmm, ESR – 85 mm in 1st hour.
- ❖ PBF   - Microcytic, hypochromic and fragmented RBC.
- ❖ Prothrombin time   - 30 sec (Control 12).
- ❖ APTT   - 60 sec (Control 32).
- ❖ Fibrinogen   - 0.05 g/L (1.5 to 4.0 g).

QUESTIONS

a. Mention four pathological conditions present in the above blood picture.
b. Give three possible causes of hematological abnormality.

CASE NO. 102

A school teacher aged 29 years is complaining of persistent puerperal bleeding for 2 months, following normal delivery. For the last 10 days, she is suffering from continuous fever, headache, weakness, bodyache and malaise.

On examination, appearance—pale and ill-looking, anemia—severe, BP—90/60 mm Hg, pulse—110/min, low volume, temperature—102°F. JVP—raised. Heart sounds—muffled. Lungs—normal. No organomegaly.

Investigations

- ❖ Full blood count   - Hb – 5.3 g/dL, WBC – 15,700/cmm, poly – 60%, lympho – 37%, eosinophil – 3%, platelets – 1, 20,000/cmm, ESR – 115 mm in 1st hr.
- ❖ Blood film   - Microcytic and hypochromic.
- ❖ Urine   - Plenty of pus cells, protein (++) and no growth in culture.
- ❖ Chest X-ray   - Cardiomegaly with oligemic lungs.
- ❖ ECG   - Low voltage tracing, heart rate 120/min.
- ❖ USG of abdomen   - Normal.

QUESTIONS

a. What is your diagnosis that explains the above diagnosis?
b. Suggest three diagnostically useful investigations.
c. What is the likely cause of puerperal bleeding?

CASE NO. 103

An old man aged 78 years, who was in good health throughout his life, presented with severe bruising in different parts of the body after minimal trauma for the last 10 months.

On examination, looks—well. Multiple bruises and ecchymoses are seen in different parts of the body. BP—145/90 mm Hg, pulse—76/min. No other physical findings.

Investigations

- ❖ Full blood count   - Hb – 13.1 g/dL, WBC – 7,700/cmm, poly – 56%, lympho – 41%, mono – 3%, platelets – 3,00,000/cmm, ESR – 47 mm in 1st hour.
- ❖ Prothrombin time   - 12 sec (Control 12 sec).
- ❖ APTT   - 35 sec (Control 36 sec).

QUESTIONS

a. Suggest five possible causes.
b. Mention one investigation to find out the underlying pathology.

CASE NO. 104

A young lady is complaining of severe difficulty in breathing, restlessness, compression in chest and feeling of impending death. She had similar attacks previously. She was hospitalized and was given 28% oxygen, nebulized salbutamol and injection aminophylline. But her dyspnea did not improve.

Investigations

- ❖ Full blood count   - Hb – 12.2 g/dL, WBC – 5,000/cmm, poly – 64%, lympho – 36%, ESR – 30 mm in 1st hr, platelets – 1,95,000/cmm.
- ❖ Chest X-ray   - Hypertranslucent lung fields.
- ❖ ECG   - Sinus tachycardia.
- ❖ Echocardiogram   - Mitral valve prolapse.
- ❖ Serum electrolytes   - Sodium 137 mmol/L. Chloride 99 mmol/L. Potassium 4.7 mmol/L. HCO_3 31 mmol/L.
- ❖ PH   - 7.65.
- ❖ Arterial blood gases   - $PaCO_2$ 2.5 kPa (normal 4.4 to 6.1). PaO_2 15.5 kPa (normal 12 to 15).

QUESTIONS

a. What is the likely diagnosis?
b. How would you treat this lady?

CASE NO. 105

A 46-year-old man was admitted in the emergency following an attack of shallow, feeble respiration and unconsciousness. No history is available from the attendant.

On examination, the patient is dyspneic, cyanosis—present, central. BP—90/60 mm Hg, pulse—110/min, respiratory rate—10/min. Heart and lungs—normal.

Investigations

- ❖ ECG   - Sinus tachycardia.
- ❖ Chest X-ray   - Normal.

Three minutes after receiving an intravenous drug, his condition improved significantly.

QUESTIONS

a. What two diagnoses are possible in such case?
b. Name the diseases and the drugs used in such cases.

CASE NO. 106

A female aged 21-years has been suffering from high grade continued fever, headache, bodyache and malaise for 3 weeks. She noticed multiple red spots and small bruises in different parts of the body recently.

On examination, the patient is pale, ill-looking and apathetic, anemia—mild, BP—90/60 mm Hg, multiple purpuric spots and bruises are present. Spleen—palpable, 2 cm. No other physical findings.

Investigations

❖ Full blood count	- Hb – 10.6 g/dL, WBC – 10,700/cmm, poly – 59%, lympho – 38% eosinophil – 3%, platelets – 45,000/cmm, ESR – 70 mm in 1st hr.
❖ Blood film	- Microcytic and hypochromic.
❖ Urine	- Pus cells are a few, protein (++).
❖ Urine C/S	- No growth.
❖ Chest X-ray	- Normal.

QUESTIONS

a. What is your diagnosis?
b. Suggest two diagnostically useful investigations.

CASE NO. 107

A 70-year-old man has been suffering from fever, cough, weight loss and occasional hemoptysis for 2 months. He was admitted in the hospital with the history of convulsion, followed by uncosnsciousness. He is a known diabetic and hypertensive, also heavy smoker.

On examination, the patient is ill-looking. Generalized clubbing—present, BP—110/80 mm Hg, pulse—90/min. Fever—99.3°F. Neck rigidity—slight, no Kernig's sign.

No response to painful stimuli. Plantar- extensor on both sides.

Investigations

❖ Full blood count	- Hb – 10.2 g/dL, WBC – 5,000/cmm, poly – 64%, lympho – 36%, ESR – 70 mm in 1st hr, platelets – 1,95,000/cmm.
❖ Random blood glucose	- 3.9 mmol/L.
❖ Serum electrolytes	- Sodium 117 mmol/L. Chloride 87 mmol/L. Potassium 4.7 mmol/L. HCO_3 21 mmol/L.
❖ Urea	- 1.8 mmol/L (normal 2.5 to 6.6).
❖ Creatinine	- 1 mg/dL (normal 0.68 to 1.36).
❖ LFT	- All normal.
❖ ECG	- Old inferior myocardial infarction.

■ QUESTIONS

a. What is the likely diagnosis?
b. What three tests should be done?
c. What single most therapy should be given initially?

■ CASE NO. 108

A 12-year-old girl is admitted in the hospital following convulsion, shortness of breath and headache.

One week before, she was suffering from fever, abdominal pain, vomiting and diarrhea.

On examination, the patient looks very ill. Anemia—moderate, temperature—38.2°C, BP—155/100 mm Hg, pulse—112/min, respiratory rate—28/min. No other physical findings.

Investigations

❖ Full blood count	- Hb – 8.3 g/dL, WBC – 13,800/cmm, poly – 70%, lympho – 29%, mono – 1%, platelets – 50,000/cmm, ESR – 70 mm in 1st hr.
❖ MCV	- 106 fl (normal 76 to 96).
❖ Reticulocytes	- 12.4% (normal 0.2 to 2).
❖ Calcium	- 1.84 mmol/L (normal 2.12 to 2.62).
❖ Phosphate	- 2.9 mmol/L (normal 0.5 to 1.4).
❖ Urea	- 29.6 mmol/L (normal 2.5 to 6.6).
❖ Creatinine	- 6.1 mg/dL (normal 0.68 to 1.36).
❖ Urine	- Few pus cells, protein (++), RBC cast (+).

■ QUESTIONS

a. What is the most likely diagnosis?
b. List three diagnostically useful investigations.

■ CASE NO. 109

A 61-year-old female, known hypertensive and diabetic noticed some blisters and bullous lesions on dorsum of the hands and face, which are more marked on exposure to sunlight and minor trauma.

On examination, anemia—mild, edema—mild, pitting. Multiple bullous lesions are present on dorsum of both hands, with few ruptured bullae. BP—125/75 mm Hg, pulse—70/min, regular.

Liver—just palpable, non-tender, soft in consistency. Spleen—just palpable. No other physical findings.

Investigations

❖ Full blood count	- Hb – 9.4 g/dL, WBC – 19,700/cmm, poly – 60%, lympho – 40%, platelets – 2, 15,000/cmm, ESR – 45 mm in 1st hr.
❖ Bilirubin	- 15 μmol/L (normal <17).

* SGOT   - 35 IU/L (normal 10 to 45).
* SGPT   - 27 IU/L (normal 10 to 50).
* Alkaline phosphatase - 60 IU/L (normal 40 to 125).
* Total protein   - 56 g/L (normal 60 to 80).
* Albumin   - 24 g/L (normal 35 to 50).
* Serum γGT   - 152 IU/L (normal 5 to 55).
* Serum iron   - 30 µmol/L (normal 10 to 28).
* TIBC   - 75 µmol/L (normal 45 to 72).

QUESTIONS

a. What is the likely diagnosis?
b. Mention two investigations.
c. What two advices would you give to the patient?

CASE NO. 110

A 57-year-old male, smoker, known hypertensive, presented with the complaints of headache, dizziness, lack of concentration and insomnia for 10 months. No history of past illness.

On examination, the patient looks obese; face is plethoric with red eyes. BP—160/110 mm Hg, pulse—82/min.

Investigations

* Full blood count   - Hb – 18.5 g/dL, WBC – 9,750/cmm, poly – 65%, lympho – 35%,
                         platelets – 4,70,000/cmm, RBC – 8.3 million/cmm,
                         ESR – 1 mm in 1st hr.
* RBS   - 6.5 mmol/L.
* Urea   - 23 mg/dL (normal 20 to 40).
* Creatinine   - 117 µmol/L (normal 70 to 168).
* Chest X-ray   - Heart slightly enlarged in TD.
* USG of abdomen   - Normal.
* ECG   - LVH.

QUESTIONS

a. What is your diagnosis?
b. Suggest two further investigations.
c. What single treatment should be given?

CASE NO. 111

A 42-year-old patient has been suffering from chronic pancreatitis for 5 years. She is admitted in the emergency department with severe acute abdominal pain, vomiting, diarrhea and tetany for one day.

Investigations

- ❖ Full blood count   - Hb – 14.3 g/dL, WBC – 15,000/cmm, poly – 80%, lympho – 20%, ESR – 50 mm in 1st hr, platelets – 1,95,000/cmm.
- ❖ Serum amylase   - 399 Somogy unit (normal 50 to 300).
- ❖ Calcium   - 2.20 mmol/L (normal 2.15 to 2.65).
- ❖ Phosphate   - 0.88 mmol/L (normal 0.8 to 1.4).
- ❖ Albumin   - 30 g/L (normal 35 to 50).
- ❖ Serum electrolytes   - Sodium 127 mmol/L. Chloride 87 mmol/L. Potassium 2.7 mmol/L. HCO_3 25 mmol/L.
- ❖ ECG   - Prolonged QT interval.

Her electrolytes are corrected, but tetany is persistent.

QUESTIONS

a. What is the probable cause of her tetany at presentation?
b. What is the likely cause of persistent tetany?

CASE NO. 112

A young patient who was suffering from nephrotic syndrome, develops severe pain in the left loin and hematuria. He was always in good health.

On examination, face is puffy with baggy eyelids. Anemia—mild. BP—130/85 mm Hg, pulse—88/min, edema—pitting. No other physical findings.

Investigations

- ❖ Full blood count   - Hb – 9.3 g/dL, WBC – 14,600/cmm, poly – 54%, lympho – 45%, mono – 1%, platelets – 1,50,000/cmm,   ESR – 55 mm in 1st hr.
- ❖ Urine   - Red cells (++++), proteinuria (+++).
- ❖ Total urine protein   - 6.90 g/24 h.
- ❖ Serum electrolytes   - Sodium 138 mmol/L. Potassium 4.2 mmol/L. Bicarbonate 26 mmol/L. Chloride 98 mmol/L.
- ❖ Urea   - 30 mg/dL.
- ❖ Creatinine   - 1.31 mg/dL.
- ❖ Albumin   - 18 g/L.

QUESTIONS

a. What is the likely diagnosis?
b. What is the alternative diagnosis?
c. Mention three diagnostically useful investigations.

CASE NO. 113

A housewife aged 42 years has been suffering from schizophrenia for long time and she is on antipsychotic drugs. Recently, she is taking little food, but complaining of polyuria and polydipsia. On the day of admission, she had some quarrel with her husband which was followed by an epileptic fit. One hour later, she is found to be semiconscious.

On examination, the patient has poor response to painful stimulus, no neck rigidity. Urinary bladder—hugely distended.

Investigations

❖ Full blood count   - Hb – 11.5 g/dL, WBC – 8,700/cmm, poly – 67%, lympho – 33%, platelets – 2,30,000/cmm, ESR – 35 mm in 1st hour.
❖ Serum electrolytes   - Sodium 120 mmol/L. Potassium 3.1 mmol/l. Chloride 87 mmol/L. Bicarbonate 19 mmol/L.
❖ Urea   - 3.5 mmol/L (normal 2.5 to 6.6).
❖ RBS   - 3.9 mmol/L.

QUESTIONS

a. What simple immediate therapy should be given?
b. What is the cause of epileptic fit?
c. What is the diagnosis?
d. What single other treatment should be given?

CASE NO. 114

A 55-year-old patient has been suffering from chronic renal failure for 6 years. He is on regular hemodialysis. For the last 6 months, he is complaining of generalized bone pain, backache, weakness, pain in the epigastrium, nausea, vomiting and constipation. He used to take tablet calcium, vitamin D, B complex and aluminum hydroxide.

Investigations

❖ Full blood count   - Hb – 7.1 g/dL, WBC – 13,000/cmm, poly – 59%, lympho – 41%, ESR – 98 mm in 1st hr, platelets – 1,95,000/cmm.
❖ Urea   - 9.2 mmol/L (normal 2.5 to 6.6).
❖ Creatinine   - 3.7 mg/dL (normal 0.68 to 1.36).
❖ Calcium   - 3.5 mmol/L (normal 2.15 to 2.65).
❖ Phosphate   - 2.6 mmol/L (normal 0.8 to 1.4)
❖ Alkaline phosphatase - 350 IU/L (normal 20 to 100).
❖ Uric acid   - 8 mg/dL.

QUESTIONS

a. What is the most likely diagnosis?
b. Suggest three tests to confirm your diagnosis.
c. What treatment should be given?
d. What is cause of bone pain?

CASE NO. 115

A 9-year-old school going boy is admitted in the surgical unit for severe acute abdominal pain, nausea and vomiting for 2 days. On the 2nd day of admission, there are multiple angioedema on face, trunk and thigh, but no history of itching.

He had similar attack four times, for which he was admitted in the hospital and treated conservatively.

Investigations

- Full blood count   - Hb – 10.9 g/dL, WBC – 9,800/cmm, poly – 65%, lympho – 31%, eosinophil – 4%, ESR – 25 mm in 1st hr.
- RBS   - 7.1 mmol/L.
- Urea   - 29 mg/dL.
- Creatinine   - 1.2 mg/dL.
- Plain abdomen X-ray - Subacute intestinal obstruction.
- Serum amylase   - 370 Somogyi units (normal <300).

QUESTIONS

a. What is the likely diagnosis?
b. Suggest two investigations that will help your diagnosis.

CASE NO. 116

A housewife aged 55 years is complaining of lethargy, weight gain and weakness for 10 months.

On examination, the patient looks obese, face—moon-like and plethoric, multiple striae are present, BP—140/100 mm Hg, pulse 96/min. Heart and lung—normal

A long synacthen test (1 mg depot synacthen SC) is carried out, which shows the following results:

Time (h)	Glucose (mmol/L)
0	160
1/2	158
1	175
4	280
8	390
24	845

QUESTIONS

a. What additional history do you like to take?
b. What is the most likely diagnosis?
c. Suggest two further diagnostically useful investigations.

CASE NO. 117

A 48-year-old man was suffering from polycythemia rubra vera. After therapy, he was feeling better. Recent blood count is done, which shows the following results:

❖ Full blood count   - Hb – 14.5 g/dL, WBC – 14,700/cmm, poly – 55%, lympho – 35%, myelocyte – 4%, metamyelocyte – 6%, nucleated RBC–5% platelets – 4,35,000/cmm, ESR – 1 mm in 1st hr.
❖ MCV   - 65 fl (normal 76 to 95).
❖ MCH   - 22 pg (normal 27 to 32).

QUESTIONS

a. What hematological abnormalities are present here?
b. Mention two causes of such abnormalities.
c. What treatment he had received?

CASE NO. 118

A middle aged lady, living alone, had been suffering from alteration of bowel habit, insomnia and weakness for 3 years. For the last 5 months, she has been suffering from polydipsia and polyuria.

On examination, the patient is obese, BP—100/70 mm Hg, pulse—60/min, edema—present, non-pitting.

Investigations

❖ Full blood count   - Hb – 11.1 g/dL, WBC – 9,000/cmm, poly – 63%, lympho – 37%, ESR – 60 mm in 1st hr, platelets – 2,95,000/cmm.
❖ Urine   - Mild proteinuria, no glycosuria, few pus cells.
❖ Fasting blood sugar   - 5.1 mmol/L.
❖ Urea   - 9.3 mg/dL.
❖ Creatinine   - 1.2 mg/dL.
❖ Serum electrolytes   - Sodium 125 mmol/L. Chloride 85 mmol/L. Potassium 4.8 mmol/L. HCO_3 25 mmol/L.
❖ USG of renal system   - Both the kidneys are slightly enlarged.

After 8 hour water deprivation test		
Time	Plasma osmolality (mOsmol/kg – Normal 285 to 295)	Urinary osmolality (mOsmol/kg)
08 AM	301	225
11 AM	310	230
02 PM	323	228
04 PM	339	236
After 20 µg desmopressin intranasally at 4 PM	338	245

QUESTIONS

a. What is the diagnosis?
b. What additional history will you take to find out the cause?

CASE NO. 119

A man aged 60 years is admitted in the hospital with the complaints of fever for 6 months. The fever is low grade, continuous, mostly with evening rise and associated with night sweating. He is also complaining of headache mostly in the occipital and temporal region, weakness, tiredness and substantial weight loss for 3 months. For the last 2 months, he is having pain and stiffness involving the neck, both shoulder joints and knee joints, frequent backache with morning stiffness.

On examination, the patient is cachexic and very ill, anemia—moderate, BP—100/60 mm Hg, pulse—110/min. All the joints are very tender, muscles also tender on mild palpation.

Investigations

❖ Full blood count	- Hb – 8.1 g/dL, WBC – 9,800/cmm, poly – 61%, lympho – 35%, eosinophil – 4%, ESR – 140 mm in 1st hr.
❖ CRP	- 47 mg/dL (normal <10).
❖ PBF	- Normocytic and normochromic.
❖ SGPT	- 35 IU/L (normal 5 to 40).
❖ SGOT	- 32 IU/L (normal 10 to 40).
❖ Alkaline phosphatase	- 260 IU/L (normal 20 to 100).
❖ γGT	- 49 IU/L (normal 5 to 30).
❖ Chest X-ray	- Heart slightly enlarged.
❖ Blood and urine culture	- No growth.
❖ MT	- 03 mm.
❖ USG of abdomen	- Liver is slightly enlarged.
❖ CT scan of brain	- Normal.

QUESTIONS

a. What diagnosis would you consider first?
b. Suggest one investigation to confirm your diagnosis.
c. Mention four differential diagnoses.

CASE NO. 120

An elderly lady is admitted in the hospital with the complaints of anorexia, weakness, irregular bowel habit and occasional pain in the abdomen for 7 months.

On examination, BP—160/100 mm Hg, pulse—80/min. Tenderness in the epigastric region. No organomegaly. Heart, lung—normal. No other physical findings.

Investigations

❖ Full blood count	- Hb – 14.3 g/dL, WBC – 11,900/cmm, poly – 52%, lympho – 43%, mono – 4%, eosinophil – 1%, platelets – 4,88,000/cmm, ESR – 10 mm in 1st hr.

❖ Chest X-ray - Normal.
❖ Serum electrolytes - Sodium 136 mmol/L. Potassium 3.1 mmol/L
Chloride 113 mmol/L. Bicarbonate 21 mmol/L.
❖ Urea - 6.7 mmol/L (normal 2.5 to 6.7).
❖ Calcium - 3.01 mmol/L (normal 2.20 to 2.67).
❖ Phosphate - 0.8 mmol/L (normal 0.8 to 1.5).
❖ Albumin - 43 g/L (normal 35 to 50).
❖ Alkaline phosphatase - 235 IU/L (normal 25 to 100).

QUESTIONS

a. What is the probable diagnosis?
b. List five investigations which would assist in the diagnosis.

CASE NO. 121

An elderly male is hospitalized with frequent headache, irritability, confusion, drowsiness and urinary incontinence for 10 days. He has been suffering from hypertension for 10 years and diabetes mellitus for 5 years. In his past history, he had an attack of fall from roof, followed by loss of consciousness, from which he recovered completely.

On examination, the patient is ill looking and emaciated. BP—150/95 mm Hg, pulse—56/min. No findings in general examination. Neck rigidity—slight. Neurological examination—muscle tone is increased in right lower limb, slightly reduced in right upper limb. Reflexes—right knee and elbow—exaggerated. Other reflexes are normal. Plantar—both extensors. Pupil—unequal, react to light.

QUESTIONS

a. What is your likely diagnosis?
b. Suggest one investigation to confirm the diagnosis.

CASE NO. 122

An woman aged 70 years presented with backache and tingling in both lower limbs with girdle pain for 6 months. Recently, she is also complaining of severe anorexia, marked loss of weight and severe backache.

On examination, the patient looks emaciated, anemia—moderate. No other physical findings.

Investigations

❖ Full blood count - Hb – 9.9 g/dL, WBC – 2,900/cmm, poly – 51%, lympho – 46%,
eosinophil – 3%, ESR – 110 mm in 1st hr, platelets – 1,20,000/cmm.
❖ MCV - 90 fl (normal 76 to 96).
❖ MCHC - 31 g/dL (normal 32 to 36).

QUESTIONS

a. Give three likely diagnoses.
b. Mention three further investigations each aiming at confirming each diagnosis.

CASE NO. 123

A 59-year-old man presented with polyuria, polydipsia, weakness, dizziness, headache, blackout, vomiting and generalized bodyache for 2 months. He is also complaining of marked loss of weight for the last one month. There is no significant past medical history.

On examination, anemia—severe, liver—enlarged, 2 cm, non-tender, firm in consistency. No splenomegly. Bony tenderness over sternum—present.

Investigations

* Full blood count — Hb – 5.8 g/dL, WBC – 2,800/cmm, poly – 59%, lympho – 31%, ESR – 140 mm in 1st hr, platelets – 25,000/cmm, myelocyte – 3%, myeloblast – 4%, metamyelocyte – 4%, nucleated RBC – few.
* PBF — Normocytic and normochromic.
* Urine — Proteinuria (++), RBC cast (++).
* Urea — 15.0 mmol/L (normal 2.5 to 6.6).
* Creatinine — 4.1 mg/dL (normal 0.68 to 1.36).
* Uric acid — 8.1 mg/dL.
* Calcium — 3.1 mmol/L.
* Alkaline phosphatase — 84 IU/L (normal 20 to 100).
* Total protein — 85 g/L (normal 55 to 75).
* Albumin — 30 g/L (normal 35 to 50).

QUESTIONS

a. What is the diagnosis?
b. Suggest one investigation to confirm your diagnosis.
c. What two additional investigations should be done?

CASE NO. 124

A 72-year-old, retired, teacher is hospitalized in the emergency department with central chest pain, nausea and shortness of breath for one day.

On examination, the patient is dyspneic, unable to lie flat. BP—85/60 mm Hg, pulse—54/min, regular. JVP—raised, 2 cm, normal wave form. ECG shows acute inferior myocardial infarction.

He was treated in CCU with injection streptokinase. After few hours, he felt dizzy, followed by syncopal attack. The nurse on duty found that his pulse—40/min, regular. BP—90/55 mm Hg.

QUESTIONS

a. What two diagnoses would you consider?
b. What next investigation would you perform?
c. What treatment should be started immediately?

CASE NO. 125

A 40-year-old, businessman, alcoholic and heavy smoker, having long standing psychiatric problem, was hospitalized following an attack of seizure. No significant past medical history.

On examination, the patients looks drowsy. BP—125/85 mm Hg, pulse—96/min, no neck rigidity, no focal neurological sign. Heart, lungs—normal.

Investigations

❖ RBS	- 4.1 mmol/L.
❖ Serum electrolytes	- Sodium 116 mmol/L. Potassium 3.0 mmol/L. Chloride 73 mmol/L. Bicarbonate 18 mmol/L.
❖ Urea	- 6.7 mmol/L (normal 2.5 to 6.7).
❖ Creatinine	- 120 µmol/L (normal 50 to 120).
❖ Calcium	- 2.00 mmol/L (normal 2.2 to 2.7).
❖ CT scan of brain	- Normal.

QUESTIONS

a. What are the two most likely diagnoses?
b. What two investigations do you suggest?

CASE NO. 126

A 60-year-old man presented with weakness, weight loss, palpitation and occasional fainting attack for 2 months. In his past history, peptic ulcer surgery was done 5 years back.

On examination, the patient is pale looking, emaciated, anemia—moderate. No jaundice. BP—105/60 mm Hg, pulse—84/min. No other physical findings.

Investigations

❖ Full blood count	- Hb – 8.9 g/dL, WBC – 4,800/cmm, poly – 65%, lympho – 35%, ESR – 40 mm in 1st hr, platelets – 2,25,000/cmm.
❖ PBF	- Macrocytic and microcytic.
❖ MCHC	- 25 g/dL.
❖ Urine	- Glycosuria (++).
❖ Glucose tolerance test shows:	

Time	Glucose (mmol/L)
0 hours	6.3 mmol/L
30 minute	13.0 mmol/L
60 minutes	10.3 mmol/L
90 minutes	2.3 mmol/L
120 minutes	3.0 mmol/L

QUESTIONS

a. What does this GTT suggest?
b. Suggest one cause of this GTT.
c. What is the cause of fainting?
d. What are the likely causes of anemia?

CASE NO. 127

A young lady aged 30 years, recently married, quarrelled with her husband and took some tablets with an intention of committing suicide. Few hours later, she became drowsy and was hospitalized. Her husband could not mention the name of the tablet.

After supportive and symptomatic treatment, she made a good recovery and was discharged from the hospital on her request. However, after 5 days, she became confused, irritable and violent. One sedative was given by a local physician, but she became deeply unconscious and was hospitalized again.

On examination, Jaundice—moderate. BP—95/60 mm Hg, pulse—90/min, low volume. Liver—just papable.

Neck rigidity—absent, reflexes—difficult to elicit, plantar—extensor on both sides.

Investigations

* Full blood count   - Hb – 12.4 g/dL, WBC – 15,900/cmm, poly – 68%, lympho – 32%, ESR – 73 mm in 1st hr, platelets – 1,90,000/cmm.
* Serum Bilirubin   - 130 µmol/L (normal 2 to 17).
* ALT   - 200 IU/L (normal 5 to 40).
* AST   - 150 IU/L (normal 10 to 40).
* Alkaline phosphatase - 110 IU/L (normal 20 to 100).
* Blood urea   - 15 mg/dL (normal 9 to 11).
* Serum creatinine   - 1.6 mg/dL (normal 0.68 to 1.36).

QUESTIONS

a. What drug she took?
b. What is the cause of jaundice?
c. Mention three causes of coma.
d. Suggest three useful investigations.

CASE NO. 128

A student aged 16 years, presented with severe weight loss, weakness, gross acanthosis nigricans and persistent glycosuria. He has been suffering from diabetes mellitus for 6 months. Both parents are diabetic.

As a part of investigations, an insulin tolerance test is carried out, which shows the following result:

Time (min)	Glucose (mmol/L)
0 (insulin 0.15 IU/kg)	10.4
15	7.4
30 (insulin 0.3 IU/kg)	7.2
45	4.7
60	3.9
75	3.7
90	5.8
120	8.7

QUESTIONS

a. What inferences can be drawn from these findings?
b. What is the cause of such result?

CASE NO. 129

A 12-year-old girl is admitted in emergency with the complaints of high grade fever, restlessness, incoherent talk and confused state for 1 day. One hour after admission, she became unconscious with incontinence of urine.

On examination, the patient looks pale, sweaty and tachypneic. BP—80/60 mm Hg, pulse—118/min. No response to painful stimuli. Plantar—extensor on both sides.

Investigations

❖ Full blood count   - Hb – 11.9 g/dL, WBC – 6,000/cmm, poly – 68%, lympho – 32%, ESR – 40 mm in 1st hr, platelets – 2,25,000/cmm.
❖ Random blood sugar - 4.4 mmol/L.
❖ Urea   - 6.3 mmol/L.
❖ Creatinine   - 1.3 mg/dL.
❖ Bicarbonate   - 10 mmol/L.
❖ CSF study   - Pressure 50 mm of H_2O (normal 50 to 180).
Cells – 4/cmm, all are lymphocytes (normal 0 to 4).
Protein 0.5 g/L (normal 0.15 to 0.4 g/L).
Glucose 3.3 mmol/L (2.5 to 4 mmol/L).
❖ Arterial blood gases - PaO_2 12.6 kPa (normal 11.2 to 14).
$PaCO_2$ 3.2 kPa (normal 4.7 to 6). pH 7.08 (normal 7.35 to 7.45).
HCO_3 16 mmol/L (normal 22 to 30).

QUESTIONS

a. What is the likely diagnosis?
b. Suggest three investigations.

CASE NO. 130

A 60-year-old man is complaining of progressive weakness first starting in left arm, then left leg, then right leg and right arm for the period of 2 years. He has recent incontinence of urine. Examination of the nervous system shows -

Muscle tone –increased in both upper and lower limbs. Muscle power –diminished in both upper and lower limbs. Reflexes—biceps absent on both sides, triceps—exaggerated both knee and ankles—exaggerated. Plantar –extensor on both sides.

QUESTIONS

a. What diagnosis will you consider first?
b. Suggest three differential diagnoses.
c. What physical sign will you see?
d. Suggest two investigations.

CASE NO. 131

A lady aged 69 years presented with weakness, loss of weight, loss of appetite and intractable pruritus for 6 months. She was always in good health.

On examination, the patient looks ill and emaciated, anemia—mild, jaundice—mild. BP—105/65 mm Hg, pulse—86/min, liver—enlarged, 3 cm, non-tender, firm in consistency. Spleen—enlarged, 5 cm.

Investigations

* Full blood count — Hb – 10.8 g/dL, WBC – 29,000/cmm, neutrophils – 32%, lymphocytes – 62%, monocytes – 4%, eosinophils – 2%, platelets – 89,000/cmm.
* Reticulocytes — 4.4% (normal 0.2 to 2).
* PBF — Normocytic and normochromic, spherocytes (+++), smudge cells.
* PCV — 0.35 (normal 0.35 to 0.47).
* MCV — 85 fl (normal 76 to 96).
* Bilirubin — 38 μmol/L (normal 2 to 17).
* SGPT — 69 IU/L (normal 5 to 40).
* Alkaline phosphatase - 94 IU/L (normal 20 to 100).
* USG of abdomen — hepatosplenomegaly and para-aortic lymphadenopathy.

QUESTIONS

a. What is the most likely underlying diagnosis?
b. Mention two causes of anemia.
c. Suggest two further investigations.

CASE NO. 132

A previously well school-going boy aged 15 years was admitted in a surgical ward with acute abdominal pain, vomiting and constipation for 2 days. On inquiry, it was found that he has substantial weight loss for the last 3 months.

On examination, the patient is emaciated and ill, BP—85/65 mm Hg, pulse—110/min, low volume. Tongue—dry.

Investigations

❖ Full blood count	- Hb – 13.4 g/dL, WBC – 15,700/cmm, poly – 85%, lympho – 15%.
❖ Abdomen X-ray	- Plenty of gas shadow and fluid level.
❖ Chest X-ray	- Normal.
❖ Serum electrolytes	- Sodium 120 mmol/L. Potassium 4.8 mmol/L. Chloride 97 mmol/L. Bicarbonate 8.9 mmol/L.
❖ Urea	- 7.5 mmol/L.
❖ Creatinine	- 1.3 mg/dL.

QUESTIONS

a. What is the most likely diagnosis?
b. What two investigations should be done immediately?

CASE NO. 133

A 56-year-old lady is hospitalized with the complaints of weakness, loss of appetite, palpitation and severe pain in both knee joints for 6 months. She is also complaining of occasional syncopal attacks.

On examination, she looks pigmented and emaciated. Anemia—moderate, No jaundice. No edema. BP—100/60 mm Hg on lying, 85/50 mm Hg on standing, pulse—120/min, low volume, irregularly irrugudar. Liver—palpable, 4 cm, non-tender, firm in consistency. No splenomegaly.

Investigations

❖ Full blood count	- Hb – 8.3 g/dL, WBC – 6,800/cmm, poly – 63%, lympho – 31%, eosinophil – 4%, monocyte – 2%, ESR – 80 mm in 1st hr.
❖ Serum electrolytes	- Sodium 123 mmol/L. Potassium 4.7 mmol/L. Chloride 92 mmol/L.
❖ Serum urea	- 10 mg/dL.
❖ Serum creatinine	- 1.2 mg/dL.
❖ RBS	- 13.1 mmol/L.
❖ Chest X-ray	- Cardiomegaly.
❖ ECG	- Multiple ventricular ectopics.
❖ Serum cortisol	- 110 nmol/L (normal 170 to 720).
❖ TSH	- 0.12 mIU/L (normal 0.5 to 5.1).

QUESTIONS

a. What is your diagnosis?
b. Suggest two further investigations to confirm your diagnosis.
c. What is the likely cause of arthritis?
d. What is the likely cause of cardiac problem?

CASE NO. 134

A 27-year young lady is complaining of flitting arthritis involving all the bigger joints, low grade fever, malaise and weakness for 3 months.

On examination, looks ill, anemia—mild, lymphadenopathy in the cervical and axillary region, which are discrete, soft and non-tender. Spleen—just palpable. All big joints—tender, but not swollen.

Investigations

❖ Full blood count	- Hb – 11.7 g/dL, WBC – 9,700/cmm, poly – 57%, lympho – 42%, mono – 1%, platelets – 1,10,000/cmm, ESR – 80 mm in 1st hr.
❖ RA test	- Positive (1:16).
❖ VDRL	- Positive.
❖ ASO titer	- 400 IU/L (normal <200).
❖ Chest X-ray	- Normal.
❖ MT	- 01.

QUESTIONS

a. Give a possible diagnosis.
b. Mention three essential investigations.

CASE NO. 135

A man aged 60 years, smoker and alcoholic, presented with the complaints of low back pain, weakness, tiredness, difficulty in climbing stairs and raising himself up from sitting for 2 months.

On examination, BP—155/100 mm Hg, pulse—82/min. Tenderness on both SI joints, wasting of both thigh muscles.

Investigations

❖ Full blood count	- Hb – 12.4 g/dL, WBC – 7,700/cmm, poly – 64%, lympho – 36%, ESR – 12 mm in 1st h, platelets – 3,80,000/cmm.
❖ Electrolytes	- Sodium 140 mmol/L. Potassium 3.1 mmol/L. Chloride 101 mmol/L. Bicarbonate 28 mmol/L.
❖ Urea	- 7.7 mmol/L.
❖ Serum cortisol	- 1000 nmol/L at 8.00 am.

A low dose and a high dose dexamethasone suppression tests were done, which shows the following results:

❖ No change after 0.25 µg synacthen.
❖ After 8 mg dexamethasone daily for 2 days, serum cortisol is 960 nmol/L.

QUESTIONS

a. Give two possible diagnoses.
b. Suggest four further investigations which would provide diagnostic information.
c. Mention three causes for his difficulty in climbing stairs.
d. Mention two causes to account for his back pain.

CASE NO. 136

A lawyer aged 53 years, smoker, presented with weakness, tiredness, lethargy, dizziness, vertigo and irritability for 5 months. For the last 3 months, he experiences weakness of both legs and difficulty in walking. He had cholecystectomy 10 years back and partial gastrectomy 5 years back.

On examination, the patients looks pale, anemia—severe, jaundice—moderate, BP—95/60 mm Hg. Liver—just palpable. No splenomegaly. Heart—apex is shifted, in the left 8th intercostal space, 10 cm from mid-line, heaving. Heart sounds—soft. In lower limbs—muscle power and tone are markedly diminished, knee and ankle jerks—absent, plantar—extensor on both sides. Gait—marked ataxia is present.

Investigations

❖ Full blood count   - Hb – 6.7 g/dL, WBC – 3,800/cmm, poly – 61%, lympho – 37%,
                            eosinophil – 2%, ESR – 30 mm in 1st h, platelets – 1,10,000/cmm.
❖ MCV   - 110 fl (normal 76 to 96).
❖ Chest X-ray   - Heart enlarged in TD.
❖ RBS   - 7.8 mmol/L.
❖ Serum bilirubin   - 100 µmol/L (normal 2 to 17).
❖ SGPT   - 39 IU/L (normal 5 to 40).
❖ SGOT   - 42 IU/L (normal 10 to 40).
❖ Alkaline phosphatase - 160 IU/L (normal 20 to 100).
❖ CT scan of brain   - Normal.

QUESTIONS

a. What is your diagnosis?
b. Suggest two investigations to confirm your diagnosis.
c. What two physical signs would you look for?

CASE NO. 137

A man aged 64 years, presented with the history of nausea, weakness, weight loss and difficulty in standing from sitting for 3 months.

On examination, the patient is pale and emaciated. Ankle edema—present, pitting. BP—170/105 mm Hg, pulse—100/min.

Investigations

- ❖ Full blood count - Hb – 7.7 g/dL, WBC – 16,700/cmm, poly – 58%, lympho – 40%, mono – 2%, platelets – 1,70,000/cmm, ESR – 70 mm in 1st hr.
- ❖ Blood film - Normocytic and normochromic.
- ❖ Urea - 48.8 mmol/L (normal 2.5 to 6.6).
- ❖ Creatinine - 700 μmol/L (normal 60 to 120).
- ❖ Serum electrolytes - Sodium 140 mmol/L. Potassium 5.6 mmol/L. Bicarbonate 20 mmol/L. Chloride 96 mmol/L.
- ❖ Arterial blood gases - PaO_2 12.6 kPa (normal 11.2 to 14). $PaCO_2$ 5.2 kPa (normal 4.7 to 6). pH 7.5 (normal 7.35 to 7.45).

▐ QUESTIONS

a. What acid-base disturbance is shown?
b. What is the likely diagnosis?
c. Suggest two possible causes of such findings.

▐ CASE NO. 138

A student of 20-year-old, previously well, presented with difficulty in breathing and severe restrosternal chest pain on climbing stairs. He took rest and was feeling comfortable. When he tried to climb stairs again, there was recurrence of the same symptoms. No significant past medical illness.

On examination, BP—100/70 mm Hg, pulse—110/min. Heart sounds—normal. Lung—clear. An abnormal sound is heard over the precordium, maximum at the left lower sternal edge. ECG—sinus tachycardia with poor R-wave progression.

▐ QUESTIONS

a. What is the likely diagnosis?
b. What immediate investigation would you suggest?

▐ CASE NO. 139

A 12-year-old school going boy, who has been suffering from hemophilia, was admitted with severe pain in the left side of his back. The pain is dull, constant and radiates to the left side of abdomen and left groin. He also complains of persistent hematuria for few days. Usual dose of anti-hemophilic factor was given along with analgesic, but his symptoms were not relieved and hematuria is persistent.

On examination, BP—90/50 mm Hg, pulse—120/min, tenderness in left iliac fossa. His left leg is in flexon, extension of the left knee is painful.

Reduced sensation over the anterior thigh and medial area of the left leg.

Investigations

❖ Full blood count	- Hb – 8.5 g/dL, WBC – 18,700/cmm, poly – 81%, lympho – 19%, platelets – 3,00,000/cmm, ESR – 35 mm in 1st hr.
❖ MCV	- 71 fl (normal 76 to 96).
❖ Prothrombin time	- 13 sec (Control 12).
❖ APTT	- 74 sec (Control 34 sec).

QUESTIONS

a. Mention two differential diagnoses for his pain.
b. What is the cause of neurological signs?
c. Give three causes of his failure to respond to treatment.
d. Mention one investigation that should be done immediately.

CASE NO. 140

A school teacher aged 34 years, known case of chronic liver disease with ascites, was admitted in the emergency department with severe watery diarrhea for several times.

On examination, anemia—mild BP—70/55 mm Hg, pulse—110/min, regular and low volume, dehydration—present, ascites—huge, spleen- just palpable

Investigations

❖ Full blood count	- Hb – 10.7 g/dL, WBC – 10,700/cmm, poly – 69%, lympho – 31%, platelets – 3,70,000/cmm, ESR – 40 mm in 1st hr.
❖ Serum electrolytes	- Sodium 120 mmol/L.Potassium 3.1 mmol/l. Bicarbonate 10 mmol/L. Chloride 110 mmol/L.
❖ Arterial blood gases	- PaO_2 12.6 kPa (normal 11.2 to 14), $PaCO_2$ 2.2 kPa (normal 4.7 to 6), pH 7.38 (normal 7.35 to 7.45).

QUESTIONS

a. What metabolic abnormalities are present?
b. Suggest one serious complication that may occur in such case.
c. Suggest two mechanisms of these abnormalities.

CASE NO. 141

A 28-year-old insulin-dependent diabetic is treated with broad spectrum antibiotic for sore throat. However, she remains ill for few weeks and hospitalized for repeated vomiting, headache and fever.

On examination, the patient looks ill, BP—90/60 mm Hg, pulse—120/min, temperature—100.2°F.

Neck rigidity—present. CBC, RBS, electrolytes, urea, creatinine, chest X-ray—all normal. Lumbar puncture and CSF study shows the following results:

❖ Pressure	- 74 cm of H_2O (normal 50 to 180).
❖ Cells	- 100 cells/cmm, 60% lymphocytes.

❖ Gm stain   - No organism seen.
❖ Protein   - 1.0 g/L (normal 0.15 to 0.40).
❖ Sugar   - 5 mmol/L (simultaneous blood sugar 22 mmol/L).

QUESTIONS

a. Give four possible diagnoses.
b. Mention four further investigations on CSF.
c. Suggest four other investigations which will help in diagnosis.

CASE NO. 142

A labor aged 32-year-old, smoker, presented with extreme weakness, paralysis of both legs, difficulty in speech and deglutition for one day. He had this type of attack several times, especially while he was going to his duty in the morning. His symptoms were improved by giving potassium therapy.

On examination, BP—150/60 mm Hg, pulse—124/min. Heart and lungs—normal.

Muscles—grade 3 weaknesses. Muscle tone—diminished. All the reflexes—absent. Planter—equivocal.

No sensory loss. No other physical findings.

QUESTIONS

a. What two differential diagnoses would you consider?
b. What is the likely diagnosis and why?
c. What history would you take in relation to the weakness?

CASE NO. 143

A 50-year-old man was suffering from bronchial carcinoma. A lobectomy was performed. Three days after operation, suddenly he developed breathlessness, heaviness, pain and compression in the chest.

On examination, the patient is dyspneic, cyanosis—present, central. BP—95/70 mm Hg, pulse—120/min, low volume. Respiratory rate 30/min.

❖ ECG   - Normal.
❖ Arterial blood gases - PaO_2 7.3 kPa (normal 11.2 to 14). $PaCO_2$ 3.9 kPa (normal 4.7 to 6). pH 7.43 (normal 7.35 to 7.45).

QUESTIONS

a. Mention three possible differential diagnoses.
b. Mention three investigations that should be done immediately.

CASE NO. 144

A 25-year-old female is admitted in the hospital with difficulty in breathing, right sided chest pain, dry cough and occasional hemoptysis for one month. She is a known case of VSD, not closed surgically.

On examination, she looks ill, face—puffy, BP—90/60 mm Hg, pulse—120/min and irregular, edema—pitting and moderate. JVP—engorged, pulsatile. Liver—enlarged, 5 cm, tender, soft in consistency.

QUESTIONS

a. What is the cause of her heart failure?
b. What caused her condition to deteriorate recently?
c. What is the cause of her hemoptysis?
d. What is the present diagnosis?
e. What specific treatment may be offered to the patient?

CASE NO. 145

A 70-year-old man was admitted in the emergency due to repeated vomiting, diarrhea and confusion for 12 hours. He passed only 250 mL of urine in the following 24 hours. He was always in good health.

On examination, the patient ill-looking, anxious, BP—85/60 mm Hg, pulse—110/min, low volume. Tongue—dry. No other physical findings.

Investigations

* Serum electrolytes   - Sodium 117 mmol/L.
                          Potassium 3.1 mmol/L.
                          Chloride 87 mmol/L.
                          Bicarbonate 11 mmol/L.
* RBS   - 5 mmol/L.
* Urea   - 6.50 mmol/L (normal 2.5 to 6.6).
* Creatinine   - 450 µmol/L (normal 60 to 120).

QUESTIONS

a. What is your diagnosis?
b. Why urea is relatively low?
c. What is the most important treatment would you start now?

CASE NO. 146

A man aged 60 years has been suffering from chronic liver disease with HCV positive. He was previously alcoholic, but stopped now. Following an episode of TIA and severe headache, he was hospitalized.

On examination, Liver—enlarged, 5 cm, firm, non-tender and irregular. Spleen—just palpable. Ascites—moderate. Few spider angiomas—present.

Investigations

* Full blood count   - Hb – 18.7 g/dL, WBC – 14,700/cmm, poly – 56%, lympho – 44%, platelets – 1,50,000/cmm, RBC – 8.2 million/cmm, ESR – 47 mm in 1st hr.

- PBF   - Macrocytic and normochromic.
- PCV   - 0.58 (normal 0.40 to 0.54).
- Total protein   - 40 g/L (normal 62 to 80).
- Albumin   - 20 g/L (normal 35 to 50).
- Prothrombin time   - 30 sec (control 12).

QUESTIONS

a. What is the likely diagnosis?
b. Suggest an alternative diagnosis.
c. Mention four diagnostically useful investigations.

CASE NO. 147

A lady aged 60 years was hospitalized because of severe anemia. Six units of blood were transfused. No cause was found and she was discharged from the hospital with iron and vitamins. However, she returned after 5 months with the same complains.

On examination, anemia—severe, edema—present and pitting. Jaundice—mild.
This time, blood pictures shows the following results:

- Full blood count   - Hb – 4.9 g/dL, WBC – 4,000/cmm, poly – 39%, lympho – 48%, monocyte – 12%, eosinophil – 1%, platelets – 90,000/cmm, ESR – 140 mm in 1st hr.
- MCV   - 101 fl (normal 76 to 96).
- Reticulocyte   - 7.2% (normal 0.2 to 2).
- PBF   - Anisopoikilocytosis, macrocytosis, microcytosis, hypochromia and hypogranular neutrophil.
- Bone marrow   - Normal cellularity. Lymphoid and megakaryocyte – normal. Erythropoiesis – normocellular and dyserythropoietic. Plasma cell – 18%. Iron stain – normal stainable iron present.

QUESTIONS

a. What is your diagnosis?
b. What other findings may be found in bone marrow?

CASE NO. 148

A housewife aged 36 years presented with severe hirsutism, oligomenorrhea and obesity for 2 years.

On examination, she is obese, BP—140/90 mm Hg, pulse—98/min, few linear white striae are present in the trunk and thigh. No other physical findings.

Investigations

- Full blood count   - Hb – 14.1 g/dL, WBC – 10,700/cmm, poly – 60%, lympho – 38%, mono – 2%, platelets – 3,60,000/cmm, ESR – 32 mm in 1st hr.
- Chest X-ray   - Normal.

❖ 9 AM cortisol	- 480 nmol/L (normal 170 to 700).
❖ 9 AM testosterone	- 5.6 nmol/L (normal 0.9 to 3.1).
❖ LH	- 7.2 IU/L (normal 2.5 to 21).
❖ FSH	- 2.8 IU/L (normal 1 to 10).
❖ Prolactin	- 380 IU/L (normal <360).
❖ SHBG	- 22 nmol/L (normal 46 to 110).
❖ After	- 0.5 mg dexamethasone 6 hourly for 48 hours:
❖ 9 AM cortisol	- <70 nmol/L.
❖ Testosterone	- 5.3 nmol/L.

QUESTIONS

a. What is the most likely diagnosis?
b. What three further investigations do you suggest?

CASE NO. 149

A 52-year-old male, previously well, was admitted in a private clinic with the complains of tiredness, loss of weight, muscular weakness and vague pains in the limbs and trunk for one year. No past illness.

Investigations

❖ Full blood count	- Hb – 9.5 g/dL, WBC – 10,900/cmm, poly – 63%, lympho – 37%, platelets – 3,90,000/cmm, ESR – 30 mm in 1st hr.
❖ Urea	- 8.7 mmol/L (normal 2.5 to 6.6).
❖ Creatinine	- 150 µmol/L (normal 60 to 120).
❖ Calcium	- 2 mmol/L (normal 2.1 to 2.62).
❖ Serum phosphate	- 0.8 mmol/L (normal 0.8 to 1.4).
❖ Alkaline phosphatase -	200 IU/L (normal 30 to 100).
❖ Serum albumin	- 40 g/L (normal 2 to 17).
❖ Serum electrolytes	- Sodium 137 mmol/L. Potassium 2.9 mmol/L. Chloride 117 mmol/L. Bicarbonate 11 mmol/L.

QUESTIONS

a. What is the likely diagnosis?
b. Suggest two likely causes of muscle weakness.
c. What is the probable cause of bone pain?
d. Suggest one biochemical test, which would confirm the diagnosis.
e. What would be the single most useful therapeutic measure?

CASE NO. 150

A 46-year-old woman is admitted in the emergency department with shortness of breath, cough, swelling of both feet and extreme weakness.

On examination, edema—pitting. Clubbing—present. JVP—raised, 3 cm. Liver—enlarged, 4 cm, tender, soft in consistency. No splenomegaly. Heart and lung—normal.

Investigations

- ❖ Vital capacity   - 2.0 L (Predicted 2.4 to 3.6).
- ❖ FEV$_1$ - 1.6 L (Predicted 2.25 to 3.25).
- ❖ Transfer factor   - 4.1 L (Predicted 5.8 to 8.7).
- ❖ Residual volume   - 1.1 L (Predicted 1.55 to 2.32).

▮ QUESTIONS

a. What pulmonary defect is present?
b. What is the likely diagnosis with the above findings?
c. Suggest five investigations to find out cause.

▮ CASE NO. 151

A housewife aged 52 years presented with weight gain, weakness, lethargy and increase in tendency to sleep for 3 years.

   On examination, she is obese, face—plethoric, BP—160/105 mm Hg, pulse—78/min. No other findings.

Investigations

- ❖ Full blood count   - Hb – 14.5 g/dL, WBC – 10,100/cmm, poly – 64%, lympho – 36%, platelets – 3,30,000/cmm, ESR – 20 mm in 1st hr.
- ❖ RBS   - 9 mmol/L.
- ❖ Chest X-ray   - Normal.
- ❖ USG of abdomen   - Hepatomegaly with fatty liver.
- ❖ Serum cortisol   - 900 nmol/L (normal 120 to 720).

   After 0.5 mg dexamethasone 6 hourly for 48 hours, 9 AM cortisol is 690 nmol/L. Then 2 mg dexamethasone 6 hourly for 48 hours, 9 AM cortisol is 150 nmol/L.

▮ QUESTIONS

a. What is the diagnosis?
b. Suggest two further investigations.

▮ CASE NO. 152

A 14-year-old school going girl was suffering from viral fever for 10 days. She noticed several small bruises on her arms and legs on the 8th day of her illness. No significant past medical history.

   She was hospitalized because of severe epistaxis and hemorrhagic bullae in her mouth.

Investigations

- ❖ Full blood count   - Hb – 11.3 g/dL, WBC – 10,700/cmm, poly – 59%, lympho – 38%, eosinophil – 3%, platelets – 30,000/cmm, ESR – 60 mm in 1st hr.
- ❖ Chest X-ray   - Normal.
- ❖ Blood film   - Normocytic and normochromic.

QUESTIONS

a. What diagnosis would you consider first?
b. Suggest two diagnostically useful investigations.
c. What alternative diagnosis should be excluded?

CASE NO. 153

A 30-year-old policeman presented with polyuria and polydipsia. No significant past medical history.

On examination, BP—110/75 mm Hg, pulse—84/min, no dehydration, no edema. No other findings. Water deprivation test is done, which shows the following results:

Osmolality	Plsama	Urine	Body weight (kg)
Basal	295	240	61
After 8 hour	305	250	59.4
After desmopressin	-	760	60

QUESTIONS

a. What is the finding in the result?
b. What is the likely diagnosis?
c. Suggest two differential diagnoses.
d. Mention five causes of the likely diagnosis.

CASE NO. 154

A 45-year-old businessman, known diabetic and mildly hypertensive, smoker, alcoholic, presented with 15 months history of frequent attacks of central abdominal pain, nausea, weight loss and occasional loose motions.

Investigations

- ❖ Full blood count   - Hb – 13.1 g/dL, WBC – 12,700/cmm, poly – 61%, lympho – 37%, eosinophil – 1%, mono – 1%, platelets – 2,98,000/cmm, ESR – 39 mm in 1st hr.
- ❖ MCV   - 102 fl (normal 76 to 96).
- ❖ Chest X-ray   - Normal.
- ❖ GGT   - 115 IU/L (normal 5 to 30 IU).
- ❖ RBS   - 12.1 mmol/L.

QUESTIONS

a. What is the likely diagnosis?
b. What is the likely cause?
c. List three investigations which would assist in the diagnosis.

CASE NO. 155

An elderly woman presented with 6 weeks history of headache, fever, irritability, weight loss and night sweating. She was hospitalized because of confusion and incoherent talk.

On examination, the patient looks emaciated and pale, anemia—moderate, BP—90/65 mm Hg, pulse—54/min.

Investigations

- ❖ Full blood count   - Hb – 8.5 g/dL, WBC – 8,700/cmm, poly – 66%, lympho – 34%, platelets – 3,50,000/cmm, ESR – 70 mm in 1st hr.
- ❖ Serum electrolytes   - Sodium 117 mmol/L. Potassium 4.9 mmol/L. Chloride 87 mmol/L. Bicarbonate 19 mmol/L.
- ❖ RBS   - 5 mmol/L.
- ❖ Urea   - 12 mmol/L (normal 2.5 to 6.6).
- ❖ Creatinine   - 150 µmol/L (normal 60 to 120).

Lumbar puncture and CSF study show the following results:
- ❖ Color   - Clear.
- ❖ Pressure   - 100 mm of H_2O (normal 50 to 180).
- ❖ Protein   - 4.7 gm/L (normal 0.15 to 0.4).
- ❖ Sugar   - 3.2 mmol/L (normal 2.8 to 4.5).
- ❖ Cells   - Total 1200/cmm, 90% lymphocytes (normal 0 to 4).

QUESTIONS

a. What is the likely diagnosis?
b. Suggest two immediate investigations.
c. Mention two causes of low sodium.

CASE NO. 156

An elderly man aged 75 years, is admitted in the hospital with headache, drowsiness and some visual disturbances. He is diabetic, controlled with insulin and hypertensive, controlled with losartan. For his eye problem, some drugs are given, the name of which he could not mention.

On examination, the patient is hyperventilating. BP—155/90 mm Hg, pulse—72/min. Respiratory rate—40/min. Neck rigidity—absent. Fundoscopy shows evidence of both hypertensive and simple diabetic retinopathy.

Investigations

- ❖ RBS   - 12.6 mmol/L.
- ❖ Serum electrolytes   - Sodium 141 mmol/L. Potassium 3.1 mmol/L. Bicarbonate 3.8 mmol/L. Chloride 125 mmol/L.
- ❖ Arterial blood gases   - $PaCO_2$ 1.94 kPa (normal 4.7 to 6).PaO_2 12 kPa (normal 11.2 to 14). pH 7.04 (normal 7.35 to 7.45).

QUESTIONS

a. Suggest a possible cause of this metabolic derangement.
b. What is the underlying metabolic abnormality?
c. Suggest two further investigations.

CASE NO. 157

A young lady aged 20 years, who was otherwise well, is admitted in emergency with the complaints of transient loss of consciousness, followed by right sided hemiparesis. There is history of occasional epistaxis in the past several times.

No neck rigidity. All reflexes on right side—exaggerated. Plantar—extensor on right side. CVS, respiratory system and abdomen—normal.

Investigations

❖ Full blood count — Hb – 8.5 g/dL, WBC – 9,700/cmm, poly – 63%, lympho – 37%, platelets – 90,000/cmm, ESR – 105 mm in 1st hr.
❖ Prothrombin time — 18 sec (control 12).
❖ APTT — 60 sec (control 30).
❖ APTT plus normal plasma — 50 sec
❖ Serum fibrinogen — 2.9 (normal 1.5 to 4).

QUESTIONS

a. What is the likely diagnosis?
b. Suggest three investigations to find out cause.

CASE NO. 158

A lady aged 39 years, housewife, has been suffering from breathlessness, occasional dry cough and weight loss for 2 years. He was hospitalized one year back due to severe breathlessness and improved.

Her lung function test shows:
❖ VC — 2.33 L (Predicted 2.4 to 3.6).
❖ FEV_1 — 1.35 L (Predicted 2.25 to 3.25)
❖ RV — 2.89 L (Predicted 1.5 to 2.32).
❖ FRC — 3.56 L (Predicted 2.17 to 3.25).
❖ TLC — 5.89 L (Predicted 3.96 to 5.66).
❖ TLCO — 4.7 mmol/min/kPa (Predicted 5.8 to 8.7).

QUESTIONS

a. What is the lung function test?
b. What is the most likely diagnosis?
c. Suggest two possible causes.

CASE NO. 159

A young girl aged 18 years is admitted in the hospital with the complaints of generalized weakness, difficulty in swallowing, difficulty in breathing and double vision. She was suffering from upper respiratory infection with fever 10 days back. She was suffering from chicken pox at the age of 8.

Muscle tone and power—diminished in upper and lower limbs.

All reflexes—diminished. Plantar—equivocal on both sides.

Investigations

❖ Full blood count	-	Hb – 11.4 g/dL, WBC – 8,700/cmm, poly – 62%, lympho – 34%, mono – 5%, ESR – 40 mm in 1st hr.
❖ Chest X-ray	-	Normal.
❖ PEFR	-	210/min (Predicted 390 to 500).
❖ FEV$_1$	-	1.6 L (Predicted 2.25 to 3.25).
❖ FVC	-	2.1 L (Predicted 2.4 to 3.6).
❖ Arterial blood gases		PaO$_2$ 10.1 kPa (normal 11.2 to 14). PaCO$_2$ 6.7 kPa (normal 4.7 to 6).

QUESTIONS

a. What two investigations are urgently required?
b. What abnormality is present?
c. What three diagnoses would you consider?

CASE NO. 160

A businessman aged 48 years is admitted in the emergency with the complaints of severe breathlessness, compression in the chest, cough with little mucoid expectoration and severe exhaustion.

Investigations

❖ Arterial gases	-	PaO$_2$ 8.02 kPa (normal 11.2 to 14). PaCO$_2$ 2.9 kPa (normal 4.7 to 6).
❖ pH	-	7.39 (normal 7.35 to 7.45).
❖ Bicarbonate	-	13 mmol/L (normal 22 to 30).
❖ Saturation of O$_2$	-	89%.

QUESTIONS

a. Mention four possible causes.
b. Suggest three further investigations.

CASE NO. 161

A 59-year-old woman, nondiabetic and nonhypertensive, presented with chest pain, bodyache, cough, weight loss and occasional fever for 2 months. She was suffering from breast cancer, treated by mastectomy, followed by radiotherapy and chemotherapy.

Investigations

- ❖ Full blood count — Hb – 11.4 g/dL, WBC – 23,700/cmm, poly – 84%, lympho – 6%, metamyelocytes – 4%, myelocytes – 4%, promyelocytes – 2%, platelets – 80,000/cmm, ESR – 10 mm in 1st hr.
- ❖ MCV — 87 fl (normal 76 to 96).
- ❖ Chest X-ray — Absent left breast shadow.

QUESTIONS

a. What abnormality is present?
b. What is the underlying diagnosis?
c. Suggest two essential investigations.

CASE NO. 162

A 53-year-old man has been suffering from bronchial asthma since his childhood. For the last 20 years, he used to take prednisolone by himself to relieve his symptoms. Recently, he is on inhaler only. For the last 10 days, he is suffering from fever, pain in the throat, cough, headache and severe respiratory distress. He is hospitalized, after an attack of severe vomiting, diarrhea, diffuse abdominal pain, followed by unconsciousness.

On examination, the patient is dyspneic and pale, BP—90/55 mm Hg, pulse—102/min, dehydration—present, slight response to painful stimuli. Heart—normal. Lungs—few rhonchi in both lungs field. Neck rigidity—absent. Plantar—extensor on both sides.

Investigations

- ❖ Full blood count — Hb – 9.8 g/dL, WBC – 18,700/cmm, poly – 81%, lympho – 19%, platelets – 2,55,000/cmm. ESR – 35 mm in 1st hr.
- ❖ Serum electrolytes — Sodium 120 mmol/L. Potassium 4.8 mmol/L. Chloride 87 mmol/L. Bicarbonate 20 mmol/L.
- ❖ RBS — 3.9 mmol/L.
- ❖ Urea — 13 mmol/L (normal 2.5 to 6.6).
- ❖ Creatinine — 140 µmol/L (normal 60 to 120).
- ❖ Chest X-ray — COPD.
- ❖ CT scan of brain — Mild cerebral atrophy.

QUESTIONS

a. What is the likely diagnosis?
b. Suggest two immediate investigations.

CASE NO. 163

A 31-year-old labor has been suffering from low grade, continuous fever, polyarthralgia, headache, lethargy and anorexia for 10 days. On the sixth day of illness, he noticed multiple maculopapular rashes on the trunk and extremities, which are non-itchy.

On examination, BP—110/65 mm Hg, pulse—90/min. Liver and spleen—just palpable, multiple faint maculopapular rashes are present all over the body.

Investigations

- ❖ Full blood count — Hb – 13.4 g/dL, WBC – 14,300/cmm, poly – 38%, lympho – 19%, reactive lymphocytes – 20%, platelets – 2,10,000/cmm, ESR – 10 mm in 1st hr.
- ❖ Blood film — Agglutination (++), polychromasia (++).
- ❖ PCV — 0.44 (normal 0.40 to 0.54).
- ❖ MCV — 93 fl (normal 76 to 96).

▧ QUESTIONS

a. Suggest four possible diagnoses.
b. Suggest four diagnostically helpful investigations.

▧ CASE NO. 164

A 21-year-old young man has been suffering from high grade, irregular fever, and pain in the throat, dry cough, severe headache and frequent vomiting for 2 weeks. For the last 5 days, he noticed high colored urine. One day before admission, he suffered from diarrhea several times, scanty urine and puffiness of face.

On examination, face- puffy, anemia—severe, jaundice—mild. Edema—mild, pitting. BP—80/50 mm Hg, pulse—120/min, dehydration—present, moderate.

Investigations

- ❖ Full blood count — Hb – 5.8 g/dL, WBC – 14,700/cmm, poly – 77%, lympho – 23%, platelets – 1,30,000/cmm, ESR – 55 mm in 1st hr.
- ❖ PBF — Macrocytosis.
- ❖ Reticulocytes — 7% (normal 0.2 to 2).
- ❖ Serum bilirubin — 79 μmol/L (normal 2 to 17).
- ❖ SGPT — 41 IU/L (normal 5 to 40).
- ❖ Serum electrolytes — Sodium 129 mmol/L. Potassium 3.1 mmol/L. Chloride 90 mmol/L. Bicarbonate 23 mmol/L.
- ❖ RBS — 4.9 mmol/L.
- ❖ Urea — 23 mmol/L (normal 2.5 to 6.7).
- ❖ Creatinine — 270 μmol/L (normal 50 to 120).

▧ QUESTIONS

a. What is your diagnosis?
b. What treatment will you start immediately?
c. Suggest one alternative diagnosis.

CASE NO. 165

An 11-year-old school going girl presented with weakness, shortness of breath with mild exertion and occasional dry cough for 2 years. Stature—short, cyanosis—present, central.

Investigations

- Full blood count - Hb – 21.4 g/dL, WBC – 15,300/cmm, poly – 48%, lympho – 45%, eosinophil – 4%, mono – 3%, RBC – 7.5 million/cmm, ESR – 1 mm in 1st hr. platelets – 5,80,000/cmm.
- Arterial blood gases PaO$_2$ 5.7 kPa (normal 11.2 to 14), PaCO$_2$ 5.2 kPa (normal 4.7 to 6).

QUESTIONS

a. What two physical signs would you look for?
b. List two possible causes for the above findings.
c. Suggest two diagnostically helpful investigations.

CASE NO. 166

A 49-year-old man presented with bilateral renal colic, frequency of micturition and polyuria with passage of small stone during micturition.

Investigations

- Urine - Plenty of RBC.
- KUB X-ray - Bilateral renal stone.
- Calcium - 3.97 mmol/L (normal 2.1 to 2.62).
- Phosphate - 1.22 mmol/L (normal 0.8 to 1.4).
- Albumin - 38 g/L (normal 35 to 50).
- Total urinary calcium - 8.5 mmol/24h (normal <7).
  Following 10 days of 100 mg hydrocortisone every 8 hours, fasting calcium was 2.47 mmol/L.

QUESTIONS

a. Suggest three possible causes for these findings.
b. What disease can be excluded with this test?

CASE NO. 167

A housewife aged 49 years was hospitalized following an attack of unconsciousness. According to the relative's statement, the patient was feeling unwell with loss of appetite, lack of interest, constipation and weight gain for the last 9 months. No significant past medical history.

On examination, BP—170/105 mm Hg, pulse—54/min, no response to painful stimulation. No neck rigidity, no Kernig's sign. Plantar—extensor on both sides. Heart and lungs—normal.

Investigations

- ❖ Full blood count   - Hb – 8.7 g/dL, WBC – 19,300/cmm, poly – 83%, lympho – 17%, platelets – 2,35,000/cmm, ESR – 41 mm in 1st hr.
- ❖ PBF   - Macrocytosis and normochromic.
- ❖ Serum bilirubin   - 29 mmol/L (normal 2 to 17).
- ❖ SGPT   - 41 IU/L (normal 5 to 40).
- ❖ Alkaline phosphatase - 95 IU/L (normal 20 to 100).
- ❖ Serum electrolytes   - Sodium 119 mmol/L. Potassium 4.1 mmol/L. Chloride 90 mmol/L. Bicarbonate 24 mmol/L.
- ❖ RBS   - 6.9 mmol/L.
- ❖ Urea   - 8.3 mmol/L (normal 2.5 to 6.7).
- ❖ Creatinine   - 110 µmol/L (normal 50 to 120).
- ❖ ECG   - Heart rate 54/min and T-inversion in V_1 to V_6.
- ❖ Chest X-ray   - Cardiomegaly.
- ❖ CT scan of brain   - Normal.

QUESTIONS

a. What is your diagnosis?
b. Suggest two immediate investigations.

CASE NO. 168

A 60-year-old man was hospitalized following an attack of acute myocardial infarction. He received injection streptokinase and aspirin.

After 1 week, there is bleeding from nose, gum and multiple bruising on the legs and trunk.

Investigations

- ❖ Full blood count   - Hb – 10.7 g/dL, WBC – 11,300/cmm, poly – 53%, lympho – 45%, eosinophil – 2%, platelets – 35,000/cmm, ESR – 41 mm in 1st hr.
- ❖ PBF   - Polychromasia (++).
- ❖ PT   - 21 sec (control 13 sec).
- ❖ APTT   - 57 sec (control 35 sec).

QUESTIONS

a. What is the likely hematological diagnosis?
b. Mention three investigations which would be diagnostically useful.

CASE NO. 169

A 12-year-old girl presented with short stature. Her mother mentioned that there is ejection of milk from both of the breasts of the girl, sometimes with squeezing and sometimes spontaneously.

No other physical findings.

Investigations

- Full blood count — Hb – 13.9 g/dL, WBC – 7,900/cmm, poly – 53%, lympho – 46%, mono – 1%, ESR – 20 mm in 1st hr.
- RBS — 5.3 mmol/L.
- Skull X-ray — Pituitary fossa is enlarged.
- Growth hormone — 10 ng/mL (normal <10 ng/mL).
- Cortisol 9 AM — 590 nmol/L (normal 170 to 720).
- FT_3 — 0.9 pmol/L (normal 1.2 to 3.1).
- FT_4 — 32 pmol/L (normal 65 to 145).
- TSH — 50 mIU/L (normal 0.8 to 3.6).
- Prolactin — 2500 mU/L (normal <360).

QUESTIONS

a. What is the likely diagnosis?
b. What treatment would you give?

CASE NO. 170

A 60-year-old man is complaining of breathlessness, cough with profuse mucoid expectoration, weight loss and anorexia for one year. He was a heavy smoker, but stopped smoking recently.

On examination, BP—95/65 mm Hg, pulse—108/min, cyanosis—absent. Lungs—few rhonchi in both lungs.

Lung function test shows the following results:

- Vital capacity — 2.11 (Predicted 3.9 to 5.01).
- FEV_1 — 1.61 (Predicted 2.3 to 3.61).
- Total lung capacity — 4.61 (Predicted 5.6 to 7.51).
- Transfer factor — 7.7 (Predicted 26).

QUESTIONS

a. What abnormality is seen here?
b. Mention three possible causes.

CASE NO. 171

A 19-year-old student is hospitalized with the complains of repeated vomiting and severe abdominal pain for 12 hours. He is on no drugs.

Investigations

- Full blood count — Hb – 15.4 g/dL, WBC – 10,800/cmm, poly – 58%, lympho – 38%, mono – 3%, ESR – 30 mm in 1st hr.
- RBS — 7.3 mmol/L.

❖ Serum electrolytes   - Sodium 138 mmol/L.
                           Chloride 99 mmol/L.
                           Potassium 7.8 mmol/L.
                           Bicarbonate 25 mmol/L.
❖ Urea   - 21 mg/dL (normal 9 to 11).
❖ Creatinine   - 1.3 mg/dL (normal 0.68 to 1.36).
❖ ECG   - Normal.
❖ USG of abdomen   - Full of gas, no other abnormality.

QUESTIONS

a. What abnormality is unusual here?
b. Explain the abnormality.
c. What further investigation would you suggest?

CASE NO. 172

An executive engineer aged 52 years was admitted in the hospital with the complaints of right sided pleuritic chest pain and hemoptysis.

On examination, anemia—severe, spleen—just palpable. No hepatomegaly.

Investigations

❖ Full blood count   - Hb – 7.1 g/dL, WBC – 12,300/cmm, poly – 58%, lympho – 32%, mono – 4%, basophils – 6%, platelets – 10,90,000/mm³, ESR – 110 mm in 1st hr.
❖ PCV   - 0.27 (normal 0.40 to 0.54).
❖ MCV   - 72 fl (normal 76 to 96).
❖ Ferritin   - 12 µg/L (normal 20 to 300).

QUESTIONS

a. Suggest two possible diagnoses.
b. List two further helpful investigations.
c. What is the cause of chest pain?
d. What one physical sign would you look for?

CASE NO. 173

A 29-year-old, single female presented with pain in the epigastrium, anorexia, nausea and constipation for 9 months. For the last 6 months, she is also complaining of recurrent attack of headache, sweating, insomnia and palpitation.

On examination, BP—185/120 mm Hg, pulse—110/min. A small goiter, irregular, nodular, non-tender and hard in consistency, no bruit.

Investigations

* ❖ Full blood count - Hb – 11.7 g/dL, WBC – 9,800/cmm, poly – 59%, lympho – 40%, mono – 1%, ESR – 33 mm in 1st hr.
* ❖ Urine - Normal.
* ❖ RBS - 8.3 mmol/L.
* ❖ Serum electrolytes - Sodium 142 mmol/L. Chloride 100 mmol/L. Potassium 4.8 mmol/L. Bicarbonate 23 mmol/L.
* ❖ Urea - 30 mg/dL (normal 9 to 11).
* ❖ Creatinine - 1.1 mg/dL (normal 0.68 to 1.36).
* ❖ Calcium - 13.6 mg/dL (normal 8.8 to 10.8).
* ❖ ECG - LVH.
* ❖ Chest PAV X-ray - Heart enlarged in TD.

QUESTIONS

a. What is your diagnosis?
b. Suggest four investigations.

CASE NO. 174

A 15-year-old girl is investigated for short stature. Her pubertal development is absent.

On examination, BP—90/55 mm Hg, pulse—84/min, anemia—absent, jaundice—absent. No other physical findings, apart from short stature.

Combined anterior pituitary function test is done (insulin: 0.15 IU/kg iv, TRH: 200 μg IV, LHRH: 100 μg IV).

Time (min)	Glucose mmol/L	Cortisol nmol/L	GH mU/L	TSH mU/L	LH IU/L	FSH IU/L
0	4.6	370	<1	0.5	>25	>50
15	2.1	410	18	10.2	>25	>50
30	0.8	470	24	12.2	>25	>50
45	2.9	660	16	10	>25	>50
60	3.8	588	8	6.8	>25	>50
90	4.1	475	4	4	>25	>50

QUESTIONS

a. Suggest a probable diagnosis.
b. Mention one confirmatory investigation.

CASE NO. 175

A 32-year-old lady presented with anorexia, nausea, vomiting and severe pain in right hypochondrium for 2 weeks. She also noticed high colored urine and rapid abdominal distension for 10 days.

She has been suffering from systemic lupus erythematosus (SLE) for 3 years which is well controlled with prednisolone. Her menstruation is irregular with frequent menorrhagia. She had three miscarriages in the past.

On examination, the patient is pale, anemia—moderate, jaundice—mild, edema—absent. BP—90/55 mm Hg, pulse—72/min. Liver—enlarged, 9 cm, tender, soft in consistency. No splenomegaly. Ascites—moderate.

QUESTIONS

a. What is your likely diagnosis?
b. Suggest three differential diagnoses.
c. Suggest four investigations for your diagnosis.

CASE NO. 176

A 30-year-old divorced lady is complaining of feeling unwell and weakness for few months. For the last 6 weeks, she is suffering from flitting arthritis involving the bigger joints, hands and feet joints, morning stiffness lasting for few minutes, fever and insomnia.

On examination, anemia—moderate, BP—100/60 mm Hg, pulse—82/min. Joints—tender, but not swollen.

Investigations

❖ Full blood count	- Hb – 8.1 g/dL, WBC – 9,300/cmm, poly – 58%, lympho – 42%, ESR – 110 mm in 1st hr, platelets – 1,10,000/cmm.
❖ MCV	- 87 fl (normal 76 to 96).
❖ Chest X-ray	- Normal.
❖ RA test	- Negative
❖ VDRL	- Positive.
❖ TPHA	- Negative

QUESTIONS

a. What is the likely diagnosis?
b. List two useful diagnostic investigations.

CASE NO. 177

A 12-year-old school going boy has been suffering from difficulty in walking, abnormality in speech and abnormal movement in right hand for 3 years.

On examination—tremor during catching some object. Speech—scanning, nystagmus in right eye, horizontal.

Muscle tone and power—diminished on right side. Gait—wide based. Plantar—equivocal.

Investigations

* Full blood count — Hb – 18.6 g/dL, WBC – 11,800/cmm, poly – 65%, lympho – 35%, platelets – 2,30,000/cmm, ESR – 20 mm in 1st hr.
* PCV — 0.56 (normal 0.40 to 0.54).
* Chest X-ray — Normal.
* Serum electrolytes — Sodium 144 mmol/L.
  Chloride 97 mmol/L.
  Potassium 4.1 mmol/L.
  Bicarbonate 25 mmol/L.

QUESTIONS

a. What is your diagnosis?
b. Suggest one confirmatory investigation.

CASE NO. 178

A 40-year-old truck driver required 14 units of blood transfusion due to profuse bleeding, following a road traffic accident. He was feeling better. After few days, he is suffering from fever, bodyache, pain in the throat and maculopapular skin rashes, no itching.

Investigations

* Full blood count — Hb – 11.1 g/dL, WBC – 3,700/cmm, poly – 40%, lympho – 59%, eosinophil – 1%, ESR – 40 mm in 1st hr, platelets – 48,000/cmm.
* PCV — 0.30 (normal 0.40 to 0.54).
* MCV — 74 fl (normal 76 to 96).

QUESTIONS

a. What diagnosis would you consider first?
b. Suggest five investigations for your diagnosis.
c. Suggest three further investigations which would help to find out the cause of the above blood picture.
d. Mention two causes of the present problem.

CASE NO. 179

A 25-year-old female is complaining of excessive thirst, weakness, polyuria, nocturia and insomnia for 6 months.

On examination, BP—165/115 mm Hg in both hands, pulse—108/min, high volume. Heart—apex is shifted, heaving.

Muscle tone and power—diminished, all reflexes—diminished. Plantar—difficult to elicit. Sensory—intact.

Investigations

❖ Full blood count	- Hb – 12.7 g/dL, WBC – 6,800/cmm, poly – 60%, lympho – 39%, mono – 1%, ESR – 20 mm in 1st hr.
❖ Urea	- 38 mg/dL (normal 9 to 11).
❖ Creatinine	- 1.2 mg/dL (normal 0.68 to 1.36).
❖ Serum electrolytes	- Sodium 148 mmol/L. Chloride 107 mmol/L. Potassium 3.1 mmol/L. Bicarbonate 27 mmol/L.
❖ RBS	- 9.3 mmol/L.
❖ ECG	- Sinus tachycardia and LVH.
❖ Chest X-ray	- Cardiomegaly, left ventricular type.
❖ Cholesterol	- 5.9 mmol/L (normal 3.7 to 7.8).
❖ Triglyceride	- 1.9 mmol/L (normal 0.8 to 2.1).

QUESTIONS

a. What is your diagnosis?
b. Suggest three investigations to confirm your diagnosis.

CASE NO. 180

A lady, who is suffering from rheumatoid arthritis for a long time, presented with weakness, lethargy, loss of appetite and high colored urine for 2 months.

On examination, the patient is pale and emaciated, anemia—severe, jaundice—mild, edema—mild and pitting. All joints of hands—deformity is present.

Investigations

❖ Full blood count	- Hb – 6.1 g/dL, WBC – 9,700/cmm, poly – 61%, lympho – 37%, monocyte – 2%, ESR – 80 mm in 1st hr, platelets – 1,48,000/cmm.
❖ PCV	- 0.37 (normal 0.35 to 0.47).
❖ MCV	- 104 fl (normal 76 to 96).
❖ Reticulocytes	- 6.8% (normal 0.2 to 2).
❖ Blood film	- Fragmented RBC present and Heinz body – present.

QUESTIONS

a. What is the hematological diagnosis?
b. What is the likely cause?

CASE NO. 181

A 20-year-old young lady presented with hirsutism, amenorrhea and occasional oligomenorrhea since the age of 14 years.

On examination, the patient is obese and depressed, hirsutism—present. BP—130/80 mm Hg, pulse—80/min. Few linear striae—present. No other physical findings.

QUESTIONS

a. Suggest four differential diagnoses.
b. Suggest one single investigation which will help in the diagnosis.
c. Mention six common investigations of such case.

CASE NO. 182

A 46-year-old engineer presented with the complaints of frequent diarrhea, weakness, weight loss and severe difficulty in rising from the chair for 6 months.

On examination, the patient looks emaciated, anemia—moderate, BP—100/60 mm Hg. Muscles of both thighs—wasting present, power and tone—diminished. All reflexes—diminished. Sensory—diminished.

Investigations

* Full blood count   - Hb – 9.4 g/dL, WBC – 4,700/cmm, poly – 68%, lympho – 32%, ESR – 100 mm in 1st hr.
* MCV   - 101 fl (normal 76 to 96).
* PBF   - Microcytic, normochromic and hypochromic, few pencil cells.
* Chest X-ray   - Normal.
* Urea   - 6.7 mmol/L (normal 9 to 11).
* Serum calcium   - 1.76 mmol/L (normal 2.1 to 2.62).
* Serum phosphate   - 0.96 mmol/L (normal 0.8 to 1.4).
* Alkaline phosphatase - 155 IU/L (normal 20 to 100).
* Albumin   - 31 g/L (normal 35 to 50).

QUESTIONS

a. Suggest a likely cause for these findings.
b. Mention three investigations which would be diagnostically useful.
c. Mention the cause of muscular weakness.

CASE NO. 183

A 41-year-old businessman presented with fever, sore throat, headache, bleeding from gum and multiple red spots in the body for one month.

On examination, the patient looks toxic and very ill, anemia—severe. Temperature—38.7°C. Multiple purpuric spots, bruises and ecchymoses are present in different parts of the body.

Investigations

* Full blood count   - Hb – 5.4 g/dL, WBC – 1,000/cmm, poly – 10%, lympho – 90%, ESR – 20 mm in 1st hr, platelets – 30,000/cmm.
* PBF   - Macrocytosis and microcytosis, anisopoikilocytosis.
* Chest X-ray   - Normal.

❖ RBS   - 4.1 mmol/L.
❖ S. creatinine - 1.4 mg/dL.
❖ Serum electrolytes - Sodium 139 mmol/L. Chloride 100 mmol/L.
                   Potassium 3.9 mmol/L. Bicarbonate 26 mmol/L.
❖ Prothrombin time - 30 sec (control 11 sec).
❖ APTT   - 50 sec (control 30 sec).
❖ Bone marrow study - Grossly hypercellular, Myeloid/erythroid ratio—increased,
                   megakaryocytes—scanty, Granulopoiesis—grossly
                   hyper-reactive with blast cells and promyelocyte.

QUESTIONS

a. What is your diagnosis?
b. Suggest two further investigations.
c. What is the prognosis?

CASE NO. 184

A middle-aged patient, known hypertensive and impaired glucose tolerance (IGT), presented with weight gain, lethargy and weakness for 7 months.

He is obese, face—puffy, edema—absent. BP—150/95 mm Hg.

Oral glucose tolerance test and simultaneous growth hormone shows:

Time (min)	Glucose (mmol/L)	GH (mU/L)
0	5.5	7.9
30	10.6	14.7
60	11.5	18.1
90	8.9	14.2
120	8.8	9.4

QUESTIONS

a. What is the likely cause?
b. Mention three other possible causes of such GTT.

CASE NO. 185

A 29-year-old housewife, mother of three children, has been suffering from severe weakness, loss of weight, vertigo, loss of appetite and amenorrhea for one year after delivery of last baby.

She is also complaining of intolerance to cold, lethargy, polyuria and increased tendency to sleep for 8 months.

On examination, the patient looks pale and emaciated, BP—90/60 mm Hg standing and 80/50 mm Hg lying.

Investigations

❖ Full blood count	-	Hb – 12.4 g/dL, WBC – 6,300/cmm, poly – 57%, lympho – 41%, mono – 2%, ESR – 60 mm in 1st hr, platelets – 2,75,000/cmm.
❖ Chest X-ray	-	Normal.
❖ RBS	-	4.1 mmol/L.
❖ Urine	-	Normal.
❖ Serum creatinine	-	1.4 mg/dL.
❖ Serum electrolytes	-	Sodium 130 mmol/L. Chloride 98 mmol/L. Potassium 3.9 mmol/L. Bicarbonate 26 mmol/L.
❖ Serum bilirubin	-	27 µmol/L (normal 2 to 17).
❖ SGOT	-	44 IU/L (normal 10 to 40).
❖ SGPT	-	36 IU/L (normal 5 to 40).
❖ Total protein	-	75 g/L (normal 50 to 75).
❖ Serum albumin	-	40 g/L (normal 35 to 50).

QUESTIONS

a. What is the likely diagnosis?
b. Suggest five investigations.

CASE NO. 186

A man aged 64 years, diabetic, nonhypertensive, had an attack of CVA 3 years back, from which he recovered completely. One year back, he had an attack of myocardial infarction with complete recovery.

He is now complaining of multiple bruising in different parts of the body and occasional gum bleeding for 2 months.

On examination, BP—125/80 mm Hg, pulse—70/min. Multiple purpura and ecchymoses—present. Heart, lungs and abdomen—normal.

Investigations

❖ Full blood count	-	Hb – 13.4 g/dL, WBC – 12,100/cmm, poly – 70%, lympho – 25%, mono – 5%, ESR – 20 mm in 1st hr, platelets – 3,75,000/cmm.
❖ PT	-	15 sec (control 13).
❖ APTT	-	46 sec (control 36).
❖ TT	-	12 sec (control 12).
❖ Bleeding time	-	14.5 minutes (normal <8.5 min).

QUESTIONS

a. Give one possible cause for the above findings.
b. What treatment would you give?

CASE NO. 187

A man aged 45 years presented with difficulty in deglutition, sudden vertigo, vomiting, difficulty in speech, double vision and weakness in the left side of body for 12 hours. He is non-diabetic, but hypertensive, took antihypertensive irregularly.

On examination, BP—160/100 mm Hg, pulse—94/min.

Dysarthria—present. Muscle tone and reflexes—diminished in left side.

Ataxia—present, left side. Nystagmus—present in left eye.

Investigations

❖ Full blood count	- Hb – 13.4 g/dL, WBC – 14,000/cmm, poly – 59%, lympho – 41%, ESR – 20 mm in 1st hr, platelets – 2,98,000/cmm.
❖ Serum bilirubin	- 20 mmol/L (normal 2 to 17).
❖ SGOT	- 54 IU/L (normal 10 to 40).
❖ SGPT	- 34 IU/L (normal 5 to 40).
❖ Total protein	- 73 g/L (nomral 50 to 75).
❖ Serum albumin	- 39 g/L (normal 35 to 50).
❖ Chest X-ray	- Normal.
❖ RBS	- 6.1 mmol/L.
❖ Serum electrolytes	- Sodium 128 mmol/L. Chloride 95 mmol/L. Potassium 3.2 mmol/L. Bicarbonate 29 mmol/L.

QUESTIONS

a. What is your diagnosis?
b. Suggest one investigation to confirm your diagnosis.
c. Mention two physical findings you should look for.

CASE NO. 188

A 60-year-old woman presented with heaviness in the chest, palpitation, breathlessness on exertion, severe generalized muscular pain, polyarthralgia with stiffness of all joints for 9 months. She also noticed gradual abdominal distension for 6 months.

On examination, the patient looks obese, pale, anemia—moderate. BP—150/100 mm Hg, pulse—56/min, ascites—moderate. No organomegaly.

Investigations

❖ Full blood count	- Hb – 9.2 g/dL, WBC – 7,700/cmm, poly – 65%, lympho – 30%, mono – 5%, ESR – 50 mm in 1st hr.
❖ MCV	- 102 fl (normal 76 to 96).
❖ PBF	- Macrocytic and normochromic.
❖ ECG	- Sinus tachycardia and T inversion in all chest leads.
❖ Chest X-ray	- Cardiomegaly with clear margin.

❖ Serum electrolytes   - Sodium 126 mmol/L.
                                       Chloride 94 mmol/L.
                                       Potassium 3.8 mmol/L.
                                       Bicarbonate 27 mmol/L.
❖ Cholesterol   - 8.9 mmol/L (normal 3.7 to 7.8).
❖ Triglyceride   - 6.4 mmol/L (normal 0.8 to 2.1).
❖ CPK   - 560 IU/L (normal 10 to 79).

QUESTIONS

a. What is the likely diagnosis?
b. Mention one single investigation to confirm your diagnosis.

CASE NO. 189

A 45-year-old housewife has been suffering from severe muscular pain, polyarthritis, fever, loss of weight and loss of appetite for the last 3 years. She is also complaining of difficulty in deglutition and occasional diarrhea for 1 year.

On examination, the patient looks emaciated, alopecia—present. Anemia—moderate. Difficulty in opening the mouth. Few mouth ulcers are present, tender. Skin—pigmented, thick. Heliotrope rash over both eyelids.

Muscles are very tender, both the knee joints are swollen and tender.

QUESTIONS

a. What is your diagnosis?
b. Suggest three investigations.
c. Mention one investigation to confirm your diagnosis.

CASE NO. 190

An elderly lady of 65 years is complaining of difficulty in deglutition, retrosternal discomfort, loss of appetite and weight loss for 3 months.

On examination, the patient is cachexic, anemia—moderate, BP—120/75 mm Hg, face—swollen and puffy. Few erythematous eruptions are noted on the back of her hands.

Investigations

❖ Full blood count   - Hb – 7.9 g/dL, WBC – 4,700/cmm, poly – 62%, lympho – 38%,
                                     ESR – 120 mm in 1st hr, platelets – 3,15,000/cmm.
❖ Serum bilirubin   - 20 µmol/L (normal 2 to 17).
❖ SGOT   - 124 IU/L (normal 10 to 40).
❖ SGPT   - 94 IU/L (normal 5 to 40).
❖ Total protein   - 53 g/L (normal 50 to 75).
❖ Serum albumin   - 29 g/L (normal 35 to 50).
❖ Chest X-ray   - Normal.

QUESTIONS

a. List four essential investigations.
b. What is the most likely diagnosis?

CASE NO. 191

A 37-year-old male presented with the complains of recurrent headache, nausea, vomiting and retrosternal discomfort for the last one year. He is also complaining of palpitation and sweating during the attack, which used to improve after taking rest.

On questioning, the patient mentioned that these symptoms are not related to exertion, but precipitated by emotion and following micturition.

On examination, BP—180/120 mm Hg, pulse—124/min, regular.

Investigations

❖ Full blood count - Hb – 13.4 g/dL, WBC – 7,800/cmm, poly – 61%, lympho – 37%,
                      mono – 2%, ESR – 20 mm in 1st hr.
❖ RBS   - 11.3 mmol/L.
❖ ECG   - Sinus tachycardia and LVH.
❖ Chest X-ray   - Cardiomegaly, left ventricular type.
❖ Serum electrolytes - Sodium 146 mmol/L.
                      Chloride 100 mmol/L.
                      Potassium 3.8 mmol/L.
                      Bicarbonate 23 mmol/L.
❖ Cholesterol   - 6.9 mmol/L (normal 3.7 to 7.8).
❖ Triglyceride   - 2.4 mmol/L (normal 0.8 to 2.1).
❖ Urea   - 38 mg/dL.
❖ Creatinine   - 1.2 mg/dL.

QUESTIONS

a. What is the likely diagnosis?
b. Suggest three investigations.

CASE NO. 192

A mother brought her 19-year-old college going girl for weight loss and amenorrhea for the last 8 months. On asking, the girl mentioned that she is having frequent backache, generalized bodyache, intolerance to cold and constipation for the same duration.

On examination, she is emaciated, anemia—mild, no jaundice, no edema. BP—90/55 mm Hg, pulse—56/min. Heart, lungs and abdomen—normal.

Investigations

- ❖ Full blood count — Hb – 10.7 g/dL, WBC – 7,800/cmm, poly – 57%, lympho – 41%, mono – 2%, ESR – 33 mm in 1st hr.
- ❖ RBS — 5.3 mmol/L.
- ❖ Serum electrolytes — Sodium 133 mmol/L.
  Chloride 97 mmol/L.
  Potassium 3.8 mmol/L.
  Bicarbonate 24 mmol/L.
- ❖ Urea — 30 mg/dL.
- ❖ Creatinine — 1.1 mg/dL.
- ❖ Chest X-ray PAV — Normal.
- ❖ FT_3 — 0.9 pmol/L (normal 1.2 to 3.1).
- ❖ FT_4 — 72 pmol/L (normal 65 to 145).
- ❖ TSH — 3.6 mIU/L (normal 0.8 to 3.6).
- ❖ LH — 1.2 IU/L (normal 2.5 to 21).
- ❖ FSH — 0.8 IU/L (normal 1 to 10).
- ❖ Prolactin — 210 mU/L (normal <360).

QUESTIONS

a. What is your diagnosis?
b. Suggest the line of treatment.

CASE NO. 193

A 50-year-old female is admitted in the hospital with severe abdominal pain, diarrhea, vomiting and wheezing. On inquiry, the patient mentioned that there is recurrent attack of nausea, vomiting, diarrhea, flushing of face and respiratory distress for the last one year.

On examination, face—plethoric with red eyes. BP—85/55 mm Hg, pulse—124/min, regular.

Liver—enlarged, 6 cm, irregular, non-tender, firm in consistency. No Splenomegaly.

Pansystolic murmur in left lower parasternal area, multiple rhonchi in both lung fields.

QUESTIONS

a. What is the likely diagnosis?
b. Suggest three investigations.

CASE NO. 194

A 19-year-old girl presented with occasional palpitation, insomnia, weakness and chest pain. She has persistent amenorrhea.

On examination, the patient is short. BP—150/100 mm Hg, pulse—100/min.

Heart—systolic murmur in left second space, near the sternum.

Investigations

- ❖ Full blood count   - Hb – 11.9 g/dL, WBC – 7,800/cmm, poly – 59%, lympho – 39%,
                           mono – 2%, ESR – 33 mm in 1st hr.
- ❖ RBS   - 5.3 mmol/L.
- ❖ Serum electrolytes   - Sodium 143 mmol/L.
                           Chloride 100 mmol/L.
                           Potassium 4.3 mmol/L.
                           Bicarbonate 24 mmol/L.
- ❖ Urea   - 37 mg/dL.
- ❖ Creatinine   - 1.2 mg/dL.
- ❖ TSH   - 3.1 mIU/L (normal 0.8 to 3.6).
- ❖ LH   - 39 IU/L (normal 2.5 to 21).
- ❖ FSH   - 20.8 IU/L (normal 1 to 10).
- ❖ Prolactin   - 415 mU/L (normal <360).
- ❖ Estrogen   - 18 pmol/L (normal 500 to 1100 pmol/L).

QUESTIONS

a. What is the likely diagnosis?
b. Mention one investigation to confirm your diagnosis.
c. What is the cause of murmur?

CASE NO. 195

A 33-year-old housewife, nonhypertensive and non-diabetic, presented with pain with blurring of vision in right eye, weakness of left leg and difficulty in speech for 10 days.

Six months back, she was suffering from complete weakness of both lower limbs, which recovered completely after 2 weeks. She used to take oral contraceptive pills for long time, but stopped recently.

On examination, BP—110/80 mm Hg, pulse—90/min. Speech—scanning.

Muscle tone—increased in left lower limb, but power is diminished in the same limb.

Reflex—left knee and ankle are exaggerated, with plantar extensor.

Horizontal nystagmus—present in right eye.

Fundoscopy—normal in both eyes.

QUESTIONS

a. What is your diagnosis?
b. Mention one investigation to confirm your diagnosis.
c. What is the cause of ocular problem?

CASE NO. 196

A 60-year-old retired officer, nonhypertensive and non-diabetic, is hospitalized because of marked weight loss and anorexia for 5 months. Though the patient does not complain of anything, his wife mentioned that he is behaving abnormally for the last 10 months. There is loss of appetite, sometimes keeps the food in mouth, disturbance in memory, forgetfulness, also frequently very angry for unnecessary reasons.

Recently, his wife noticed that the patient has disturbance in sleep, sometimes walking at night aimlessly, difficulty in micturition and defecation, occasionally involuntary passes stool and urine.

On examination, anemia—mild, BP—140/95 mm Hg, pulse—60/min, occasional resting tremor in right hand.

The patient is uncooperative. Muscle tone, power, reflexes—normal.

Investigations

- ❖ Full blood count   - Hb – 9.9 g/dL, WBC – 5,800/cmm, poly – 54%, lympho – 43%, mono – 3%, ESR – 43 mm in 1st hr.
- ❖ RBS   - 4.3 mmol/L.
- ❖ Serum electrolytes   - Sodium 139 mmol/L.
  Chloride 99 mmol/L.
  Potassium 3.5 mmol/L.
  Bicarbonate 26 mmol/L.
- ❖ Urea   - 40 mg/dL.
- ❖ Creatinine   - 1.1 mg/dL.
- ❖ TSH   - 3.8 mIU/L (normal 0.8 to 3.6).
- ❖ Chest X-ray   - Normal.
- ❖ USG of abdomen   - Mild enlargement of prostate.
- ❖ CT scan of brain   - Diffuse cerebral atrophy.

QUESTIONS

a. What is the likely diagnosis?
b. Suggest two differential diagnoses.

CASE NO. 197

A 50-year-old man was admitted in the hospital with difficulty in walking, slurring of speech and urinary incontinence for 8 months.

His wife mentioned that the patient has severe disturbance in memory, confusion, disorientation, irrelevant talking and twitching of muscles of face.

Neurological examination shows: HPF—disorientation in time and space. Speech—dysarthria, scanning. Resting tremor in both hands, few myoclonus noted in the face. Rigidity—present, cog-wheel type. Reflexes—all exaggerated. Plantar—difficult to elicit for rigidity. Eye—horizontal nystagmus in both eyes.Gait—wide based.

QUESTIONS

a. Suggest three investigations.
b. Mention three differential diagnoses.
c. What is the most probable diagnosis?

CASE NO. 198

A 60-year-old male was suffering from UTI and is on antibiotic for one week. His condition is not improving. On the seventh day of illness, he developed abdominal pain, vomiting and frequent bloody diarrhea. He has been suffering from recurrent peptic ulcer disease which is well controlled with omeprazole.

On examination, BP—80/60 mm Hg, pulse—112/min, low volume, dehydration—severe. Abdomen—diffuse tenderness, more on left side. No organomegaly. No other physical findings.

QUESTIONS

a. What is the likely diagnosis?
b. What three investigations should be done to confirm the diagnosis?
c. Suggest the line of management.

CASE NO. 199

A 66-year-old businessman, hypertensive, smoker is admitted in the hospital with severe bloody diarrhea, abdominal cramps and extreme weakness for 48 hours. He was resuscitated and four units of blood transfusion were given. After 3 days, again there is diarrhea with fresh blood per rectum. He had four attacks in the past within 2 years.

He is a known patient of chronic duodenal ulcer for which he used to take ranitidine, omeprazole and also antacids frequently.

On examination, looks pale, anemia—moderate, BP—160/65 mm Hg, pulse—90/min. Abdomen—tenderness in the epigastrium. No organomegaly.

Heart—ejection systolic murmur in left sternal edge.

Investigations

❖ Full blood count	- Hb – 8.1 g/dL, WBC – 15,800/cmm, poly – 64%, lympho – 32%, mono – 4%, ESR – 23 mm in 1st hr.
❖ RBS	- 4.3 mmol/L.
❖ Serum electrolytes	- Sodium 137 mmol/L. Chloride 99 mmol/L. Potassium 3.4 mmol/L. Bicarbonate 28 mmol/L.
❖ Urea	- 36 mg/dL.
❖ Creatinine	- 1.2 mg/dL.
❖ Chest X-ray	- Heart enlarged in TD.
❖ USG of abdomen	- Normal.
❖ Endoscopy	- Normal.
❖ Sigmoidoscopy	- Normal.

QUESTIONS

a. Suggest three differential diagnoses.
b. Mention three investigations.
c. What is the most likely diagnosis?

CASE NO. 200

An 11-year-old boy was suffering from hemophilia which was well controlled with frequent transfusion of factor VIII. Three days ago, there was persistent bleeding following extraction of a tooth. Factor VIII, fresh blood and fresh frozen plasma were given, but the bleeding did not stop.

QUESTIONS

a. What are the three possible causes of failure of treatment?
b. How to treat such case?

CASE NO. 201

A 20-year-old young man was hospitalized following an attack of right sided weakness, severe headache, drowsiness and vomiting for 8 hours. On questioning, it was found that he has been suffering from low grade, continuous fever, weight loss, polyarthralgia and loss of appetite for the last 3 months.

On examination, the patient looks ill and emaciated. Anemia—moderate, jaundice—absent. BP—85/65 mm Hg, pulse—120/min, temperature—38.1°C.

Liver and spleen—not palpable. Neck stiffness—mild. No Kernig's sign.

Heart—soft first heart sound and mid diastolic murmur in mitral area.

Muscle power—diminished in both upper and lower limbs, in right side, but muscle tone is increased.

All reflexes on right side—increased. Plantar—extensor on right side, normal on left side.

A diagnosis of cardiovascular disease (CVD) with right sided hemiplegia is done.

QUESTIONS

a. Mention two differential diagnoses of his problem.
b. Suggest four investigations for your diagnosis.

CASE NO. 202

A 31-year-old office clerk has been suffering from fever, malaise, bodyache, headache, nausea and vomiting for 3 days. He is hospitalized because of confusion, drowsiness, incoherent and unintelligible talk, speech disturbance and one attack of convulsion.

On examination, the patient is uncooperative. BP—125/95 mm Hg, pulse—112/min, temperature—38.8°C. Neck rigidity—slight. No Kernig's sign. Disturbance of memory—present with disorientation in time and space.

Fundoscopy—normal.

Investigations

- ❖ Full blood count   - Hb – 13.6 g/dL, WBC – 4,800/cmm, poly – 44%, lympho – 54%, mono – 2%, ESR – 28 mm in 1st hr.
- ❖ RBS   - 5.3 mmol/L.
- ❖ Serum electrolytes   - Sodium 140 mmol/L. Chloride 100 mmol/L. Potassium 3.9 mmol/L. Bicarbonate 26 mmol/L.
- ❖ Urea   - 40 mg/dL.
- ❖ Creatinine   - 1.1 mg/dL.

QUESTIONS

a. Suggest four investigations.
b. What is the likely diagnosis?
c. Mention three differential diagnoses.

CASE NO. 203

A 14-year-old school going girl has been suffering from frequent attack of low grade continuous fever, mostly with evening rise and occasional night sweating for the last 2 years. She is also complaining of polyarthralgia, weakness, loss of appetite, mouth ulcer and weight loss for the same duration.

Previous records reveal that few cervical lymph nodes were found, Find needle aspiration cytology (FNAC) shows reactive hyperplasia, hemoglobin 8.2 g/dL and ESR is >100, done several times. Blood and urine culture were negative.

One full course of anti-Koch's therapy for 6 months was given, but no response.

On examination, the patient looks emaciated, pale, anemia—moderate. No jaundice.

Few bilateral cervical lymphadenopathy, discrete, firm, non-tender.

Liver and spleen—just palpable. No ascites.

Heart—pansystolic murmur in left lower parasternal area.

Investigations

- ❖ Full blood count — Hb – 8.6 g/dL, WBC – 4,300/cmm, poly – 48%, lympho – 50%, platelets – 1,10,000/cmm, mono – 2%, ESR – 108 mm in 1st hr.
- ❖ RBS — 6.3 mmol/L.
- ❖ Urea — 46 mg/dL.
- ❖ Creatinine — 1.3 mg/dL.
- ❖ Chest X-ray — Heart slightly enlarged in TD.
- ❖ Blood for C/S — No growth.
- ❖ MT — 12 mm.
- ❖ Urine — Protein (+), few pus cells, no growth on C/S.

QUESTIONS

a. What is the likely diagnosis?
b. What is the diagnosis of cardiac problem?
c. Suggest three investigations.

CASE NO. 204

A 60-year-old man presented with cough with occasional hemoptysis, marked weight loss, polyuria, polydipsia, anorexia, nausea and constipation for 2 months. He is hospitalized, because of confusion and acute abdominal pain. He is non-diabetic, non-hypertensive, heavy smoker. No significant past medical history.

Investigations

- ❖ Full blood count - Hb – 9 g/dL, WBC – 6,300/cmm, poly – 54%, lympho – 43%, mono – 3%, ESR – 30 mm in 1st hr.
- ❖ FBS - 6.3 mmol/L.
- ❖ Serum electrolytes - Sodium 121 mmol/l. Chloride 81 mmol/L. Potassium 3.9 mmol/l. Bicarbonate 29 mmol/l.
- ❖ Urea - 2.2 mmol/L.
- ❖ Creatinine - 1 mg/dL.
- ❖ Serum calcium - 3.2 mmol/L. (normal 2.1 to 2.62)
- ❖ CPK - 432 IU/L (normal 17 to 148)
- ❖ CXR - Irregular opacity in the right apex.
- ❖ CT scan of brain - Mild cerebral atrophy.
- ❖ MT - 10 mm.

QUESTIONS

a. Mention the likely diagnosis.
b. Suggest two further investigations.

CASE NO. 205

A 12-year-old girl presented in the rheumatology clinic with the complains of fever, weakness, loss of weight and polyarthritis for 7 months. Initially, the pain started in the right wrist, followed by left wrist, then knees, ankle joints and both shoulders. After one week of these symptoms, she feels stiffness of neck, associated with sore throat.

On examination, the patient looks pale and cachexic, anemia—mild, no jaundice. BP—100/60 mm Hg, pulse—116/min, temperature—38°C.

Cervical lymphadenopathy on both sides, also few left axillary lymphadenopathy, non-tender, soft in consistency and discrete. Liver and spleen—just palpable. Heart and lungs—normal. All joints—tender.

Investigations

- ❖ Full blood count - Hb – 9.2 g/dL, WBC – 16,300/cmm, poly – 74%, lympho – 26%, ESR – 90 mm in 1st hr.
- ❖ CXR - Normal.
- ❖ USG of abdomen - Splenomegaly and hepatomegaly.
- ❖ ASO titer - 300 IU/L.
- ❖ MT - 10 mm.

QUESTIONS

a. What is the most likely diagnosis?
b. Suggest one differential diagnosis.
c. Mention three investigations.

CASE NO. 206

A 35-year-old office clerk, smoker, non-diabetic and nonhypertensive, presented with fever, weight loss, headache and occasional loose motion for one month. Fever is low grade, continuous, occasionally with chill and rigor, subsides with sweating.

On examination, the patient is pale and emaciated. Anemia—severe, jaundice—mild. Few palpable axillary and cervical lymph nodes, soft, non-tender and discrete. Temperature—38.4°C.

Liver—enlarged, 4 cm and non-tender, firm in consistency. Spleen—enlarged, 14 cm. Heart—systolic flow murmur present in pulmonary area. Lungs—clear.

Investigations

❖ Full blood count	-	Hb – 7.9 g/dL, WBC – 1,800/cmm, poly – 41%, lympho – 48%, mono – 11%, platelets – 1,00,000/cmm, ESR – 30 mm in 1st hr.
❖ PBF	-	Normocytic and normochromic.
❖ FBS	-	6.3 mmol/L.
❖ Urea	-	2.8 mmol/L.
❖ Creatinine	-	1.3 mg/dL.
❖ Chest X-ray	-	Normal.
❖ USG of abdomen	-	Hepatosplenomegaly.
❖ Serum albumin	-	23 g/L (normal 35 to 50).

QUESTIONS

a. What is the likely diagnosis?
b. Suggest four further investigations.
c. Suggest two differential diagnoses.

CASE NO. 207

A 21-year-old student is complaining of high grade, continuous fever with chill and rigor, profuse sweating, loss of appetite and weakness for 9 days. Two weeks ago, he suffered from urethritis.

On examination, the patient looks toxic and depressed. BP—90/60 mm Hg, pulse –124/min, temperature—39.8°C. jaundice—mild.

Liver—just palpable, tender. No splenomegaly.

Investigations

❖ Full blood count	-	Hb – 12.9 g/dL, WBC – 18,800/cmm, poly – 86%, lympho – 13%, mono – 1%, platelets – 1,80,000/cmm, ESR – 60 mm in 1st hr.
❖ FBS	-	6.3 mmol/L.
❖ Chest X-ray	-	Right dome slightly elevated.
❖ Urine	-	Few pus cells.
❖ Bilirubin	-	25 µmol/L (normal 2 to 17).
❖ SGPT	-	49 IU/L (normal 10 to 40).
❖ Alkaline phosphatase	-	310 IU/L (normal 25 to 100).
❖ Serum albumin	-	27 g/L (normal 35 to 50).

QUESTIONS

a. What is the likely diagnosis?
b. What single investigation is helpful for your diagnosis?
c. Suggest four further investigations.

CASE NO. 208

A 34-year-old housewife is hospitalized in the emergency, following an attack of syncope and mild convulsion with breathlessness. On questioning, she complains of low grade fever, polyarthritis involving the joints of hands, knees, shoulders and both elbow for the last 6 months. She is also complaining of dry cough, breathlessness on exertion and skin rash on legs for 2 months.

On examination, she is ill looking and emaciated. Jaundice –mild. Edema—mild, pitting.

BP—90/50 mm Hg, pulse—98/min, low volume. JVP—raised, 4 cm. Few small red nodules—in the shin of both leg, mildly tender.

Right supraclavicular lymph nodes—present,variable in size, discrete, non-tender, firm in consistency.

Precordium—apex in left sixth intercostal space, in anterior axillary line, thrusting in nature.

First and second heart sounds—soft, third heart sound in apical area.

Liver—enlarged, 3 cm, tender, soft, smooth.

Investigations

- ❖ Full blood count - Hb – 12.1 g/dL, WBC – 10,800/cmm, poly – 76%, lympho – 20%, mono – 4%, platelets – 2,80,000/cmm, ESR – 40 mm in 1st hr.
- ❖ FBS - 6.1 mmol/L.
- ❖ Chest X-ray - Cardiomegaly with reticulonodular shadow in both lungs.
- ❖ Bilirubin - 23 μmol/L (normal 2 to 17).
- ❖ SGPT - 56 IU/L (normal 10 to 40).
- ❖ Alkaline phosphatase - 160 IU/L (normal 25 to 100).
- ❖ Serum albumin - 37 g/L (normal 35 to 50).
- ❖ Echocardiography - Dilated cardiomyopathy.

QUESTIONS

a. What is the likely diagnosis compatible with the above picture?
b. What is the likely cause of cardiac abnormality?
c. Suggest five further investigations.

CASE NO. 209

A 62-year-old man, non-diabetic, nonhypertensive, presented with weakness, difficulty in rising from sitting, diffuse bone pain and polyuria for 4 months. No significant past medical history.

On examination, anemia—mild, BP—105/70 mm Hg, corneal arcus—present, proximal muscles—weak. No other physical findings.

Investigations

* Full blood count — Hb – 11.1 g/dL, WBC – 4,800/cmm, poly – 56%, lympho – 43%, mono – 1%, platelets – 2,87,000/cmm, ESR – 70 mm in 1st hr.
* Urine — Proteinuria (+++), glucose (+++).
* RBS — 7.1 mmol/L.
* Serum albumin — 32 g/L. (normal 35 to 50)
* Serum electrolytes — Sodium 137 mmol/L. Chloride 110 mmol/L. Potassium 3 mmol/L. Bicarbonate 13 mmol/L.
* Urea — 4.5 mmol/L.
* Creatinine — 1.06 mg/dL.
* Serum calcium — 2 mmol/L (normal 2.1 to 2.62).
* CPK — 132 IU/L (normal 17 to 148).

QUESTIONS

a. What is the likely diagnosis?
b. Suggest three further investigations.

CASE NO. 210

A 51-year-old man, previous heavy smoker, complains of shortness of breath on mild exertion, anorexia, fatigue and abdominal distension for 2 months. He had been suffering from frequent dry cough and breathlessness for 20 years. Two years before, CABG was done due to three vessels coronary artery blockage.

On examination, BP—130/60 mm Hg, pulse—120/min and low volume. Edema—mild, pitting. JVP—raised, 5 cm.

Chest—barrel shaped.Breath sounds-normal vesicular. No added sounds.

Heart—both first and second sounds are soft. Third heart sound—present.

Liver—3 cm, tender,soft in consistency. No splenomegly. Ascites—moderate.

Investigations

* Full blood count — Hb – 13.2 g/dL, WBC – 4,900/cmm, poly – 56%, lympho – 43%, mono – 1%, platelets – 2,75,000/cmm, ESR – 70 mm in 1st hr.
* RBS — 7.1 mmol/L.
* Serum albumin — 30 g/L (normal 35 to 50).
* Serum electrolytes — Sodium 140 mmol/L. Chloride 108 mmol/L. Potassium 3.9 mmol/L. Bicarbonate 23 mmol/l.
* Urea — 5.5 mmol/L.
* Creatinine — 1.08 mg/dL.
* Bilirubin — 27 μmol/L (normal 2 to 17).
* SGPT — 59 IU/L (normal 10 to 40).
* Alkaline phosphatase — 105 IU/L (normal 25 to 100).
* Chest X-ray — Normal.
* USG of abdomen — Hepatomegaly with ascites.

QUESTIONS

a. What is the most likely diagnosis?
b. Suggest three further investigations.
c. Suggest one definitive investigation.

CASE NO. 211

A 31-year-old lady presented with pleuritic left sided chest pain, multiple skin rashes in different parts of body, low grade fever and polyarthralgia for 5 months. She is taking phenytoin for the last 2 years, because of repeated convulsion.

On examination, the patients looks pale and cachexic. Anemia—moderate. No jaundice, no edema.

Multiple erythematous skin rashes – present in the whole body. Spleen – just palpable.
Chest – pleural rub in left lower part of chest.

Investigations

❖ Full blood count	- Hb – 9.2 g/dL, WBC – 3,900/cmm, poly – 46%, lympho – 53%, mono – 1%, platelets – 1,00,000/cmm, ESR – 95 mm in 1st hr.
❖ RBS	- 8.1 mmol/L.
❖ Chest X-ray	- Pneumonitis in left side.
❖ ECG	- Normal.

QUESTIONS

a. What is the most likely diagnosis?
b. Suggest three further investigations
c. Suggest one definitive investigation.

CASE NO. 212

A 47-year-old housewife is admitted in the emergency with severe acute abdominal pain, nausea and several episodes of vomiting and diarrhea for 36 hours. She also complains of tenesmus, with occasional fresh blood in the stool. She has been suffering from systemic sclerosis for the last 4 years.

On examination, she is ill looking and toxic. Skin—pigmented, tight with some vitiligo. BP—80/60 mm Hg, pulse—112/m, low volume.

Abdomen—distended, diffusely tender, bowel sounds—increased. No organomegaly.

Investigations

❖ Full blood count	- Hb – 10.2 g/dL, WBC – 13,900/cmm, poly – 76%, lympho – 24%, platelets – 2,00,000/cmm, ESR – 90 mm in 1st hr.
❖ RBS	- 4.1 mmol/L.
❖ Serum electrolytes	- Sodium 130 mmol/L. Chloride 90 mmol/L. Potassium 3.1 mmol/L. Bicarbonate 28 mmol/L.
❖ Urea	- 7.5 mmol/L.
❖ Creatinine	- 1.02 mg/dL.
❖ Chest X-ray	- Reticulonodular shadow with right small subdiaphragmatic free air.

▌QUESTIONS

a. What is your diagnosis?
b. Suggest three further investigations.
c. Suggest one differential diagnosis.
d. Suggest very essential single treatment immediately to be given.

▌CASE NO. 213

A 30-year-old male, presented with persistent bleeding, following extraction of one tooth. He has been suffering from mitral stenosis with atrial fibrillation. One year back, he had an attack of TIA. He is taking aspirin, digoxin and diuretic.

Investigations

❖ Full blood count   - Hb – 13.2 g/dL, WBC – 15,900/cmm, poly – 70%, lympho – 30%, platelets – 8,70,000/cmm, ESR – 95 mm in 1st hr.
❖ RBS   - 5.1 mmol/L.
❖ PBF   - Normal.
❖ Prothrombin time   - 13 sec (control 12).
❖ APTT   - 39 sec (normal 32 to 37).
❖ Thrombin time   - 12 sec (normal 11 to 12).
❖ Bleeding time   - 12 sec (normal 3 to 9).
❖ Chest X-ray   - Mitral valvular disease.

▌QUESTIONS

a. What is your diagnosis?
b. What advice would you give to this patient?

▌CASE NO. 214

A 31-year-old farmer, living in a remote area, is under treatment for multibacillary leprosy for 6 months. Recently, he is complaining of weakness, loss of appetite and bluish coloration of the skin.

On examination, the patient looks pale and ill, malnourished and cyanosed. Anemia—severe. No jaundice. BP—90/50 mm Hg, pulse—60/min. Skin—few crusted lesions over the trunk and both arms, some oozing are present.

Investigations

❖ Full blood count   - Hb – 7.1 g/dL, WBC – 11,100/cmm, poly – 66%, lympho – 34%, platelets – 2,20,000/cmm, ESR – 50 mm in 1st hr.
❖ MCV   - 110 fl (normal 76 to 96).
❖ Blood film   - Polychromasia, macrocytosis anisopoikilocytosis, few fragmented red cells.
❖ Reticulocyte   - 6% (normal 0.2 to 2).

❖ RBS   - 4.1 mmol/L.
❖ Serum electrolytes   - Sodium 139 mmol/L. Chloride 90 mmol/L.
                                  Potassium 3.8 mmol/L. Bicarbonate 28 mmol/L.
❖ Urea   - 6.5 mmol/L.
❖ Creatinine   - 1.3 mg/dL.

QUESTIONS

a. What is the likely cause of the above blood picture?
b. What additional morphological feature in the blood film would be helpful diagnostically?
c. What test should be done to find out the cause of cyanosis?
d. Mention three causes of anemia.

CASE NO. 215

A 43-year-old man, smoker, non-diabetic and nonhypertensive, working in a textile mill, presented with breathlessness, cough and occasional tightness in the chest for 10 years. Initially, these symptoms were intermittent, more marked when he was in his workplace, and he felt comfortable while at rest and holidays. For the last one year, his symptoms are progressively increasing during mild activity, but relieved with salbutamol and beclomethasone inhaler and while he is at home.

    On examination of the patient at his house, no physical findings.

Investigations

❖ Full blood count   - Hb – 12.1 g/dL, WBC – 6,100/cmm, poly – 50%, lympho – 40%,
                               eosinophil – 10%, platelets – 3,20,000/cmm, ESR – 10 mm in 1st hr.
❖ Chest X-ray   - Hypertranslucent lungs.
❖ Spirometry   - Suggestive of obstructive airway disease and reversibility test
                               shows 10% increase of FEV_1.

QUESTIONS

a. What is the most probable diagnosis?
b. Suggest one alternative likely diagnosis?
c. Mention three investigations helpful for your diagnosis.
d. Suggest three lines of management.

CASE NO. 216

A 13-year-old boy has been suffering from severe weakness, polyuria, nocturia, weight loss and cramps in legs since his childhood. No history of diarrhea or vomiting. Father notices that his son feels extreme tiredness with minor activity or sports. Also, he is not doing well at school and occasional tetany like attack occurs frequently.

    On examination, BP—110/75 mm Hg, pulse—76/min, muscle power and tone— diminished, all reflexes—diminished. Planter—equivocal.

Investigations

❖ Full blood count   - Hb – 12.2 g/dL, WBC – 9,000/cmm, poly – 55%, lympho – 45%, platelets – 3,90,000/cmm, ESR – 32 mm in 1st hr.

❖ RBS   - 5.1 mmol/L.

❖ Urine   - Protein (+).

❖ Serum creatinine   - 1.1 mg/dL.

❖ Serum electrolytes   - Sodium 140 mmol/L. Chloride 84 mmol/L. Potassium 2.5 mmol/L. Bicarbonate 39 mmol/L.

❖ Surum calcium   - 2.2 mmol/L (normal 2.1 to 2.62)

❖ Surum magnesium   - 0.6 mmol/L (normal >0.8).

❖ USG of abdomen   - Normal.

❖ Chest X-ray   - Normal.

▐ QUESTIONS

a. What is your diagnosis?
b. Suggest two further investigations.
c. Suggest two differential diagnoses.

▐ CASE NO. 217

A 36-year-old labor presented with weakness, weight loss, anorexia, constipation and occasional vomiting. He has been suffering from indigestion and dyspepsia for long time. He used to take antacid, omeprazole, ranitidine. No significant past medical history.

On examination, the patient is pale, dehydrated and emaciated. Anemia—moderate, no jaundice. BP—90/75 mm Hg, pulse—96/min, low volume. Muscles—generalized wasting. Muscle power and tone—diminished, reflexes—diminished, planter—flexor on both sides.

Investigations

❖ Full blood count   - Hb – 9.2 g/dL, WBC – 6,200/cmm, poly – 55%, lympho – 45%, platelets – 3,90,000/cmm, ESR – 22 mm in 1st hr.

❖ RBS   - 4.1 mmol/L.

❖ Serum creatinine   - 110 µmol/L (normal 55 to 125).

❖ Serum urea   - 12.3 mmol/L (normal 2.5 to 6.6).

❖ Serum electrolytes   - Sodium 131 mmol/L. Chloride 81 mmol/L. Potassium 2.2 mmol/L. Bicarbonate 37 mmol/L.

❖ USG of abdomen   - Full of gas.

▐ QUESTIONS

a. What one history will clarify the diagnosis?
b. What metabolic abnormality is seen here?
c. What is the likely diagnosis?
d. Suggest one investigation which will confirm your diagnosis.

CASE NO. 218

A woman aged 46-year-old, presented with severe pain in right hypochondrium and right loin for 3 days. She was treated with analgesic, but pain continued with disturbance of sleep.

She was afebrile. There was tenderness in the right hypochondrium and right loin. Initial investigation—Chest X-ray and abdomen are normal. WBC—26,700/cmm, poly—90%, lympho—10%.

After 5 days, the pain is more severe which radiates to the right loin, groin and inner thigh.

On examination, the patient is very toxic, ill looking, lying with right leg flexed. Temperature—40°C, right loin and groin—very tender.

Right leg and calf—red, swollen and tender.

QUESTIONS

a. What is the probable initial diagnosis?
b. What is the subsequent diagnosis?
c. Suggest one single clinical sign for your diagnosis.
d. What single and simple investigation would you suggest?
e. Explain two causes of the signs of right leg.

CASE NO. 219

An elderly gentleman of 65 years, nonhypertensive, but diabetic, which is well controlled with insulin, presented with mouth ulcers, multiple blisters involving the face, trunk and back of the body. There are also few ulcers in his genitals.

On examination, he is emaciated, moderately anemic. There are multiple bullae, few ruptured with ulceration and crust formation in the upper part of body, also multiple ulcers with oozing are present in his genitals. Few ulcers with eroded margin in the mouth.

QUESTIONS

a. What is the most likely diagnosis?
b. Mention three differential diagnoses.
c. Mention one investigation to confirm your diagnosis.

CASE NO. 220

A 30-year-old housewife, presented with frequency of micturition and dysuria, low grade fever, weakness and loss of appetite for about 2 months. She is also complaining of arthralgia and generalized bodyache for the same duration. She was treated with one course of broad-spectrum antibiotic, which had not helped.

On examination, she is ill looking and pale, mildly anemic, no jaundice, no edema. Temperature—37.9°C. Pulse —100/min, BP—95/65 mm Hg.

Her abdomen is soft with mild suprapubic tenderness. Rest of the clinical examination was normal.

Investigations

- ❖ Full blood count   - Hb – 10.2 g/dL, WBC – 10,800/cmm, poly – 60%, lympho – 40%, platelets – 2,20,000/cmm, ESR – 70 mm in 1st hr.
- ❖ Chest X-ray   - Normal.
- ❖ USG of abdomen   - Normal.
- ❖ Random blood sugar - 4.8 mmol/L.
- ❖ Urine   - Proteinuria (+), pus cells – plenty.
- ❖ Urine C/S   - No growth.

▌QUESTIONS

a. Mention two differential diagnoses.
b. Mention three investigations for your diagnosis.

▌CASE NO. 221

A 56-year-old lady, nonhypertensive, non-diabetic was admitted with confusion, cough with purulent expectoration and high grade continued fever for 6 days.

Investigations

- ❖ Full blood count   - Hb – 12.2 g/dL, WBC – 17,800/cmm, poly – 82%, lympho – 18%, platelets – 3,20,000/cmm, ESR – 70 mm in 1st hr.
- ❖ Chest X-ray   - Consolidation (right).
- ❖ RBS   - 6.1 mmol/L.
- ❖ Serum creatinine   - 110 µmol/L (normal 55 to 125).
- ❖ Serum urea   - 8.3 mmol/L (normal 2.5 to 6.6).
- ❖ Serum electrolytes   - Sodium 111 mmol/L. Chloride 71 mmol/L. Potassium 3.2 mmol/L. Bicarbonate 32 mmol/L.
- ❖ Urine   - Proteinuria (+), pus cells – few.

She was treated with infusion of 3% hypertonic sodium chloride, antibiotics and nebulized salbutamol. Her condition deteriorated, there were two episodes of fits, followed by coma.

▌QUESTIONS

a. What is the possible cause of her deterioration?
b. Mention one investigation at this stage.

▌CASE NO. 222

A 58-year-old lady presented in the emergency with severe pain in both loin for one hour. She was suffering from malaise, weakness, loss of weight, thirst and polyuria for 3 weeks. She has a long history of chronic arthritis and recurrent urinary tract infections. Her sister and brother are sufferer of rheumatoid arthritis.

On examination, BP—160/95 mm Hg, pulse—76/min. Tenderness in both loin. Muscle power and tone—diminished, all reflexes—normal.

Investigations

- ❖ Full blood count – Hb – 9.2 g/dL, WBC – 6,000/cmm, poly – 62%, lympho – 38%, platelets – 3,20,000/cmm, ESR – 60 mm in 1st hr.
- ❖ Chest X-ray – Normal.
- ❖ RBS – 6.7 mmol/L.
- ❖ Serum creatinine – 310 µmol/L (normal 55 to 125).
- ❖ Serum urea – 9.3 mmol/L (normal 2.5 to 6.6).
- ❖ Serum electrolytes – Sodium 117 mmol/L, Chloride 77 mmol/L, Potassium 3.0 mmol/L, Bicarbonate 32 mmol/L.
- ❖ Urine – Proteinuria (+), few casts and plenty of pus cells, no growth, on culture.
- ❖ USG of abdomen – Normal.
- ❖ Plain X-ray KUB – Normal.

QUESTIONS

a. What is the most likely diagnosis?
b. Mention three investigations for your diagnosis.
c. Mention four important steps of management.

CASE NO. 223

A 55-year-old male, service holder, hypertensive, non-diabetic, smoker was admitted in the hospital with severe respiratory distress, dry cough, chest pain and low grade fever for 15 days. He was suffering from bronchial asthma, which is well controlled with salbutamol inhaler.

There is no other significant past medical history, apart from appendicectomy, done 3 years back.

On examination, he is ill looking and dyspneic. Anemia—severe, no jaundice. Edema—mild. BP—170/95 mm Hg, pulse—86/min. JVP was not raised.

Heart—normal, chest—few rhonchi in both lung fields. Examination of other systems reveal no abnormality.

Investigations

- ❖ Full blood count – Hb – 8.2 g/dL, WBC – 11,800/cmm, poly – 62%, lympho – 18%, mono – 5%, eosinophil – 15%, platelets – 2,20,000/cmm, ESR – 100 mm in 1st hr.
- ❖ Chest X-ray – Increased translucency in both lung fields.
- ❖ RBS – 6.1 mmol/L.
- ❖ Serum creatinine – 410 µmol/L (normal 55 to 125).
- ❖ Serum urea – 9.3 mmol/L (normal 2.5 to 6.6).
- ❖ Serum electrolytes – Sodium 131 mmol/L, Chloride 71 mmol/L. Potassium 4.9 mmol/L, Bicarbonate 34 mmol/L.
- ❖ Urine – Proteinuria (++), RBC – few.
- ❖ USG of abdomen – Both kidneys measured 12.5 cm.
- ❖ Plain X-ray KUB – Normal.

QUESTIONS

a. Mention three differential diagnoses.
b. What is the most likely diagnosis?
c. Mention four investigations.

CASE NO. 224

An elderly gentleman is admitted with right sided pleuritic chest pain, cough and mild breathlessness. There is tender left calf with swelling of foot.

Investigations

❖ Full blood count	-	Hb – 13 g/dL, WBC – 15,800/cmm, poly – 82%, lympho – 18%, platelets – 2,30,000/cmm, ESR – 30 mm in 1st hr.
❖ Chest X-ray	-	Small consolidation in right lung.
❖ RBS	-	6.1 mmol/L.
❖ Serum creatinine	-	110 µmol/L (normal 55 to 125).
❖ Serum urea	-	4.3 mmol/L (normal 2.5 to 6.6).
❖ USG of abdomen	-	Mild hepatomegaly with small right-sided pleural effusion.
❖ Doppler ultrasound	-	Deep vein thrombosis of left leg.

Low molecular weight heparin and a broad-spectrum antibiotic were started. Five days later, investigations show the following findings:

❖ Full blood count	-	Hb – 12.8 g/dL, WBC – 10,800/cmm, poly – 72%, lympho – 28%, platelets – 35,000/cmm.
❖ APTT	-	36 sec (normal 32 to 37).
❖ Prothrombin time	-	12.5 mmol/L (control 12).

QUESTIONS

a. What is the most likely explanation of the hematological abnormality?
b. What is the next management of such case?

CASE NO. 225

A housewife aged 33 years was referred for the management of her uncontrolled diabetes mellitus and hypertension. She was suffering from depression for long-time. In addition to insulin, atenolol and valsartan, she was taking sertraline and alprazolam. Both of her parents are diabetic and hypertensive.

On examination, she is very obese, round face with a few facial acne. Edema—mild. Few linear striae are present in the trunk. BP—165/95 mm Hg, pulse—70/min. JVP was not raised.

An initial diagnosis was Cushing's syndrome.

Investigations

❖ Full blood count	-	Hb – 11.2 g/dL, WBC – 7,800/cmm, poly – 60%, lympho – 36%, mono – 3%, eosinophil – 1%, platelets – 2,25,000/cmm, ESR – 10 mm in 1st hr.
❖ Chest X-ray	-	Normal.
❖ RBS	-	16 mmol/L.
❖ Serum creatinine	-	90 µmol/L (normal 55 to 125).
❖ Serum urea	-	4.3 mmol/L (normal 2.5 to 6.6).
❖ Serum electrolytes	-	Sodium 141 mmol/L, Chloride 100 mmol/L. Potassium 3.4 mmol/L, Bicarbonate 28 mmol/L.
❖ Urine	-	Glucose (+++).
❖ Serum cortisol	-	Morning – 840 nmol/L, midnight – 960 nmol/L
❖ USG of abdomen	-	Normal.
❖ CT scan of abdomen	-	Normal.
❖ MRI of brain	-	Normal.

An overnight dexamethasone suppression test showed failure of suppression of cortisol.

QUESTIONS

a. What is the likely diagnosis?
b. What next investigation would you suggest?

CASE NO. 226

A 57-year-old male, smoker, labor, known diabetic for 20 years, on oral hypoglycemic drug, presented with extreme weakness, nausea, insomnia and polyuria for 2 months.

In his past medical history, cholecystectomy was done 7 years back. Pneumonia, 2 times in the past 6 months.

On examination, he is ill looking, puffy face, mildly anemic. Pulse—90/min, BP—155/95 mm Hg. Examination of other systems reveal no abnormality. Fundoscopy reveals evidence of background diabetic retinopathy.

Investigations

❖ Full blood count	-	Hb – 11 g/dL, WBC – 5,800/cmm, poly – 58%, lympho – 36%, mono – 5%, eosinophil – 1%, platelets – 2,90,000/cmm, ESR – 20 mm in 1st hr.
❖ Chest X-ray	-	Normal.
❖ RBS	-	11 mmol/L.
❖ Serum creatinine	-	190 µmol/L (normal 55 to 125).
❖ Serum urea	-	7.3 mmol/L (normal 2.5 to 6.6).
❖ Serum electrolytes	-	Sodium 138 mmol/L, Chloride 98 mmol/L. Potassium 3.9 mmol/L, Bicarbonate 28 mmol/L.
❖ Urine	-	Proteinuria (+++).
❖ USG of abdomen	-	Normal.

QUESTIONS

a. What is your clinical diagnosis?
b. Mention one drug for the management of the patient.

CASE NO. 227

A 47-year clerk, non-smoker, presented with anorexia, pain in upper abdomen and weakness for 2 months. He has no significant history of past illness. In his family history, father and grandmother were suffering from type 2 diabetes mellitus.

On examination, he is obese, BP—145/90 mm Hg, pulse—76/min.

Tenderness in right upper quadrant and epigastric region. Liver—just palpable, no evidence of CLD. Other systems reveal no abnormality.

Investigations

- Full blood count   - Hb – 13 g/dL, WBC – 6,800/cmm, poly—63%, lympho – 33%,
                             mono – 3%, eosinophil – 1%, platelets – 4,20,000/cmm,
                             ESR – 30 mm in 1st hr.
- Chest X-ray   - Normal.
- RBS   - 14.2 mmol/L.
- Serum creatinine   - 95 μmol/L (normal 55 to 125).
- S. urea   - 4.3 mmol/L (normal 2.5 to 6.6).
- Urine   - Normal.
- Serum bilirubin   - 11 mmol/L (normal 2 to 17).
- SGPT   - 103 IU/L (normal 10 to 40).
- Alkaline phosphatase - 104 IU/L (normal 25 to 100).
- G-GT   - 80 IU/L (normal 4 to 35).
- Serum albumin   - 40 g/L (normal 37 to 49).
- Serum cholesterol   - 9.9 mmol/L (normal 3.7 to 7.8).
- Serum triglyceride   - 3.4 mmol/L (normal 0.8 to 2.1).
- USG of abdomen   - Mildly enlarged, homogenous echogenic liver.
- HbsAg   - Negative.
- Anti-HCV   - Negative.

QUESTIONS

a. What is your clinical diagnosis?
b. Mention three lines of management.
c. What further investigation would you suggest?

CASE NO. 228

A 39-year-old man, teacher, is admitted in the emergency with a history of generalized headache, confusion, severe dry cough, polydipsia and polyuria, weakness of left arm and left leg. Following an attack of generalized seizures, he was hospitalized in emergency. He used to smoke 20 cigarettes per day.

On examination, the patient is confused and dehydrated. BP—145/90 mm Hg, pulse—76/min, temperature 37.8°C. Few lymph nodes are palpable on both sides of neck, firm and non-tender. Both parotids are enlarged.

Spleen is just palpable, no hepatomegaly.

There is right lower motor neuron facial nerve palsy, both eyes are red. Fundoscopy and the remaining cranial nerves appeared normal.

There is left-sided hemiparesis with left extensor plantar and brisk reflexes.

Investigations

❖ Full blood count   - Hb – 11.8 g/dL, WBC – 6,300/cmm, poly – 74%, lympho – 20%, eosinophil – 4%, mono – 4%, platelets – 2,20,000/cmm, ESR – 50 mm in 1st hr.
❖ Chest X-ray   - Reticulonodular shadow in both lungs.
❖ RBS   - 6.2 mmol/L.
❖ Serum creatinine   - 97 µmol/L (normal 55 to 125).
❖ Serum urea   - 5.3 mmol/L (normal 2.5 to 6.6).
❖ USG of abdomen   - Splenomegaly with few para-aortic lymph nodes.
❖ CT scan of brain   - Small right sided cerebral infarct.

QUESTIONS

a. Mention four differential diagnoses.
b. What is the most likely diagnosis with the above picture?
c. Mention four further investigations to confirm your diagnosis.

CASE NO. 229

A 22-year-old University student was admitted with severe respiratory distress, weakness and difficulty in eating. Two days after admission, his condition deteriorated and he was transferred to ICU. On query, it was found that he had history of occasional fatigue and weakness, which was worse at the end of the day for the last few months.

On examination, the patient is orthopneic, central cyanosis is present. BP—105/60 mm Hg, pulse—98/min, respiratory rate—30/min. Examination of heart and lungs are normal.

There is bilateral ptosis. Muscle power and tone—diminished in all four limbs. All reflexes—diminished.

Investigations

❖ Full blood count   - Hb – 13.7 g/dL, WBC – 9,800/cmm, poly – 66%, lympho – 30%. mono – 3%, eosinophil – 1%, platelets – 3,70,000/cmm, ESR – 40 mm in 1st hr.
❖ Chest X-ray   - Normal.
❖ RBS   - 7.2 mmol/L.
❖ S. electrolytes   - Sodium 141 mmol/L, Chloride 100 mmol/L. Potassium 3.4 mmol/L, Bicarbonate 28 mmol/L.
❖ Serum creatinine   - 95 µmol/L (normal 55 to 125).
❖ Serum urea   - 4.3 mmol/L (normal 2.5 to 6.6).
❖ Serum calcium   - 2.3 mmol/L (normal 2.20 to 2.67).

QUESTIONS

a. What is the cause of deterioration of this patient?
b. What is the ideal therapeutic management at this stage?
c. Mention two further investigations.

CASE NO. 230

A 42-year-old man presented with 9 months history of frequent sneezing, headache and ear ache. There is also occasional epistaxis. For the last few weeks, he is also suffering from low grade fever, weakness and loss of weight. His grandmother was suffering from bronchial asthma, otherwise, there is no significant illness in his family.

On examination, he is emaciated and pale looking, moderately anemic. BP3105/60 mm Hg, pulse—68/min, respiratory rate—20/min.

A few purpuric rashes in both legs. Nose—hypertrophic turbinate with crust in both noses.

Investigations

❖ Full blood count	-	Hb – 10.7 g/dl, WBC – 19,800/cmm, poly – 66%, lympho – 30%, mono – 3%, eosinophil – 1%, platelets – 4,70,000/cmm, ESR – 60 mm in 1st hr.
❖ Chest X-ray	-	Few opacities in the apex of both lungs.
❖ X-ray PNS	-	Maxillary sinusitis.
❖ RBS	-	7.2 mmol/L.
❖ Serum electrolytes	-	Sodium 141 mmol/L, Chloride 100 mmol/L. Potassium 3.4 mmol/L, Bicarbonate 28 mmol/L.
❖ Serum creatinine	-	95 µmol/L (normal 55 to 125).
❖ Serum urea	-	4.3 mmol/L (normal 2.5 to 6.6).

QUESTIONS

a. What is the likely diagnosis?
b. Mention one alternative diagnosis.
c. Mention two further investigations.

CASE NO. 231

A 69-year elderly man, hypertensive, diabetic, is suffering from ischemic heart disease. He was on ARB, oral hypoglycemic and isosorbide mononitrate, aspirin. Following a syncopal attack, ECG shows complete heart block. He had a VVI single chamber permanent pacemaker implanted and was discharged from the hospital. After few days, he is complaining of frequent dizziness and 3 attacks of syncope.

QUESTIONS

a. Mention four probable causes of his syncope.
b. What is the most likely cause you should consider first?
c. How to treat such case?

CASE NO. 232

A housewife aged 49 years presented with moderate to severe dyspnea, dry cough, occasional fever, weight loss and night sweats. Initially, her symptoms were intermittent, worse in the evening, but for the last 4 weeks, her symptoms become more severe and progressively increasing. There was no previous history of breathlessness, also there is no family history of such illness.

Her husband has a farm, where she was occasionally working.

On examination, she is emaciated and pale looking, moderately anemic. Cyanosis—present, no jaundice, no clubbing. JVP—normal. BP—100/70 mm Hg, pulse—98/min, respiratory rate—28/min. Heart and lungs are normal. No other physical findings.

Investigations

- Full blood count - Hb – 10.7 g/dL, WBC – 6,800/cmm, poly – 61%, lympho – 35%, mono – 3%, eosinophil – 1%, platelets – 3,900,000/cmm, ESR – 10 mm in 1st hr.
- Chest X-ray - Reticulonodular shadow in upper and mid zones.
- RBS - 7.2 mmol/L.
- ECG - Normal.

QUESTIONS

a. Mention two differential diagnoses.
b. What is the most likely diagnosis?
c. Mention three investigations.

CASE NO. 233

A 19-year-old student, obese, presented with delayed puberty. He noticed sparse body hair, underdeveloped penis with small testes.

Apart from short stature and small testes, few pubic and axillary hair, no other physical findings.

Investigations

- Full blood count - Hb – 12.7 g/dL, WBC – 7,800/cmm, poly – 59%, lympho – 40%, eosinophil – 1%, platelets – 3,10,000/cmm, ESR – 09 mm in 1st hr.
- Chest X-ray - Normal.
- FBS - 4.2 mmol/L.
- USG of testes - Both are small.
- FSH - 0.80 U/L (normal 1 to 6).
- LH - 1.1 U/L (normal 2.5 to 21).
- Testosterone - 4.5 nmol/L (normal 9 to 35).
- TSH - 0.6 mIU/L (normal 0.8 to 3.6).

QUESTIONS

a. What is the likely diagnosis?
b. What further history would you like to take?
c. Mention one further investigation.

CASE NO. 234

An elderly woman presented with severe sharp pain in the middle of her back and difficulty in walking, weakness and pain in both lower limbs. She also complains of difficulty in standing from squatting.

On examination, she is emaciated, moderately anemic. BP—160/70 mm Hg, pulse—68/min. Tenderness over the thoracic spine. Also both limbs are tender. No other physical findings.

Investigations

❖ Full blood count	- Hb – 11.6 g/dL, WBC – 7,000/cmm, poly – 69%, lympho – 30%, eosinophil – 1%, platelets – 3,90,000/cmm, ESR – 25 mm in 1st hr.
❖ RBS	- 7.2 mmol/L.
❖ ECG	- Normal.
❖ Serum electrolytes	- Sodium 138 mmol/L, Chloride 100 mmol/L. Potassium 4.1 mmol/L, Bicarbonate 28 mmol/L.
❖ Serum creatinine	- 105 µmol/L (normal 55 to 125).
❖ Serum urea	- 5.3 mmol/L (normal 2.5 to 6.6).
❖ Serum calcium	- 2.0 mmol/L (normal 2.20 to 2.67).
❖ Serum phosphate	- 0.6 mmol/L (normal 0.8 to 1.4).
❖ Serum alkaline phosphatase	- 240 IU/L (normal 45 to 105).
❖ Serum parathormone	- 9.5 pmol/L (0.5 to 5.4).
❖ X-ray of spine	- Partial collapse of T11 vertebrae.

QUESTIONS

a. What is the likely diagnosis?
b. Mention two further investigations.

CASE NO. 235

A 34-year-old labor presented with continuous fever, malaise, headache, bodyache and dry cough for 9 days. Amoxiclav and cough syrup were prescribed by a local physician, but his condition was not improving. He is also complaining of dyspnea, vomiting and arthralgia. He noticed multiple skin rashes in the trunk for 3 days, but itching.

On examination, he looks unwell and very toxic, temperature—39°C, BP—100/70 mm Hg, pulse—108/min.

Multiple maculopapular rashes are present in the trunk. Chest examination shows fine crepitations in left side of back. Neck stiffness—present. Kernig's sign—negative.

Investigations

- ❖ Full blood count
  - Hb – 9.2 g/dL, WBC – 7,200/cmm, poly – 66%, lympho – 33%, eosinophil – 1%, platelets – 2,100,000/cmm, ESR – 25 mm in 1st hr.
- ❖ RBS
  - 7.2 mmol/L.
- ❖ Serum bilirubin
  - 31 µmol/L (normal 2 to 17).
- ❖ SGPT
  - 58 IU/L (normal 10 to 40).
- ❖ Alkaline phosphatase -
  104 IU/L (normal 25 to 100).
- ❖ Gamma-GT
  - 40 IU/L (normal 4 to 35).
- ❖ Serum albumin
  - 36 g/L (normal 37 to 49).
- ❖ Chest X-ray
  - Consolidation in left side.
- ❖ Serum electrolytes
  - Sodium 128 mmol/L, Chloride 90 mmol/L, Potassium 4.3 mmol/L.
- ❖ Serum creatinine
  - 105 µmol/L (normal 55 to 125).
- ❖ Serum urea
  - 5.3 mmol/L (normal 2.5 to 6.6).

QUESTIONS

a. What is the likely diagnosis?
b. What is the rash?
c. What is the cause of anemia?
d. Mention two investigations.

CASE NO. 236

A 66-year-old man presented with gradual onset of limb weakness, pain in muscle, loss of weight, cough and hemoptysis, associated with intermittent diplopia for 2 months.

On examination, he looks emaciated, generalized clubbing, moderately anemic. There is right sided partial ptosis and also proximal myopathy in both lower limbs.

Muscle power—diminished in lower limbs, with reduced tendon reflexes. No sensory abnormality.

Investigations

- ❖ Full blood count
  - Hb – 9.0 g/dL, WBC – 4,200/cmm, poly – 59%, lympho – 39%, eosinophil – 2%, platelets – 2,10,000/cmm, ESR – 65 mm in 1st hr.
- ❖ RBS
  - 4.2 mmol/L.
- ❖ Serum albumin
  - 26 g/L (normal 37 to 49).
- ❖ Chest X-ray
  - Consolidation in right apex.
- ❖ Serum electrolytes
  - Sodium 130 mmol/L. Chloride 92 mmol/L. Potassium 4 mmol/L.
- ❖ Serum creatinine
  - 110 µmol/L (normal 55 to 125).
- ❖ Serum urea
  - 4.3 mmol/L (normal 2.5 to 6.6).

QUESTIONS

a. What is the likely diagnosis?
b. What is the cause of hyponatremia?
c. Mention two investigations.

CASE NO. 237

A 46-year-old man was hospitalized following sudden collapse with loss of consciousness, during his morning walk. The attendant mentioned that the patient complained of severe headache and vomiting before collapse.

After query, one of his relatives informed that the patient is a heavy smoker, used to take some drugs and occasional alcohol. Also, the patient was suffering from some kidney disease.

On examination, the patient is unconscious, no response to painful stimuli, BP—120/70 mm Hg, pulse—50/min.

Heart and lungs—normal, plantar—bilateral extensor.

Blood sugar, serum electrolytes, creatinine are all normal. ECG shows sinus bradycardia.

QUESTIONS

a. What is the likely diagnosis?
b. Suggest one immediate investigation.
c. What further investigation would you suggest?
d. What is the likely problem in kidney?

CASE NO. 238

A college student aged 18 years is hospitalized because of severe repeated vomiting. His mother noticed that her son has some difficulty in walking, incoherent speech and looks more clumsy for 1 month. He was suffering from epilepsy, which is well controlled by phenytoin and sodium valproate.

On examination, he looks ill, dehydrated. Pulse—90/min, BP—110/80 mm Hg. Heart, lung and abdominal examinations were normal.

Neurological examination shows—hypotonia, muscle power is diminished in both upper and lower limbs, with slightly reduced all tendon reflexes. No sensory abnormality, ataxic gait, mild tremor of both hands, dysarthria, bilateral rapid nystagmus on lateral gaze and bilateral dysdiadochokinesia.

Investigations

❖ Full blood count	- Hb – 12.2 g/dL, WBC – 5,200/cmm, poly – 60%, lympho – 40%,
❖ RBS	- 3.2 mmol/L.
❖ SGPT	- 78 IU/L (normal 10 to 40).
❖ SGOT	- 115 IU/L (normal 45 to 105).
❖ Alkaline phosphatase	- 114 IU/L (normal 25 to 100).
❖ Gamma-GT	- 60 IU/L (normal 4 to 35).
❖ Serum albumin	- 38 g/L (normal 37 to 49).

❖ Serum electrolytes   - Sodium 133 mmol/L.
                         Chloride 90 mmol/L.
                         Potassium 3.3 mmol/L.
❖ Serum creatinine   - 105 µmol/L (normal 55 to 125).
❖ Serum urea   - 7.3 mmol/L (normal 2.5 to 6.6).
❖ CT scan of brain   - Normal.

QUESTIONS

a. What is the likely diagnosis?
b. Mention one further investigation.

CASE NO. 239

A 57-year-old man, nonhypertensive, but diabetic, was admitted in emergency with severe headache, high grade continuous fever, confusion, vertigo and photophobia. He vomited twice following admission in hospital. No history of traveling.

On examination, he is drowsy, ill looking, dehydrated. Pulse—60/min, regular. BP—90/60 mm Hg, temperature—38°C. Heart, lung and abdominal examinations were normal.

Neck stiffness—present, diplopia—present in both eyes in horizontal position. Speech—slurred.

Pupil—constricted. Gait—ataxic. Fundoscopy—normal.

Investigations

❖ Full blood count   - Hb – 11.3 g/dL, WBC – 13,200/cmm, poly – 79%, lympho – 21%.
❖ RBS   - 8.2 mmol/L.
❖ SGPT   - 38 IU/L (normal 10 to 40).
❖ SGOT   - 100 IU/L (normal 45 to 105).
❖ Alkaline phosphatase - 90 IU/L (normal 25 to 100).
❖ Gamma-GT   - 35 IU/L (normal 4 to 35).
❖ Serum albumin   - 36 g/L (normal 37 to 49).
❖ Serum electrolytes   - Sodium 137 mmol/L.
                          Chloride 90 mmol/L.
                          Potassium 3.4 mmol/L.
❖ Serum creatinine   - 100 µmol/L (normal 55 to 125).
❖ Serum urea   - 7.3 mmol/L (normal 2.5 to 6.6).
❖ CT scan of brain   - Normal.
❖ CSF study   - Cells 80/mm³, 80% neutrophil, protein – 0.8 g/L,
                          glucose – 2.8 mmol/L, Gram stain – negative.

QUESTIONS

a. What is the likely diagnosis?
b. Mention two investigations.

CASE NO. 240

A 55-year-old man presented with cough, difficulty in breathing and compression in chest for 1 month. Two weeks before, he was suffering from cough, productive of yellow sputum and fever. There was no history of night sweats or weight loss.

Investigations

❖ Full blood count	- Hb – 13.3 g/dL, WBC – 11,100/cmm, poly – 59%, lympho – 27%, mono – 1%, eosinophil – 13%, ESR – 10/h.
❖ RBS	- 7.2 mmol/L.
❖ Chest X-ray	- Diffuse perihilar opacities.
❖ Serum electrolytes	- Sodium 140 mmol/L. Chloride 102 mmol/L. Potassium 4 mmol/L.
❖ Serum creatinine	- 110 µmol/L (normal 55 to 125).
❖ Serum urea	- 4.3 mmol/L (normal 2.5 to 6.6).

QUESTIONS

a. What is the most likely diagnosis?
b. Mention three investigations.

CASE NO. 241

A school boy aged 10 years presented with occasional difficulty in breathing, polyarthritis involving large and small joints, excessive thirst and polyuria for one year. He was suffering from measles at the age of three, otherwise no significant past medical history. No history of such illness in the family.

Investigations

❖ Full blood count	- Hb – 9.0 g/dL, WBC – 3,200/cmm, poly – 59%, lympho – 39%, eosinophil – 2%, platelets – 1,10,000/cmm, ESR – 105 mm in 1st hr.
❖ RBS	- 4.2 mmol/L.
❖ Chest X-ray	- Hypertranslucent lung fields.
❖ Serum creatinine	- 110 µmol/L (normal 55 to 125).

Pulmonary function tests were done, results are:

	Actual	Predicted
❖ FEV$_1$	1.8	4.5
❖ FVC	3.7	5.6
❖ FEV$_1$/FVC	55%	80%
❖ TLC	3.9	7.2
❖ Residual volume	1.9	2.2
❖ Kco (mmol/L/kPa)	6.2	10

QUESTIONS

a. What is the diagnosis of lung function?
b. What is the cause of polyuria?
c. What is the likely diagnosis?
d. Mention two investigations.

CASE NO. 242

A 38-year-old housewife presented with fever with chill and rigor, dry cough with left sided pleuritic pain. She was always in good health. Only other history, she is on oral contraceptive pills for 6 months.

Investigations

❖ Full blood count   - Hb – 13.2 g/dL, WBC – 24,200/cmm, poly – 83%, lympho – 5%, normoblasts – 7%, myeloblasts – 3%, myelocytes – 2%, platelets – 1,48,000/cmm, ESR – 55 mm in 1st hr
❖ RBS   - 7.2 mmol/L
❖ Chest X-ray   - Consolidation in left side.

QUESTIONS

a. What is the likely diagnosis of such blood picture?
b. What further findings may be found in blood film?
c. Mention one further investigation.

CASE NO. 243

A lady aged 31 years, school teacher, is hospitalized following sudden onset of paralysis of left side of the body. She is nonhypertensive, non-diabetic, no history of head injury. There is history of three miscarriages.

On examination, she is drowsy and very ill, pulse—66/min, regular. BP—90/60 mm Hg, temperature—37°C. Heart, lungs and abdominal examinations were normal.

Neck stiffness—slight. Kernig's sign—negative.

Left sided weakness. Reflexes—all exaggerated in left side with extensor plantar. Normal on right side.

Investigations

- ❖ Full blood count — Hb – 10.2 g/dL, WBC – 3,200/cmm, poly – 70%, lympho – 30%, platelets – 88,000/cmm.
- ❖ RBS — 4.2 mmol/L.
- ❖ Serum electrolytes — Sodium 143 mmol/L.
  Chloride 100 mmol/L.
  Potassium 4.3 mmol/L.
- ❖ Serum creatinine — 105 µmol/L (normal 55 to 125).
- ❖ Serum urea — 7.3 mmol/L (normal 2.5 to 6.6).
- ❖ CT scan of brain — Infarct in right middle cerebral artery territory.
- ❖ Color Doppler echocardiogram — Small ASD.

QUESTIONS

a. What is the likely cause of her disability?
b. Mention three further investigations.
c. What is the likely cause of miscarriage?

CASE NO. 244

A 50-year-old man, office clerk, presented with high grade continuous fever, cough, breathlessness and increasing confusion for 9 days. The cough is productive with yellow sputum. He also complains of moderate diffuse abdominal pain and vomiting, which contains food materials. He is non-diabetic and nonhypertensive, smoker, used to take 15 to 20 sticks daily for long time.

On examination, he looks unwell, confused and dehydrated. Temperature 39.7°C, BP—95/60 mm Hg, pulse—110/min and regular respiratory rate—32/min.

Examination of abdomen—diffuse tenderness, no organomegaly. Auscultation of chest—few crepitations in left lower part. Heart—normal.

Neurological examination reveals incoherent talk and confusion. No other abnormality.

Investigations

- ❖ Full blood count — Hb – 12.3 g/dL, WBC – 10,200/cmm, poly – 82%, lympho – 18%,
- ❖ RBS — 7.2 mmol/L.
- ❖ Urine — Protein (++), RBC – plenty.
- ❖ SGPT — 136 IU/L (normal 10 to 40).
- ❖ SGOT — 150 IU/L (normal 45 to 105).
- ❖ Alkaline phosphatase — 109 IU/L (normal 25 to 100).
- ❖ Serum albumin — 26 g/L (normal 37 to 49).
- ❖ Serum electrolytes — Sodium 129 mmol/L.
  Chloride 97 mmol/L.
  Potassium 3.3 mmol/L.
- ❖ Chest X-ray — Consolidation in left lower zone.
- ❖ Serum creatinine — 100 µmol/L (normal 55 to 125).
- ❖ Serum urea — 7.3 mmol/L (normal 2.5 to 6.6).

QUESTIONS

a. What is the likely diagnosis?
b. Suggest three investigations to confirm your diagnosis.
c. Mention three causes of hyponatremia.
d. Mention three lines of management.

CASE NO. 245

A 49-year-old male farm worker, smoker, presented with generalized bodyache, polyarthralgia, malaise, headache, low back pain and night sweating for one month. He also complains of loss of appetite and weight loss for the same duration.

Apart from cholecystectomy done 3 years back, he was always in good health. All family members also are in good health.

On examination, he is ill looking, moderately anemic, cervical lymphadenopathy on both sides, which are non-tender, firm, discrete, movable. Few tender, red, macular lesions on his shins.

Pulse—80/min, regular; BP—110/60 mm Hg, temperature—38.9°C. Heart—soft systolic murmur at the apex.

Examination of abdomen—liver is palpable, 3 cm, non-tender, soft in consistency, spleen is palpable, 5 cm. Left testicle is tender. His lower back and limbs are tender, but movements are not restricted.

Investigations

* Full blood count — Hb – 11.3 g/dl, WBC – 2,200/cmm, poly – 42%, lympho – 58%.
* RBS — 6.2 mmol/L.
* Urine — Protein (+).
* Chest X-ray — Normal.
* Blood culture — Normal.
* Urine culture — Normal.
* USG of abdomen — Hepatosplenomegaly, enlarged left testes and scrotum.
* FNAC of lymph node - Reactive hyperplasia.
* MT — Negative.

QUESTIONS

a. What is the diagnosis?
b. Mention one investigation for your diagnosis.
c. How to manage such a case?

CASE NO. 246

An elderly man aged 66 years, presented with weakness and clumsiness of left hand, which is progressively increasing. He experienced dizziness on turning his head suddenly, also difficulty in walking with a tendency to fall. No history of headache, visual disturbance or weight loss.

On examination, he is emaciated with kyphoscoliosis. Pulse—80/min, regular, BP—110/60 mm Hg. Heart, lung and abdominal examinations were normal.

Neurological examination shows:

* Wasting of small muscles of hands, more prominent on the left.
* There is reduced power on flexion and abduction of arms.
* Muscle power is diminished in both lower limbs, muscle tone—increased.
* Reflexes—supinator and biceps reflexes on left side are absent, but present on the right. Triceps reflexes—brisk bilaterally.
* Ankle and knee reflexes—brisk bilaterally.
* Plantar—extensor on left, but the right is equivocal.
* Sensation—normal, with the exception of vibration.

QUESTIONS

a. Mention four differential diagnoses.
b. What is the most likely diagnosis?
c. Mention one single investigation to confirm your diagnosis.
d. Where is the site of lesion?

CASE NO. 247

A 25-year-old lady teacher, is referred from an obstetrician for medical consultation. Following delivery of a baby 3 months back, the patient is complaining of weakness, tiredness on mild exertion and loss of appetite. She has been breastfeeding normally and her son is well. She has one daughter, delivered by lower uterine cesarean section (LUCS).

On examination, she is mildly anemic, edema—mild, pulse—110/min, BP—145/70 mm Hg. Thyroid—mildly enlarged. Cardiovascular, respiratory and abdominal examinations are normal.

Investigations

* Full blood count   - Hb – 10.0 g/dL, WBC – 8,200/cmm, poly – 70%, lympho – 30%,
* RBS   - 11.2 mmol/L.
* S. electrolytes   - Sodium 141 mmol/L.
  Chloride 102 mmol/L.
  Potassium 3.8 mmol/L.
* Chest X-ray   - Normal.
* Serum creatinine   - 100 μmol/L (normal 55 to 125).
* Serum urea   - 6.3 mmol/L (normal 2.5 to 6.6).
* FT_3 - 6.5 pmol/L (normal 1.2 to 3.1).
* FT_4 - 172 pmol/L (normal 65 to 145).
* TSH   - 0.6 mIU/L (normal 0.8 to 3.6).

QUESTIONS

a. What is the most likely diagnosis?
b. What treatment will you give?

CASE NO. 248

An elderly man aged 70 years presented with weakness and low grade fever and some weight loss for three months. There is no significant history of past illness. He is a non-smoker, non-alcoholic and non-hypertensive.

On examination, the patient is slightly emaciated, mildly anemic. Pulse—80/min, regular, BP—110/60 mm Hg. Heart and lung—normal. Abdominal examination—just palpable liver, no splenomegaly.

Investigations

❖ Full blood count	- Hb – 11.2 g/dl, WBC – 72,000/cmm, poly – 22%, lympho – 70%, mono – 4%, eosinophil – 3%, basofil – 1%.
❖ MCV	- 112 fl.
❖ RBS	- 6.2 mmol/L.
❖ Urine	- Normal.
❖ Chest X-ray	- Normal.
❖ USG of abdomen	- Hepatosplenomegaly.
❖ Serum bilirubin	- 46 μmol/L (normal 3 to 19).
❖ SGPT	- 36 IU/L (normal 10 to 40).
❖ SGOT	- 50 IU/L (normal 45 to 105).
❖ Alkaline phosphatase	- 96 IU/L (normal 25 to 100).
❖ Serum albumin	- 39 g/L (normal 37 to 49).

QUESTIONS

a. What is the likely diagnosis?
b. Why his bilirubin is high?
c. What are the likely causes of anemia?
d. Why MCV is high?
e. Mention one investigation to find out the cause of anemia.

CASE NO. 249

A 19-year-old male student, was suffering from epilepsy, which was well controlled with sodium valproate. During the last few days, he had several attacks of convulsion and carbamazepine was added. For the last 2 days, he is suffering from high grade fever with multiple skin rashes.

On examination, he looks unwell and dehydrated. Temperature—39.7°C, BP—95/60 mm Hg, pulse—110/min, respiratory rate—32/min. Multiple, diffuse, erythematous, rashes with some blistering lesions in the trunk and abdomen, also few ulcers in oral cavity.

Examination of abdomen—diffuse tenderness, no organomegaly. Auscultation of chest—normal.

QUESTIONS

a. What is the likely diagnosis?
b. Mention one alternative diagnosis.
c. What immediate treatment is essential?

CASE NO. 250

A 60-year-old man, presented with dry cough and severe respiratory distress. He was a heavy smoker, but stopped recently. Apart from cholecystectomy and herniotomy, there is no other past medical history.

His routine investigation like blood count and other biochemistry reveal no abnormality. Respiratory function tests shows the following results:

- Vital capacity   - 2.8 (Predicted 3.9 to 5.01).
- FEV_1 - 2.4 (Predicted 3.0 to 3.61).
- RV   - 1.4 (Predicted 2.0 to 2.6).
- TLco (mmol/min/kPa)   - 6.2 (Predicted 7.4).
- Kco (mmol/min/kPa/L) - 1.7 (Predicted 1.4).

QUESTIONS

a. What does the pulmonary function test indicate?
b. Mention three differential diagnoses.
c. Mention one single investigation.

CASE NO. 251

A 61-year-old man presented with dry cough and breathlessness on moderate exertion for 9 months. Recently, he feels more breathlessness at night, which interferes with his sleep. The patient also complains of some loss of weight and feels tired, even with mild usual activity.

He is a heavy smoker, used to take 20 to 30 cigarettes/day for long time.
Respiratory function tests shows the following results:

- Vital capacity   - 2.9 (Predicted 3.8 to 5).
- FEV_1 - 2.6 (Predicted 3.2 to 4.7).
- RV   - 1.0 (Predicted 1.3 to 2.8).
- TLC   - 3.6 (Predicted 6.3 to 8.2).
- TLco (mmol/min/kPa) - 4.6 (Predicted 8.0 to 12.6).
- Kco (mmol/min/kPa)   - 1.2 (Predicted 1.2 to 2.1).

QUESTIONS

a. What is the likely diagnosis?
b. What does the pulmonary function test indicate?
c. Mention three further investigations.

CASE NO. 252

A 56-year-old lady singer, diagnosed as high grade non-Hodgkin's lymphoma. One cycle of CVP (cyclophosphamide, vincristine, prednisolone) was given. On the 4th day, she is complaining of severe vomiting, polyarthritis, extreme weakness, scanty micturition and puffy face. She was hospitalized in emergency.

On examination, she looks very ill, moderately anemic. Few cervical lymphadenopathy on both sides. Pulse—100/min, regular, BP—100/60 mm Hg. Heart and lungs are normal. Abdominal examination—just palpable liver and spleen is enlarged, 2 cm.

Investigations

❖ Full blood count   - Hb – 9.2 g/dL, WBC – 4,000/cmm, poly – 42%, lympho – 50%,
                        mono – 4%, eosinophil – 4%.
❖ RBS   - 4.2 mmol/L.
❖ Urine   - Protein (++), RBC cast (++).
❖ Chest X-ray   - Bilateral hilar lymphadenopathy.
❖ USG of abdomen   - Hepatosplenomegaly.
❖ Serum electrolytes   - Sodium 143 mmol/L.
                        Chloride 100 mmol/L.
                        Potassium 6.3 mmol/L.
                        Bicarbonate 16.2 mmol/L.
❖ Serum creatinine   - 605 µmol/L (normal 55 to 125).
❖ Serum urea   - 12.3 mmol/L (normal 2.5 to 6.6).
❖ Serum uric acid   - 12 mg/L (normal 2 to 7).

QUESTIONS

a. What is the likely diagnosis?
b. Mention two further investigations.
c. What treatment should be given?
d. What further investigation should be done before starting treatment?

CASE NO. 253

A 53-year-old typist, non-diabetic, but hypertensive which is well controlled with atenolol, presented with painful swelling, affecting the left calf.
    On examination, left calf is swollen, red and tender. Other systems reveal no abnormality.

Investigations

❖ Full blood count   - Hb – 18.2 g/dL, WBC – 8,000/cmm, poly – 90%, lympho – 10%,
                        platelets – 2,10,000/cmm.
❖ MCV   - 78 fl (normal 76 to 96).
❖ PCV   - 0.58 (normal 0.40 to 0.54).
❖ Prothrombin time   - 13 sec (control 12).
❖ APTT   - 37 (control 38).
❖ RBS   - 6.2 mmol/L.
❖ Urine   - Normal
❖ Chest X-ray   - Normal.
❖ USG of abdomen   - Normal.
❖ Serum creatinine   - 105 µmol/L (normal 55 to 125).
❖ Serum urea   - 6.3 mmol/L (normal 2.5 to 6.6).
❖ Serum uric acid   - 5 mg/L (normal 2 to 7).

QUESTIONS

a. What is the hematological abnormality?
b. Mention two investigations to confirm your diagnosis.
c. Mention three other investigations.

CASE NO. 254

A 20-year-old young male presented with severe central chest pain and breathlessness. He is suffering from severe myopia.

On examination, the patient looks distressed due to pain. He is tall, lean and thin with long and narrow face. No cyanosis. Pulse—110/min, regular and normal volume. BP—100/80 mm Hg, respiratory rate—34/min.

QUESTIONS

a. What diagnosis would you consider first?
b. Mention two urgent investigations.
c. What is the likely unified diagnosis?
d. Mention one differential diagnosis for his chest pain.

CASE NO. 255

A 15-year-old girl is hospitalized due to severe cough, respiratory distress and high grade fever. There is small amount of blood in sputum one time only. Her mother says that her daughter has been suffering from recurrent respiratory infection since her childhood and also bronchial asthma, for which she took regular inhaler. The girl also had intermittent abdominal pain and loose, bulky stool.

On examination, she is ill-looking and emaciated, moderately anemic. There is generalized clubbing.

Auscultation of chest—coarse crepitations in both lung fields, unaltered by coughing.

Abdomen—distended, generalized tenderness is present and a small, firm mass in right iliac fossa.

Investigations

❖ Full blood count	-	Hb – 9.2 g/dL, WBC – 18,000/cmm, poly – 90%, lympho – 10%, platelets – 2,30,000/cmm.
❖ Urine	-	Glucose (++).
❖ RBS	-	11 mmol/L.
❖ Chest X-ray	-	Bronchiectasis with consolidation.
❖ USG of abdomen	-	Gaseous distension.
❖ Serum creatinine	-	115 µmol/L (normal 55 to 125).
❖ Serum urea	-	6.3 mmol/L (normal 2.5 to 6.6).
❖ Serum electrolytes	-	Sodium 135 mmol/L.
		Chloride 97 mmol/L.
		Potassium 3.2 mmol/L.

QUESTIONS

a. What is the likely diagnosis?
b. What is the cause of mass in right iliac fossa?
c. What investigation should be done to confirm your diagnosis?
d. What is the likely organism that causes consolidation?

CASE NO. 256

A 67-years-elderly, retired secretary, non-hypertensive, but diabetic, well controlled on oral hypoglycemic drugs, presented with high grade fever, severe cough and breathlessness for 3 days. On query, it was found that he has been suffering from long-standing difficulty in deglutition for solid and liquid. He was also suffering from recurrent pneumonia.

On examination, the patient looks distressed due to breathlessness. Pulse—120/min, regular. BP—130/80 mm Hg, respiratory rate—30/min, temperature—39.8°C.

Investigations

* Full blood count — Hb – 12.2 g/dL, WBC – 18,000/cmm, poly – 91%, lympho – 9%.
* RBS — 9.2 mmol/L.
* Chest X-ray — Homogeneous opacity in right mid zone.

QUESTIONS

a. What is the underlying diagnosis?
b. Mention three further investigations.

CASE NO. 257

An elderly man was hospitalized due to worsening of lack of mobility. His wife mentioned that her husband had very poor memory, frequent falls and severe, progressively increasing disturbance of mobility for 3 years. He also had auditory and visual hallucinations. The patient was on syndopa (levodopa and carbidopa), selegiline and ropinirole. He is unable to tolerate small doses of neuroleptics, with marked cognitive deterioration, drowsiness and myoclonus.

On examination, the patient looks apathetic and very ill, pulse—70/min, BP—160/80 mm Hg (lying), 130/70 mm Hg (standing). Heart, lungs and abdomen—normal.

Neurological examination reveals resting tremor, bradykinesia and rigidity. Marked dementia is present.

QUESTIONS

a. What is the likely diagnosis?
b. Mention three investigations.

■ CASE NO. 258

An 18-year-old girl was referred, because of primary amenorrhea and poorly developed secondary sexual character. There is history of repair of cleft palate at the age of 6 years.

On examination, she is short, scanty axillary and pubic hair, breasts are small.

Investigations

- ❖ Full blood count   - Hb – 12 g/dL, WBC – 6,000/cmm, poly – 52%, lympho – 44%, mono – 4%.
- ❖ RBS   - 4.2 mmol/L.
- ❖ Serum creatinine   - 105 µmol/L (normal 55 to 125).
- ❖ Estradiol concentration - 80 pmol/L (normal 130 to 450).
- ❖ LH   - 2.9 mU/L (normal 3 to 10).
- ❖ FSH   - 4 mU/L (normal 3 to 10).
- ❖ Prolactin   - 400 mU/L (normal 50 to 450).

■ QUESTIONS

a. What is the endocrine abnormality?
b. What further history is helpful for diagnosis?
c. What is the underlying diagnosis?

■ CASE NO. 259

A 64-year-old man presented with confusion, difficulty in walking and urinary incontinence. There is no history of trauma. Apart from cholecystectomy and herniorrhaphy, he was always in good health.

On examination, the patient looks apathetic, pulse—74/min, regular. BP—130/80 mm Hg. Heart, lung and abdominal examinations—all normal.

Neurological examination reveals mild global cognitive dysfunction associated with ataxia. Fundoscopy—normal.

■ QUESTIONS

a. Mention two specific investigations for your diagnosis.
b. What is the likely diagnosis?
c. Mention one single management which is likely to be most helpful.

■ CASE NO. 260

A 48-year-old housewife presented with weakness, lethargy, headache, bodyache, palpitation and intolerance to heat for 5 months. She is in menopause for 2 years.

On examination; BP—140/70 mm Hg, pulse—110/min, regular. Thyroid—diffusely enlarged, firm in consistency, non-tender.

Investigations

- ❖ Serum FT$_3$ - 3.23 pmol/L (normal 1.3 to 3.5).
- ❖ Serum FT$_4$ - 13.71 pmol/L (normal 9.5 to 25.5).
- ❖ TSH   - 0.79 mIU/L (normal 0.5 to 5.1).
- ❖ Radio-iodine uptake - After 2 hours—27% (normal 5 to 15).
                                 After 24 hours—55% (normal 15 to 30).

▓ QUESTIONS

a. What is the likely diagnosis?
b. Suggest three further investigations.
c. What specific treatment would you suggest?

▓ CASE NO. 261

A 25-year-old farmer presented with high grade fever, generalized bodyache, headache, weakness and vomiting for 5 days.

On examination, he looks toxic, anemia—modarate. Temperature—39.4°C, jaundice—mild, both eyes—red, pulse—120/min, BP—80/60 mm Hg. Heart—soft heart sounds. Lungs-clear.

Abdomen—hepatomegaly, 2 cm, tender, soft in consistency. No spenomegaly. Next stiffness—present.

Investigations

- ❖ Full blood count   - Hb – 8.3 g/dL, WBC – 18,000/cmm, poly – 85%, lympho – 15%, platelets – 1,10,000/cmm.
- ❖ Prothrombin time   - 23 sec (control 12).
- ❖ APTT   - 57 (control 45).
- ❖ Biluribin   - 6 mg/dL.
- ❖ RBS   - 5.2 mmol/L.
- ❖ Urine   - Protein (++).
- ❖ Chest X-ray   - Cardiomegaly.
- ❖ USG of abdomen   - Hepatomegaly.
- ❖ Serum creatinine   - 405 μmol/L (normal 55 to 125).
- ❖ Serum urea   - 12.3 mmol/L (normal 2.5 to 6.6).
- ❖ Serum electrolytes   - Sodium 136 mmol/L.
                                 Chloride 99 mmol/L.
                                 Potassium 5.3 mmol/L.
- ❖ SGPT   - 236 IU/L (normal 10 to 40).
- ❖ SGOT   - 250 IU/L (normal 45 to 105).
- ❖ Alkaline phosphatase - 190 IU/L (normal 25 to 100).
- ❖ Serum albumin   - 33 g/L (normal 37 to 49).
- ❖ Hepatitis A, B and E   - Negative.

QUESTIONS

a. What is the likely diagnosis?
b. Mention three differential diagnoses.
c. Mention three investigations.
d. What is the hematological diagnosis?

CASE NO. 262

A 21-year-old man is hospitalized, because of severe respiratory distress and cough with frothy expectoration. He is unable to lie flat. There is history of difficulty in walking since his childhood and also difficulty in speech.

On examination, he is dyspneic, pulse—124/min, BP—80/60 mm Hg.

Heart—apex is shifted, soft heart sounds. A pansystolic murmur is present in mitral area. Lungs—coarse crepitations in both lung fields. Abdomen—hepatomegaly, 1 cm, tender, soft in consistency

Neurology examination—speech is scanning. Muscle tone and power—diminished in both lower limbs. Loss of both knee and ankle jerks, but plantar—extensor on both sides. Loss of vibration and position senses.

QUESTIONS

a. What is the cause of breathlessness?
b. What is the cardiac diagnosis?
c. What is the underlying diagnosis?

CASE NO. 263

A 19-year-old University student has been suffering from low grade continuous fever for 8 weeks. He is also complaining of weakness, loss of weight, arthralgia, dry cough and frequent night sweating.

He had measles during childhood, but otherwise he was always in good health.

On examination, he looks emaciated, toxic, moderately anemic, no jaundice, no edema. Temperature—38.7°C,

Pulse—110/min,regular. BP—150/60 mm Hg.

Heart—soft heart sounds. There is an early diastolic murmur in left lower parasternal area.

Investigations

❖ Full blood count	-	Hb – 8.9 g/dL, WBC – 14,300/cmm, poly – 80%, lympho – 20%, ESR – 90, platelets – 1,70,000/cmm.
❖ RBS	-	6.2 mmol/L.
❖ Urine	-	Protein (+), RBC cast (+), few pus cells.
❖ Chest X-ray	-	Heart is slightly enlarged.
❖ USG of abdomen	-	Splenomegaly.
❖ Urine for CS	-	Negative.
❖ Blood culture	-	Negative.

QUESTIONS

a. What diagnosis would you consider first?
b. Mention two further investigations.

CASE NO. 264

A young lady aged 32 years, 8 months pregnant, known diabetic, is hospitalized for pre-eclampsia. She is complaining of increasing ankle edema, headache, blurred vision and vomiting for the last 24 hours.

On examination, the patient looks very ill and moderately anemic, pulse—120/min, BP—190/105 mm Hg. Edema (++), pitting.

Heart—soft heart sounds. There is an early diastolic murmur in left lower parasternal area and also few crepitations in both lung bases.

Methyldopa was given for hypertension and magnesium sulfate infusion was given for pre-eclampsia. After 2 days, the patient complains of facial flushing, severe nausea and blurred vision, but headache is less. Blood pressure—100/80 mm Hg.

Attendant of the patient informed the doctor that the patient has slurring of speech and double vision and severe weakness. Few minutes later, the patient becomes drowsy, only responds to painful stimuli. BP—100/50 mm Hg, pulse—55/min.

QUESTIONS

a. What is the most likely cause of her symptoms?
b. What is your immediate management?
c. Mention two immediate investigations which will be helpful for further management.

CASE NO. 265

A female of 20 years old, recently married, was suffering from pain in the epigastrium, frequent headache and repeated vomiting. Antiemetic and omeprazole were given and she was feeling better, but noticed galactorrhea over the last 2 weeks. She has also amenorrhea for the last 6 weeks.

Her menarche started at the age of 14 years and her period is usually irregular.

On examination, she is moderately obese, anemia—mild, pulse—70/min, BP—110/60 mm Hg. Heart and lungs—normal. Abdomen—tenderness in epigastric region, no organomegaly.

Investigations

- ❖ Full blood count   - Hb – 10.3 g/dL, WBC – 9,000/cmm, poly – 65%, lympho – 30%, mono – 5%, platelets – 2,10,000/cmm.
- ❖ RBS   - 5.2 mmol/L.
- ❖ Chest X-ray   - Normal.
- ❖ USG of abdomen   - Small hepatomegaly.
- ❖ SGPT   - 36 IU/L (normal 10 to 40).
- ❖ SGOT   - 100 IU/L (normal 45 to 105).

- ❖ Alkaline phosphatase - 98 IU/L (normal 25 to 100).
- ❖ Serum albumin - 39 g/L (normal 37 to 49).
- ❖ Serum oestradiol - 132 nmol/L (130 to 600).
- ❖ Serum LH - 6.5 mU/L (2 to 20).
- ❖ Serum FSH - 3.2 mU/L (2 to 20).
- ❖ Serum prolactin - 4340 mU/L (50 to 450).
- ❖ TSH - 2.8 mU/L (0.4 to 5.0).

QUESTIONS

a. Mention two differential diagnoses.
b. Suggest one investigation.
c. What is the most likely diagnosis?
d. What single treatment is helpful?

CASE NO. 266

A 50-year-old male presented with frequent headache, polyuria, weakness, and sleep disturbance for 5 months. He was generally well before, with no previous medical history note. His father was hypertensive, died following cerebral hemorrhage.

He was a previous smoker, use to take 20 to 30 cigarettes per day, but stopped recently.

On examination, pulse—80/min, BP—160/110 mm Hg. Thyroid gland is slightly diffusely enlarged, no evidence of toxic features. Examination of other systems reveal no abnormality. Fundoscopy—normal.

Investigations

- ❖ Full blood count - Hb – 12.3 g/dL, WBC – 6,000/cmm, poly – 70%, lympho – 28%, eosinophil – 2%, platelets – 4,10,000/cmm.
- ❖ RBS - 7.2 mmol/L.
- ❖ Urine - Normal.
- ❖ Chest X-ray - Heart is slightly enlarged.
- ❖ USG of abdomen - Normal.
- ❖ Serum creatinine - 110 µmol/L (normal 55 to 125).
- ❖ Serum urea - 6.3 mmol/L (normal 2.5 to 6.6).
- ❖ Serum electrolytes - Sodium 146 mmol/L.
  Chloride 102 mmol/L.
  Potassium 2.9 mmol/L.
  Bicarbonate 36 mmol/L.

QUESTIONS

a. What is the likely diagnosis?
b. Mention two investigations to confirm your diagnosis.
c. Mention one drug to treat his hypertension.

CASE NO. 267

A 19-year-old girl, student, presented with fever and difficulty in deglutition for 3 months. The fever was high grade (highest recorded 105°F), associated with chill and rigor and subsides with paracetamol with profuse sweating. She also had oral ulcer. For these complaints, she was treated by several private practitioners and in a medical college hospital.

Laboratory investigations done before showed: Hb 10.5 g/dL, ESR 90, TC 4,000/cmm, neutrophil 63%, lymphocyte 32%, malarial parasite was absent, urine—plenty of epithelial cells, normal liver functions. Urine and blood cultures revealed no growth. ICT for malaria, CFT for kala-azar, sputum for AFB and febrile antigen were all negative. Ultrasonogram of abdomen and chest X-ray were also normal. MT—negative, ANA and anti-dsDNA—negative.

She was given many antibiotics including cefixime, ceftriaxone, amoxicillin, tetracycline, renamycin and cefuroxime, also anti-malarial treatment. But her condition did not improve. She developed cough, lost weight (from 43 to 36 kg) and became anemic (Hb came down to 7.8 g/dL with PBF showing combined deficiency anemia). FNAC of lymph node was done, which showed reactive hyperplasia.

On examination, the patient is ill-looking, moderately anemic and grossly emaciated. Lymphadenopathy involving right supraclavicular and both inguinal regions, firm, non-tender, mobile, few matted and without any sinus. Systemic examinations revealed no abnormality. A biopsy was taken from supraclavicular lymph node, which shows necrotizing lymphadenitis.

QUESTIONS

a. What diagnosis would you consider with the above finding?
b. What specific drug should be given?

CASE NO. 268

A 60-year-old, retired male, smoker, presented with pain in chest and severe backache, aggravated on movement, anorexia, nausea, constipation and frequent dizziness for 2 months. There was one attack of syncope 3 days back.

On examination, the patient looks very ill and severely anemic, edema—moderate, pitting, pulse—70/min, BP—100/50 mm Hg. JVP—raised.

Abdomen—liver is enlarged, 6 cm, tender, soft in consistency.

Heart—apex is shifted, thrusting in nature. Third heart sound is present with a systolic murmur in apical area. Examination of other systems reveal no abnormality.

Fundoscopy—few scatterd hemorrhage in both fundus.

Investigations

❖ Full blood count	-	Hb – 7.3 g/dL, WBC – 3,000/cmm, poly – 65%, lympho – 35%, platelets – 91,000/cmm, ESR – 100.
❖ RBS	-	5.2 mmol/L.
❖ Urine	-	Protein (+++)
❖ Serum creatinine	-	150 µmol/L (normal 55 to 125).
❖ Serum urea	-	8.3 mmol/L (normal 2.5 to 6.6).

❖ Serum electrolytes   - Sodium 131 mmol/L.
                          Chloride 99 mmol/L.
                          Potassium 5.3 mmol/L.
❖ Alkaline phosphatase - 190 IU/L (normal 25 to 100).
❖ Serum albumin   - 28 g/L (normal 37 to 49).
❖ Total protein   - 70 g/L (normal 45 to 60).
❖ Serum calcium   - 3.2 mmol/L (normal 2.20 to 2.67).
❖ X-ray of dorsolumbar - Diffuse osteopenia of all vertebrae and
  spine   partial collapse of D_{12} vertebra.

QUESTIONS

a. What is the likely diagnosis?
b. What is the cause of syncope?
c. Mention one investigation to confirm your diagnosis.

CASE NO. 269

A 41-year-old man presented with severe pain around his right eye and headache. These symptoms occur episodically, every 2 to 3 months. This time, pain started without any apparent precipitating event and had waken him from sleep. The pain is severe, radiated upwards over the right frontal and temporal region. Headache is associated with watering of right eye and a blocked left nostril. He vomited two times with pain, but there is no history of visual disturbance, or diplopia.

On examination, he looks distressed with flushed face, red right eye with nasal discharge. There is partial right sided ptosis and miosis, pulse—76/min, BP—100/80 mm Hg.

QUESTIONS

a. Mention two therapeutic options which will be helpful to relieve his symptoms quickly.
b. Mention two differential diagnoses.
c. Mention one drug for prevention.

CASE NO. 270

A 59-year-old male, retired, non-smoker, hypertensive and diabetic, is hospitalized in emergency with severe central chest pain and breathlessness. ECG shows extensive acute anterior myocardial infarction. He was treated properly and was feeling comfortable.

On the 3rd day, the patient again experiences chest pain, which is very severe.

On examination, pulse—120/min and regular, BP—80/70 mm Hg.

QUESTIONS

a. Mention five differential diagnoses.
b. Mention two findings in precordium, helpful for two diagnoses.
c. Mention two immediate investigations.

CASE NO. 271

A housewife aged 41 years old, presented with frequent diarrhea, epigastric discomfort, palpitation, sleep disturbance and weight loss for 6 weeks. There was no significant past medical history. She was taking occasional antacid and ranitidine by herself without consultation of doctors.

On examination, she looks slightly emaciated, moderately anemic, pulse—120/min, BP—130/50 mm Hg.

A smooth, diffusely enlarged mass was palpable over the trachea, which moves upward on swallowing. Fine tremor of both hands—present.

Abdomen—soft, non-tender with active bowel sounds.

Heart—apex is shifted, thrusting in nature. Third heart sound is present with a systolic murmur in apical area.

Examination of other systems reveal no abnormality.

Investigations

- ❖ Full blood count - Hb – 9.3 g/dL, WBC – 5,000/cmm, poly – 60%, lympho – 40%, platelets – 1,91,000/cmm, ESR – 30.
- ❖ RBS - 10.2 mmol/L.
- ❖ Urine - Sugar (+)
- ❖ Serum creatinine - 120 µmol/L (normal 55 to 125).
- ❖ Serum urea - 5.8 mmol/L (normal 2.5 to 6.6).
- ❖ Serum electrolytes - Sodium 141 mmol/L. Chloride 99 mmol/L. Potassium 4.3 mmol/L.
- ❖ Chest X-ray - Heart is slightly enlarged.
- ❖ USG of abdomen - Normal.
- ❖ FT_4 - 13 pmol/L (normal 9 to 23).
- ❖ TSH - 0.1 mU/L (normal 0.4 to 5).
- ❖ Radioiodine uptake - After 2 hours 20% (normal 5 to 15). After 24 hours 50% (normal 15 to 30).

QUESTIONS

a. What is the most likely diagnosis?
b. Mention one investigation to confirm your diagnosis

CASE NO. 272

An 18-year-old young patient presented with cough, dyspnea, headache and puffiness of face. He was unable to lie flat, because of dyspnea.

On examination, the patient looks distressed with puffy, plethoric face, redness of both eyes and periorbital edema. Pulse—106/min, regular. BP—110/70 mm Hg. Respiratory rate—30/min.

Lymphadenopathy involving cervical and axillary areas, nontender, soft in consistency, variable size and shape. JVP—engorged. Liver—just palpable, spleen—enlarged, 1 cm.

QUESTIONS

a. What is the likely cause of his symptoms?
b. What is the likely diagnosis?
c. Mention one investigation which will be helpful for your diagnosis.
d. Mention two further investigations to confirm your diagnosis.

CASE NO. 273

A 50-year-old man is hospitalized following high grade fever, cough and pleuritic right sided chest pain for 2 days. He had a renal transplantation 3 years ago. His symptoms started 2 days before, following travel abroad, with a flu-like illness with generalized arthralgia and bodyache.

His cough is productive, purulent and slightly greenish sputum with occasional hemoptysis.

He was taking prednisolone, azathioprine and cyclosporin. Because of high uric acid, allopurinol 100 mg daily was given.

On examination, the patient looks very ill and pale. Anemia—severe. No jaundice and edema, temperature—39.9°C, pulse—120/min, BP—90/60 mm Hg. Heart—normal.

Examination of chest—dull on percussion, increased vocal resonance and bronchial breathing in right lower part.

Investigations

❖ Full blood count   - Hb – 6.3 g/dL, WBC – 1,000/cmm, poly – 30%, lympho – 70%, platelets – 41,000/cmm.
❖ RBS   - 3.2 mmol/L.
❖ Serum creatinine   - 220 µmol/L (normal 55 to 125).
❖ Serum urea   - 10.3 mmol/L (normal 2.5 to 6.6).
❖ Serum electrolytes - Sodium 140 mmol/L. Chloride 100 mmol/L. Potassium 4.2 mmol/L.
❖ Chest X-ray   - Consolidation in right lung.

QUESTIONS

a. What is the likely cause of his blood picture?
b. What is the likely cause of his symptoms?
c. What treatment should be given?
d. What drug should be given for renal transplantation?

CASE NO. 274

A 41-year-old man presented with irregular jerky movements of his lower limbs and fingers for one year, which is progressively increasing. Recently, his wife noticed that the patient has developed increasing problems with concentration and became more forgetful. He was always in good health. He is a heavy smoker, used to take 25 to 30 sticks/day and also alcoholic.

On examination, he looks distressed with choreiform movement.

Neurological examination—speech is slurred. Muscle tone and power—diminished in both lower and upper limbs. Reflexes—difficult to elicit. Planter—equivocal.

QUESTIONS

a. What further history do you like to take?
b. What is the likely diagnosis?
c. Mention two investigations.

CASE NO. 275

A 58-year-old, known hypertensive and diabetic, has been suffering from chronic kidney disease. He is on regular hemodialysis for 5 years and apparently well. Five months previously, there was right sided consolidation, which was treated with broad spectrum antibiotic, from which there is complete recovery. Recently, he is complaining of generalized bodyache, tingling, numbness and joint stiffness involving his hands, arms and shoulders. He is also complaining of nausea, constipation and insomnia.

His blood pressure and diabetes mellitus are well controlled. No recent investigations are done.

QUESTIONS

a. What is the cause of his symptoms?
b. What is the specific treatment?
c. How to prevent such symptoms ?

CASE NO. 276

A 40-year-old man, presented with weakness, dizziness, loss of appetite, malaise and palpitation for 2 months. He also complains of breathlessness on mild exertion for one month.

Four years ago, he had a Starr-Edward metallic valve replacement for aortic valvular disease. He is on warfarin, but no other medication and has no other medical problem.

On examination, the patient looks pale and moderately anemic, Jaundice—moderate, edema—moderate, pitting, pulse—90/min, BP—100/70 mm Hg. JVP—raised. Abdomen –liver is enlarged, 3 cm, tender, soft in consistency.

Examination of other systems reveal no abnormality. Fundoscopy—few scattered hemorrhage in both fundus. Metallic valve is functioning well.

Investigations

* Full blood count   - Hb – 7.3 g/dL, WBC – 11,000/cmm, poly – 60%, lympho – 30%, mono – 5%, eosinophil – 5%, platelets – 2,10,000/cmm. platelets – 41,000/cmm.
* Peripheral blood film - Fragmented red cells with polychromasia.
* RBS   - 3.2 mmol/L.
* Serum creatinine   - 120 µmol/L (normal 55 to 125).
* Serum urea   - 5.3 mmol/L (normal 2.5 to 6.6).
* Serum electrolytes   - odium 140 mmol/L. Chloride 100 mmol/L. Potassium 4.2 mmol/L.
* Chest X-ray   - Consolidation in right lung.

- ❖ Serum bilirubin   - 96 µmol/L (normal 3 to 19).
- ❖ SGPT   - 36 IU/L (normal 10 to 40).
- ❖ SGOT   - 55 IU/L (normal 45 to 105).
- ❖ Alkaline phosphatase - 96 IU/L (normal 25 to 100).
- ❖ LDH   - 900 u/L (normal 10 to 250).

▉ QUESTIONS

a. What is the hematological diagnosis?
b. Mention one further investigation.
c. What is the underlying cause of such abnormality?
d. What is the cardiac diagnosis?

▉ CASE NO. 277

A 39-year-old varnish worker was hospitalized following collapse in his house. He is alcoholic and heavy smoker. His wife mentioned that after drinking something, her husband is complaining of pain in abdomen, vomiting, headache, confusion followed by sudden fall on the ground from bed. On the next day, the patient is also complaining of blurring of vision.

On examination, the patient is semiconscious, poorly responds to painful stimuli, pulse—110/min, BP—90/70 mm Hg. Temperature—37°C. Respiratory rate—24/min. No neck rigidity. Kernig's sign—negative.Pupils—dilated. Neurological examination—depressed all reflexes, plantar—equivocal. Fundoscopy—blurred disk margins

Investigations

- ❖ Full blood count   - Hb – 11.3 g/dL, WBC – 5,000/cmm, poly – 60%, lympho – 40%, platelets – 1,91,000/cmm, ESR – 30.
- ❖ RBS   - 6.2 mmol/L.
- ❖ Serum creatinine   - 110 µmol/L (normal 55 to 125).
- ❖ Serum urea   - 6.3 mmol/L (normal 2.5 to 6.6).
- ❖ Serum electrolytes   - Sodium 131 mmol/L. Chloride 96 mmol/L. Potassium 5.4 mmol/L. Bicarbonate 12 mmol/L.
- ❖ pH   - 7.21 (normal 7.35 to 7.45).
- ❖ Blood lactate   - 6 mmol/l.
- ❖ Serum amylase   - 120 IU/L (normal < 220).
- ❖ Chest X-ray   - Normal.
- ❖ USG of abdomen   - Normal.
- ❖ ECG   - Sinus tachycardia.

▉ QUESTIONS

a. What is the likely diagnosis?
b. Mention two further investigations.
c. What metabolic abnormality is present?

CASE NO. 278

A 48-year-old housewife presented with severe weakness for 2 months. She has three sons, all were delivered by LUCS. She is non-hypertensive and non-diabetic. Her only other problem is long-standing constipation, otherwise she was in good health.

On examination, she is obese, pulse—90/min, BP—130/70 mm Hg. Heart and lungs—normal. No organomegaly.

Neurological examination—muscle tone and power are all diminished. All the reflexes—diminished. No sensory abnormality. Examination of other systems are normal.

Investigations

❖ Full blood count - Hb – 12.3 g/dL, WBC – 6,000/cmm, poly – 60%, lympho – 35%, mono – 4%, eosinophil – 1%. platelets – 1,91,000/cmm, ESR – 10.
❖ RBS - 6.2 mmol/L.
❖ Serum creatinine - 100 μmol/L (normal 55 to 125).
❖ Serum urea - 8.3 mmol/L (normal 2.5 to 6.6).
❖ Serum electrolytes - Sodium 141 mmol/L. Chloride 96 mmol/L. Potassium 2.1 mmol/L. Bicarbonate 36 mmol/L.
❖ Chest X-ray - Normal.
❖ USG of abdomen - Normal.
❖ 24-hour urine potassium - 10 mmol/L (normal < 20).

QUESTIONS

a. What is the biochemical abnormality in this case?
b. Mention two differential diagnoses.

CASE NO. 279

An elderly man presented with persistent cough, breathlessness and heaviness in chest for 3 months. Cough is unproductive, but occasionally, there is slight mucoid expectoration with scanty blood stained sputum. It never wakes him from sleep. Recently, he has lost weight about 3 kg in one month. He is also complaining of loss of appetite and constipation over the last 2 weeks. He is a heavy smoker, used to take 20 to 30 cigarettes a day for long time.

On examination, he is slightly emaciated, mildly anemic, generalized clubbing with nicotine stain in fingers. Pulse—80/min, BP—105/70 mm Hg. Examination of other systems were unremarkable.

Investigations

❖ Full blood count - Hb – 11.3 g/dL, WBC – 7,000/cmm, poly – 62%, lympho – 33%, mono – 2%, eosinophil – 3%, platelets – 3,91,000/cmm, ESR – 60.
❖ RBS - 8.2 mmol/L.
❖ Serum creatinine - 120 μmol/L (normal 55 to 125).
❖ Serum urea - 5.3 mmol/L (normal 2.5 to 6.6).

- ❖ Serum electrolytes — Sodium 143 mmol/L. Chloride 102 mmol/L. Potassium 4.4 mmol/L.
- ❖ Serum calcium — 3.26 mmol/L (normal 2.0 to 2.55).
- ❖ Chest X-ray — Right hilar lymphadenopathy.
- ❖ USG of abdomen — Normal.
- ❖ ECG — Normal.

QUESTIONS

a. Mention three differential diagnoses.
b. Mention two further investigations to confirm your diagnosis.
c. What is the most likely diagnosis?

CASE NO. 280

A 47-year-old man, labor, who was working abroad, presented with low grade, continued fever, weight loss, loss of appetite, malaise and weakness for 4 months. For the last 5 days, he is suffering from confusion, visual disturbance, weakness of left arm and leg, with high continued fever. He had one attack of tonic-clonic seizure.

On examination, the patient is confused, response to painful stimulus, pulse—120/min, BP—90/70 mm Hg. Temperature—39.9°C, cervical lymphadenopathy on left side, firm, non-tender, matted, no sinus.

Neck—slightly rigid, No Kernig's sign. No focal neurological sign, planter—extensor on both sides.

Fundoscopy shows retinal pigmented scarring in right eye, normal left eye.

QUESTIONS

a. What is the likely diagnosis?
b. Mention five differential diagnoses.
c. Mention four investigations to confirm your diagnosis.

CASE NO. 281

A 20-year-old girl presented with pain in multiple joints, low grade continuous fever, weakness, loss of weight and few mouth ulcers for 3 months. Her symptoms are relieved by taking paracetamol or ibuprofen. She was always in good health, only suffering from multiple acne in the face, for which she is taking minocycline. Her sister is suffering from rheumatoid arthritis.

On examination, she looks slightly emaciated, moderately anemic. Few acne in the face, also skin rash over the nose. Cervical lymphadenopathy on right side, which are firm, discrete, non-tender.

Investigations

- ❖ Full blood count — Hb – 8.3 g/dL, WBC – 3,800/cmm, poly – 47%, lympho – 50%, mono – 2%, eosinohil – 1%, platelets – 1,91,000/cmm, ESR – 90.
- ❖ RBS — 6.2 mmol/L.

- ❖ Chest X-ray   - Normal.
- ❖ USG of abdomen   - Small splenomegaly.
- ❖ RA test   - Positive (in low titer).
- ❖ CRP   - 110 mg/L (normal < 10).
- ❖ ANA   - Positive (1:800).
- ❖ Anti-ds DNA   - Negative.

QUESTIONS

a. What is the likely diagnosis?
b. Mention one investigation to confirm your diagnosis.

CASE NO. 282

A 35-year-old male presented with recurrent oral ulcer and pain in multiple big joints for 2 years. On questioning, he mentioned that his mouth ulcer is very painful, for which it is difficult to eat. He is also complaining of occasional pain in abdomen with bloody diarrhea. Recently, there are multiple painful ulcers in scrotum. He was suffering from deep venous thrombosis in right calf, from which there is complete recovery.

On examination, he is ill-looking. Few ulcers on both sides of tongue, both eyes are red.

Both knee, ankle and elbow joints are swollen and painful. Few painful, reddish nodular lesions over the shin of both legs. Multiple ulcers in the skin of scrotum.

QUESTIONS

a. What is the likely diagnosis?
b. Mention two differential diagnoses.

CASE NO. 283

An woman aged 50 years presented with frequent dry cough for 2 years, which is more or less persistent during the day time. She also complains of occasional compression in chest, not related to exertion, no breathlessness or hemoptysis. Her cough usually disappears or becomes less frequent at night, worsen during laughing and talking. She also complains of occasional hoarseness of voice.

She is hypertensive, on ACE inhibitor lisinopril. However, because of dry cough, ACE inhibitor is discontinued but no improvement of cough.

On examination, BP—110/70 mm Hg, pulse—80/min. Heart sounds—normal, no murmur. Auscultation of chest—normal. Abdominal examination—tenderness in epigastrium. No organomegaly.

Blood count, sugar, ECG and chest radiograph—normal.

QUESTIONS

a. What is the likely diagnosis?
b. Mention one investigation.

CASE NO. 284

A 60-year-old man, known diabetic and hypertensive, has been suffering from coronary artery disease, well controlled on drugs. He is hospitalized, because of sudden collapse. His wife mentioned that the patient had an attack of cardiac arrest 2 days back, recovered fully following home resuscitation.

Chest X-ray shows cardiomegaly, ECG reveals severe ischemic changes. Echocardiogram shows severe left ventricular dysfunction.

His diabetes mellitus is well controlled with oral drug, hypertension is also well controlled with diltiazem. He is also taking aspirin, isosorbide mononitrate and simvastatin. All blood biochemistry reports—normal.

QUESTIONS

a. What is the likely cause of his collapse?
b. What is the best long-term management strategy in this case?

CASE NO. 285

A 29-year-old pregnant lady was hospitalized because of convulsion. Emergency LUCS was done. The baby, apparently looks well, no cry, pulse—40/min. ECG of baby shows complete heart block. You are called to see the baby and mother.

QUESTIONS

a. What is the likely cause of complete heart block of this baby?
b. What treatment should be given to the baby?
c. What history do you like to take from the mother?

CASE NO. 286

A 33-year-old service holder has been suffering from recurrent UTI for one year. She is feeling well with a full course of antibiotic. She is also suffering from insulin-dependent diabetes mellitus and hypertension, which are well controlled with drugs.

On examination, BP—160/95 mm Hg. Pulse—80/min, no edema, mildly anemic. Examination of other systems reveal no abnormality. Urinalysis—proteinuria (++).

QUESTIONS

a. What is the best method of preserving renal function?
b. Mention two anti-hypertensive drugs helpful in this case.
c. What is the likely diagnosis in such case?

CASE NO. 287

A 53-year-old man, farmer, has been suffering from low grade continued fever, more in evening, associated with night sweating for 3 months. He is also complaining of weakness, weight loss and fatigue for the same duration. He is non-smoker, non-hypertensive and non-diabetic. He was suffering from pulmonary tuberculosis 10 years back.

On examination, the patient looks emaciated and moderately anemic. Pulse—100/min, BP—100/70 mm Hg. Temperature—38.8°C, few purpuric spots are present in both legs. Liver—palpable, 3 cm, nontender, firm. Spleen is palpable 4 cm. Heart sounds are normal and his chest is clear.

Investigations

❖ Full blood count	-	Hb – 11.3 g/dL, WBC – 8,000/cmm, poly – 50%, lympho – 40%, mono – 5%, eosinophil – 5%, platelets – 1,10,000/cmm.
❖ Peripheral blood film	-	Fragmented red cells with polychromasia.
❖ RBS	-	3.2 mmol/L.
❖ Serum creatinine	-	120 µmol/L (normal 55 to 125).
❖ Serum urea	-	5.3 mmol/L (normal 2.5 to 6.6).
❖ Serum electrolytes	-	Sodium 140 mmol/L. Chloride 100 mmol/L. Potassium 4.2 mol/L.
❖ Chest X-ray	-	Heart is slightly enlarged.
❖ Serum bilirubin	-	18 µmol/L (normal 3 to 19).
❖ SGPT	-	96 IU/L (normal 10 to 40).
❖ SGOT	-	55 IU/L (normal 45 to 105).
❖ Alkaline phosphatase	-	105 IU/L (normal 25 to 100).
❖ Serum albumin	-	34 g/L (normal 37 to 49).
❖ Blood culture	-	Negative.
❖ Urine	-	Protein (+), red cells few.
❖ Urine C/S	-	Negative.
❖ Echocardiography	-	Small vegetation near aortic valve.

QUESTIONS

a. What diagnosis would you consider first?
b. Mention one investigation.
c. How to treat such case?

CASE NO. 288

A 44-year-old woman presented with dyspnea on exertion, weight loss, abdominal distension and swelling of both legs for 6 weeks. She has been suffering from rheumatoid arthritis, for which she is on sulfasalazine and NSAID. She has completed full course of antituberculous therapy one month back.

On examination, she looks emaciated and moderately anemic. Pulse—110/min, irregularly irregular, BP—90/65 mm Hg. Edema—bilateral and pitting. JVP—elevated.

Heart—apex beat could not be localized, heart sounds are soft, but no murmur. Abdomen—hepatomegaly, 4 cm, soft and tender. No splenomegaly. Shifting dullness—present but no fluid thrill.

Investigations

- ❖ Full blood count — Hb – 10.3 g/dL, WBC – 7,500/cmm, poly – 49%, lympho – 50%, mono – 1%, platelets – 4,10,000/cmm, ESR – 80.
- ❖ RBS — 4.2 mmol/L.
- ❖ Chest X-ray — Normal heart size and old healed lesion.
- ❖ Urine — Protein (+).

QUESTIONS

a. What is the likely diagnosis?
b. Mention one differential diagnosis.
c. Suggest three investigations.

CASE NO. 289

A 25-year-old woman, returned from Australia to Bangladesh, 3 days ago. After 2 days, suddenly she developed right sided hemiparesis and dysphasia. She had past medical history of DVT, one year back, from which there was complete recovery.

Physical examination reveals, DVT in right calf and also there is right sided hemiplegia of upper motor neuron type with dysphasia.

Routine blood count, sugar, urea, creatinine, chest X-ray and ECG are normal. CT scan of brain shows cerebral infarction involving middle cerebral artery territory on left side.

QUESTIONS

a. What is the underlying diagnosis?
b. Mention one investigation to find out the underlying diagnosis.

CASE NO. 290

A young man 29 years, smoker, non-hypertensive and non-diabetic, presented with frequent dizziness for one year, but no syncopal episode. He had two similar attacks 2 months back. During the second episode, he almost lost consciousness persisted for few minutes. His father died at the age of 34 years, due to heart attack.

ECG shows left ventricular hypertrophy. Echocardiogram reveals hypertrophic cardiomyopathy.

QUESTIONS

a. Mention two investigations which would indicate an increased risk of sudden cardiac death.
b. What is the cause of sudden death in this case?
c. What specific treatment should be given in such case?
d. What is the likely cause of death of his father?

CASE NO. 291

A 38-year-old man was hospitalized with severe head injuries in a road traffic accident and was unconscious for 24 hours. He was treated conservatively, feeling well and was discharged. Recently, he again presented with extreme weakness, polyuria and loss of weight.

Investigations

❖ Full blood count	-	Hb – 13.3 g/dL, WBC – 8,600/cmm, poly – 50%, lympho – 42%, mono – 5%, eosinophil – 3%, platelets – 3,10,000/cmm.
❖ RBS	-	6.2 mmol/L.
❖ Serum creatinine	-	120 μmol/L (normal 55 to 125).
❖ Serum urea	-	5.3 mmol/L (normal 2.5 to 6.6).
❖ Serum electrolytes	-	Sodium 160 mmol/L (N 135 to 145). Chloride 118 mmol/L (N 95 to 107). Potassium 4.1 mmol/L (N 3.5 to 5). Bicarbonate 33 mmol/L (N 23 to 32).

QUESTIONS

a. What is the likely diagnosis?
b. Mention one investigation which is helpful for your diagnosis.
c. How to treat the above biochemical abnormality?

CASE NO. 292

A 33-year-old lady presented with weakness, dizziness, palpitation and extreme fatigue for 2 months. Her symptoms are progressively increasing. For the last 10 days, she noticed bleeding from gum during brushing her teeth.

She was suffering from rheumatoid arthritis for long time and was taking disease modifying drugs.

Investigations

❖ Full blood count	-	Hb – 7.3 g/dl, WBC – 3,200/cmm, poly – 46%, lympho – 52%, eosinophil – 2%, platelets – 90,000/cmm.
❖ Peripheral blood film	-	Macrocytic anemia.
❖ RBS	-	3.8 mmol/L.
❖ Serum creatinine	-	120 μmol/L (normal 55 to 125).
❖ Serum urea	-	5.3 mmol/L (normal 2.5 to 6.6).
❖ Serum bilirubin	-	18 mmol/L (normal 3 to 19).
❖ SGPT	-	40 IU/L (normal 10 to 40).
❖ Alkaline phosphatase	-	98 IU/L (normal 25 to 100).

QUESTIONS

a. What is the hematological diagnosis?
b. Mention three causes of such abnormality.
c. Mention one physical finding which will be helpful for your diagnosis.
d. What one investigation should be done with the above blood picture?

CASE NO. 293

A 50-year-old man, non-diabetic and non-hypertensive, presented with weakness, malaise, low grade continued fever and breathlessness for 25 days. He had a Starr-Edward aortic valve replacement one month ago. He is on warfarin.

On examination, he is ill-looking, moderately anemic. Pulse—108/min, regular. BP—100/75 mm Hg. Temperature—38.2°C, splinter hemorrhage is present in right index finger.

Auscultation of heart revealed a prosthetic second heart sound, there is an early diastolic murmur in left lower parasternal area. 2-D echocardiogram—normal. Abdomen—spleen is just palpable. No hepatomegaly.

QUESTIONS

a. What two investigations should be done for the diagnosis?
b. What measures should be taken immediately?

CASE NO. 294

An elderly man presented with weakness, low grade continued fever and weight loss for 6 weeks. On query, he mentioned that for the last 2 months, he has been suffering from alternating constipation and diarrhea, night sweats and fatigue. No significant past medical history.

On examination, he is ill-looking and pale. Anemia—moderate. BP—100/60 mm Hg, Pulse—100/min, regular.

Precordial examination reveals an early diastolic murmur at left parasternal area in third intercostal space. No other abnormality on physical examination.

Investigations

- ❖ Full blood count - Hb – 9 g/dL, WBC – 14,100/cmm, poly – 79%, lympho – 21%, ESR – 110.
- ❖ RBS - 7.2 mmol/L.
- ❖ Serum creatinine - 100 μmol/L (normal 55 to 125).
- ❖ Serum urea - 8.3 mmol/L (normal 2.5 to 6.6).
- ❖ Chest X-ray - Normal.
- ❖ USG of abdomen - Doubtful mass in left lower abdomen.
- ❖ Blood culture - Positive.
- ❖ 2-D echocardiogram - Small vegetation in mitral valve.

QUESTIONS

a. What is the most likely causative organism in this case?
b. If repeated blood culture is negative, what is the likely diagnosis?
c. Mention one further investigation with negative blood culture.

CASE NO. 295

A 23-year-old male presented with severe headache, nausea and vomiting for 3 days. His headache is more on right side, throbbing in nature, associated with pain in right eye. For the last 2 days, he developed high fever, up to 105°C, associated with chill and rigor.

On examination, he looks very toxic. BP—95/65 mm Hg, Pulse—115/min and regular. Few herpetiform blister like lesions with redness in upper lip and nose.

Right eye—swollen, red, looks protruded, unable to move due to pain. Fundoscopy—papilloedema in right eye.

QUESTIONS

a. What is the likely diagnosis?
b. Mention two investigations.
c. Suggest three lines of management.

CASE NO. 296

A 24-year-old lady, recently married, is referred for weight gain and amenorrhea. Her menstruation is always irregular, sometimes occur after 3 months. Family history reveals that her father is hypertensive and diabetic, mother was suffering from thyroid disease.

On examination, she looks obese, hirsutism is present. BP—130/70 mm Hg.

Routine blood count, sugar, chest X-ray, electrolyte, urea and creatinine are normal.

Thyroid function shows:
* T_4 - 250 nmol/L (normal 55 to 144).
* T_3 - 3.9 nmol/L (normal 1.3 to 3.10).
* TSH   - 3.2 mIU/L (normal 0.35 to 5.0).

QUESTIONS

a. What is the likely diagnosis?
b. Mention one immediate investigation.
c. Mention two further investigations.

CASE NO. 297

A 19-year-old young male is hospitalized because of fever, vomiting and severe headache for 3 days. His symptoms deteriorated over the last 6 hours and no urine is passed. Following introduction of urinary catheter, 60 cc urine is collected and sent for analysis.

On examination, he looks very ill, Face—puffy. Anemia—moderate. BP—140/90 mm Hg, Pulse—100/min. Temperature—38.7°C. Edema—mild, pitting.

Investigations

* Full blood count   - Hb – 8.1 g/dL, WBC – 16,100/cmm, poly – 56%, lympho – 42%, eosinophil – 2%, platelets – 1,20,000/cmm.
* RBS   - 6 mmol/L.
* Serum electrolytes   - Sodium 132 mmol/L, Chloride 90 mmol/L, Potassium 5 mmol/L.
* Serum creatinine   - 400 µmol/L (normal 55 to 125).
* Serum urea   - 30 mmol/L (normal 2.5 to 6.6).
* Serum osmolality   - 320 mOsmol/kg.
* Urine   - Sodium 90 mmol/L. Potassium 30 mmol/L. Urea 120 mmol/L. Creatinine 7 µmol/L. Osmolality 300 mOsmol/kg.

QUESTIONS

a. What is the likely diagnosis?
b. Mention two reasons in favor of your diagnosis.

CASE NO. 298

A 40-year-old cultivator is hospitalized due to semi-consciousness, incoherent talk and convulsion. There is vomiting and diarrhea, after admission in the hospital.

On examination, he is semiconscious, but response to painful stimulus. BP—95/65 mm Hg, Pulse—120/min. Excess salivation and lacrimation.

Pupils are small, respond sluggishly. Generalized muscle weakness. Twitching of muscles are present. All reflexes—slightly exaggerated. Plantar responses—equivocal. Lungs—multiple rhonchi are audible in both lung fields. Heart—normal.

QUESTIONS

a. What is the likely diagnosis?
b. Mention five lines of management.
c. Mention five investigations.

CASE NO. 299

A 45-year-old male presented with severe generalized pain in the muscles and extreme weakness for ten days. The patient also experiences difficulty in walking, severe difficulty in standing from sitting, unable to comb his hair. In his past medical history, he is suffering from hypertension and diabetes mellitus, which are well controlled with oral drugs. Recently, his cholesterol and triglyceride level were found to be very high, for which simvastatin is prescribed.

On examination, his muscles are very tender. BP—140/90 mm Hg, Pulse—80/min. There is proximal myopathy. Muscle tone, power, sensation are all normal. Other systems reveal no abnormality.

Investigations

❖ Full blood count — Hb – 11.3 g/dL, WBC – 5,900/cmm, poly – 60%, lympho – 38%, mono – 2%, platelets – 4,91,000/cmm, ESR – 20.
❖ RBS — 8.2 mmol/L.
❖ Serum creatinine — 310 µmol/L (normal 55 to 125).
❖ Serum urea — 12.3 mmol/L (normal 2.5 to 6.6).
❖ Serum electrolytes — Sodium 139 mmol/L. Chloride 100 mmol/L. Potassium 5.6 mmol/L.
❖ Serum CPK — 1199 U/L (normal 24 to 170).
❖ Chest X-ray — Normal.
❖ USG of abdomen — Normal.

QUESTIONS

a. What is the likely diagnosis?
b. What is the cause of renal failure?
c. What immediate step should be taken for management?

CASE NO. 300

A lady aged 29 years, presented with low grade continuous fever, generalized bodyache, polyarthralgia and loss of weight for 3 months. On query, she mentioned light-headedness, dizziness and fatigue for few months. Her symptoms are progressively increasing. Recently, her appetite had reduced and she had further loss of weight.

Six months before, she had one episode of weakness and numbness of the right arm and face, persisted for almost an hour and there is also three attack of syncope. There is no other past medical history note.

On examination, she is pale and emaciated. Anemia—moderate. No jaundice, No oedema. BP—70/30 mm Hg. Pulse—90/min, low volume in right radial, very feeble in left radial. Both brachial pulses were weak, right carotid pulse was absent, left carotid is present with a thrill over it. Auscultation over carotid- bruit is present.

Both femoral pulses were easily palpable and also bruit is present over the femoral artery. Examination of other systems reveal no abnormality.

Investigations

- ❖ Full blood count - Hb – 8.3 g/dL, WBC – 6,700/cmm, poly – 49%, lympho – 57%, mono – 3%, eosinophil – 1%, platelets – 3,70,000/cmm.
- ❖ RBS - 7.9 mmol/L.
- ❖ Serum creatinine - 90 µmol/L (normal 55 to 125).
- ❖ Serum urea - 5.9 mmol/L (normal 2.5 to 6.6).
- ❖ Serum electrolytes - Sodium 138 mmol/L.
  Chloride 101 mmol/L.
  Potassium 4.3 mmol/L.
- ❖ Chest X-ray - Normal.
- ❖ Blood culture - Negative.
- ❖ Urine - Protein (+).
- ❖ Urine C/S - Negative.
- ❖ MT - 10.
- ❖ ECG - LVH.
- ❖ Echocardiography - LVH, no vegetation and no other abnormality.

QUESTIONS

a. What is the diagnosis?
b. Which investigation would you request to confirm your diagnosis?

CASE NO. 301

A lady aged 60 years, known diabetic and hypertensive, presented with shortness of breath and extreme weakness for 3 months. She was taking aspirin, insulin, amlodipine and calcium tablets regularly.

On examination, she is very pale, anemia—moderate, jaundice—mild, edema—mild and pitting.

Investigations

- ❖ Full blood count   - Hb – 6 g/dL, WBC – 3,000/cmm, poly – 50%, lympho – 56%, mono – 2%, eosinophil – 2%, platelets – 50,000/cmm. ESR 55 mm in first hr.
- ❖ MCV   - 111 fL (normal 76 to 96).
- ❖ RBS   - 8.9 mmol/L.
- ❖ Urinalysis   - Increased urobilinogen.

QUESTIONS

a. What should be the next investigation?
b. Mention one further investigation for confirmation of diagnosis.

CASE NO. 302

A farmer of 38 years, presented with generalized pigmentation. No other physical finding apart from pigmentation.

Investigations

- ❖ Chest X-ray   - Normal.
- ❖ USG of abdomen   - Normal.
- ❖ RBS   - 6.9 mmol/L.
- ❖ Serum ferritin   - 440 µg/L (normal 15 to 250).
- ❖ Serum iron   - 38 µg/L (normal 14 to 32).
- ❖ Serum iron binding   - 89 µg/L (normal 40 to 80).
  capacity

QUESTIONS

a. What further history may be helpful for the diagnosis?
b. Mention one further investigation.
c. If patient's father is a case of hemochromatosis, what investigation should be done?

CASE NO. 303

A 36-year-old, businessman, presented with pain in the abdomen, occasional diarrhea and abdominal distension for 3 months. Stool is pale and frothy. The patient is also complaining low back pain (LBP) and polyarthritis involving all the bigger joints. Patient's wife mentioned that he has developed disturbance of memory recently.

On examination, he is pigmented and emaciated. BP—80/30 mm Hg, Pulse—90/min, low volume.

He has limited vertical eye movements along with simultaneous movement of eyes and muscles of mastication.

QUESTIONS

a. What is the most likely diagnosis?
b. How do you confirm the diagnosis?

CASE NO. 304

A 27-year-old housewife has been suffering from type 1 diabetes mellitus for 3 years, which is well controlled. For the last 2 months, she has been suffering from progressive weight loss and fatigue. She has no fever and her bowel habit is normal, also appetite is good. She does not have any menstrual abnormality.

On examination, she looks emaciated and pale, anemia—severe.

Investigations

❖ Full blood count	- Hb – 6.9 g/dL, WBC – 3,000/cmm, poly – 50%, lympho – 46%, mono – 2%, eosinophil – 2%, platelets – 1,50,000/cmm. ESR 55 mm in Ist hour.
❖ MCV	- 65 fL (normal 76 to 96).
❖ PBF	- Microcytic hypochromic.
❖ RBS	- 6.9 mmol/L.
❖ HbA$_1$C	- <6.1.
❖ Urinalysis	- Normal.
❖ Chest X-ray	- Normal.
❖ USG of abdomen	- Normal.

QUESTIONS

a. What is the likely cause of weight loss and fatigue which is related to type 1 DM?
b. Mention one definitive investigation for the diagnosis.

CASE NO. 305

A 55-year-old lady presented with progressive breathlessness for 3 months.

On examination, she looks pale, anemia—severe, edema—present, pitting. BP—95/65 mmHg, pulse—120/min. Temp—37°C. JVP—raised. Chest—bilateral fine inspiratory crepitations in lower chest.

Abdomen—tenderness in right upper abdomen.
Fundoscopy—reveals hemorrhages in both fundi.

Investigations

- ❖ Full blood count   - Hb – 5.3 g/dL, WBC – 3,100/cmm, poly – 49%, lympho – 57%, mono – 3%, eosinophil – 1%, platelets – 1,10,000/cmm.
- ❖ RBS   - 7.9 mmol/L.
- ❖ MCV   - 120 fL (normal 76 to 96).
- ❖ MCH   - 32 pg (normal 27 to 32).

◼ QUESTIONS

a. What is the likely diagnosis?
b. How can you confirm the diagnosis?
c. What should be the immediate management of this patient?
d. What is the cause of breathlessness?

◼ CASE NO. 306

A 42-year-old housewife, diagnosed case of rheumatoid arthritis and is on treatment. She attended in outpatient department for follow-up. Her few routine investigation reports are as follows:

- ❖ Full blood count   - Hb – 11 g/dL, TC – 7500/cmm, platelet count 4,00,000/cmm.
- ❖ MCV   - 106 fL (normal 76 to 96).
- ❖ Serum creatinine   - 0.8 mg/dL (normal 0.68 to 1.36).
- ❖ SGPT   - 30 U/L (normal 5 to 40).

◼ QUESTIONS

a. What drug is given for her RA?
b. Why is MCV high?

◼ CASE NO. 307

A 57-year-old man is being treated for atrial fibrillation. On follow-up, he complains of tiredness and increased tendency to sleep. Clinically, he is euthyroid.

Investigations

- ❖ FT$_3$ - 0.7 nmol/L (normal 1.3 to 3.5).
- ❖ FT$_4$ - 26 pmol/L (normal 70 to 160).
- ❖ TSH   - 11.5 mU/L (normal 0.5 to 5.1).

◼ QUESTION

a. What is the diagnosis?

◼ CASE NO. 308

A 32-year-old alcoholic was found unconscious at a road side.
    On examination, patient is unconscious, poor response to painful stimuli. Temperature—35.2°C, BP—100/70 mm Hg.

Investigations

* Creatinine   - 3.2 mg/dL (normal 0.68 to 1.36).
* SGPT   - 460 U/L (normal 5 to 40).
* Gamma GT   - 40 U/L (normal 5 to 30).
* Urine dipstick for blood - +++.

QUESTION

a. What is the most likely diagnosis?

CASE NO. 309

A 70-year-old man, visited for follow-up in psychiatric department, suddenly collapsed in outpatient waiting room.

On examination, he was conscious, but unresponsive. Temperature—41°C, BP—150/100 mm Hg. Muscle rigidity is present, reflexes could not be elicited, plantar—equivocal.

QUESTION

a. What is the likely diagnosis?

CASE NO. 310

A 50-year-old man presented with the complaints of anorexia, nausea, vomiting, confusion and abdominal pain.

Investigations

* Full blood count   - Hb 10 g/dL, TC–6,500/cmm, platelet count–4,40,000/cmm, ESR–10 mm in first hr.
* Serum calcium   - 14 mg/dL (normal 9.1 to 11.6).
* Serum albumin   - 40 g/dL (normal 35 to 50).
* Serum phosphate   - 0.8 mmol/L (normal 0.8 to 1.4).
* Serum creatinine   - 1 mg/dL (normal 0.68 to 1.36).
* Skull X-ray (lateral view) - Ground glass appearance.
* Dorsal spine X-ray   - Osteoporosis.

QUESTIONS

a. What is the cause of his symtomps?
b. What is the next investigation of this patient?
c. What is the etiological diagnosis?
d. What is the most common cause of the etiological diagnosis?
e. What are the indications of surgery of this patient?

CASE NO. 311

A 60-year-old man presented with the complaints of weakness, lethargy, palpitation, polyuria and polyphagia.

Investigations

- ❖ Full blood count   - Hb – 6 g/dL, TC–3,500/cmm, platelet count – 1,40,000/cmm, ESR – 120 mm in first hr.
- ❖ PBF   - Marked rouleaux formation.
- ❖ Urine   - Protein ++, pus cell 4 to 6/HPF.
- ❖ SGPT   - 30 U/L (normal 5 to 40).
- ❖ Serum creatinine   - 3.5 mg/dL (normal 0.57 to 1.36).
- ❖ Blood urea   - 60 mg/dL (normal 15 to 40).
- ❖ L/S spine X-ray   - Lytic lesion in lumbar vertebrae.
- ❖ Skull X-ray   - Multiple lytic lesion.

QUESTIONS

a. What next investigation will you do?
b. Give six causes of his renal failure.

CASE NO. 312

A 24-year-old man presented with the complains of weakness, lethargy and palpitation. He was given repeated blood transfusion. Recently, he develops weakness of both lower limbs.

On examination, the patient is pale and severely anemic, also icteric. There is hepatosplenomegaly. All jerks in lower limbs are exaggerated.

Plantar—extensor on both sides. All sensations in lower limbs are impaired.

Investigations

- ❖ Full blood count   - Hb – 7 g/dL, WBC – 3,000/cmm, poly – 50%, lympho – 56%, mono – 2%, eosinophil – 2%, platelets – 50,000/cmm. ESR – 55 mm in first hr.
- ❖ PBF   - Microcytic hypochromic anemia and few target cells.
- ❖ Reticulocyte   - 3% (normal 0.2 to 2).
- ❖ Coombs test   - Negative.
- ❖ Hb electrophoresis   - Hb F 20%, Hb A 80%.
- ❖ CXR   - Cardiomegally.

QUESTIONS

a. What is your diagnosis?
b. What is the cause of his weakness of legs?
c. Mention one simple investigation?
d. What is the treatment option in such case ?

CASE NO. 313

A 45-year-old woman presented with the complains of cough and progressive breathlessness. On examination, she has cyanosis, clubbing and end-expiratory crepitations.

QUESTIONS

a. Give six histories from the patient.
b. Give four examination findings of this patient.

CASE NO. 314

A 19-year-old obese girl, who is suffering from tuberculosis, presented with recurrent, tender and ulcerating nodule on the calf of the lower limbs.

QUESTIONS

a. What is the most likely diagnosis?
b. How to confirm your diagnosis?

CASE NO. 315

A 59-year-old gentleman with a long history of psoriasis, presented with generalized erythroderma and severe polyarthritis for 5 days. He is treated with emolients, fluid replacement, antibiotic and other symptomatic treatment without much improvement.

QUESTION

Mention two line of further management.

CASE NO. 316

A housewife aged 31 years, presented with cyanosis of the lower limbs and clubbing of toes, not in fingers.

QUESTION

a. What is the most likely diagnosis?
b. Mention one single investigation.

CASE NO. 317

A lady aged 43 years, very pale looking, presented with the complains of tiredness and lethargy. On examination, she is having numerous depigmented areas in arms and legs.

QUESTION

What is the most likely disease accompanying this skin lesion?

CASE NO. 318

A female, housewife aged 26 years, presented with alopecia and crusted lesions around her mouth and fingers. There is history of small bowel resection a year ago for recurrent exacerbation of Crohn's disease.

QUESTIONS

a. What is your diagnosis?
b. Mention the specific treatment.

CASE NO. 319

A 51-year-old labor presented with an ulcer at the tip of nose which is shallow, irregular and painless. He returned from Middle East 2 months back.

QUESTIONS

a. What is the lesion?
b. How to confirm the diagnosis?

CASE NO. 320

A young lady presented with severe pruritic papule and vesicle on the elbow, buttock and knee, which are not responding to antihistamine, local and also systemic steroid.

QUESTIONS

a. What disease is she suffering from?
b. How to confirm your diagnosis?

CASE NO. 321

A 66-year-old, retired, gentleman, presented with sudden onset of right sided hemiplegia involving the face, arm and leg (lesser extent), homonymous hemianopia and global aphasia.

QUESTIONS

a. Where is the site of the lesion?
b. Which vessel is involved?

CASE NO. 322

A 29-year-old male, smoker, non-hypertensive, presented with severe acute asthma. He is treated with oxygen, nebulized bronchodilators, IV steroid, IV aminophylline, but there is no good response.

QUESTION

a. What is the next most appropriate drug to add?

CASE NO. 323

A young housewife presented with gradual abdominal distension and ankle edema for 6 months. All routine blood tests including blood sugar are normal, except Hb—9.5 g/dL, urine shows glycosuria (++) and proteinuria (+).

QUESTIONS

a. What one history should you ask?
b. What single investigation would you suggest?

CASE NO. 324

A male patient aged 55 years, known case of ischemic heart disease presented with 2 months history of stiffness of the fingers and few photosensitive rash. He is on anticonvulsant for 2 years for epilepsy. Examination reveals swelling of the hands and wrist joints, associated with tenderness of the metacarpophalangeal joints.

Chest X-ray shows small bilateral pleural effusion.

Investigations

❖ Full blood count   - Hb – 10.8 g/dL, WBC – 10,000/cmm, poly – 56%, lympho – 40%,
                        mono – 2%, eosinophil – 2%, platelets – 2,50,000/cmm.
                        ESR – 55 mm in first hr.
❖ ANA   - Positive.
❖ Anti-ds DNA   - Negative.

QUESTIONS

a. What is your diagnosis?
b. What is your next investigation to confirm your diagnosis?

CASE NO. 325

A 45-year-old female is admitted with an intracranial bleeding under the care of neurosurgeon. MRI shows sub-arachnoid hemorrhage and clipping of a cerebral arterial aneurysm was done successfully.

The surgical team document the following investigation results on postoperative days.

❖ Full blood count   - Hb – 10.8 g/dL, WBC – 10,000/cmm, poly – 56%, lympho – 40%,
                        mono – 2%, eosinophil – 2%, platelets – 2,50,000/cmm. ESR –
                        55 mm in first hr.
❖ Serum electrolytes - Sodium 127 mmol/L. Chloride 94 mmol/L.
                        Potassium 3.5 mmol/L.
❖ Urea   - 4.2 mmol/L.
❖ Creatinine   - 95 µmol/L.
❖ Serum osmolality - 262 mosm/L.
❖ Urine osmolality - 700 mosm/L.
❖ Urinary sodium   - 70 mmol/L.

QUESTIONS

a. What is your diagnosis?
b. Name one treatment option of this patient.

CASE NO. 326

A 34-year-old man, was hospitalized with stage IIB Hodgkin's lymphoma. His cardiac and respiratory functions were normal. ABVD (Adriamycin, Bleomycin, Vinblastine and Dacarbazine) chemotherapy regimen was started. First three cycles of the chemotherapy were well tolerated by him. After completion of the 4th cycle, he was hospitalized again with exertional dyspnea and severe dry cough. There is no fever. Chest X-ray and ECG are normal.

QUESTIONS

a. What is the most likely cause of his symptoms ?
b. Mention two further investigation.

CASE NO. 327

A 72-year-old man with pseudobulbar palsy presents with progressively increasing dysphagia. Percutaneous endoscopic gastrostomy was done for nutritional support. But, his weakness was increasing even with good nutrition.

QUESTIONS

a. What is your diagnosis?
b. What investigation will support your diagnosis?

CASE NO. 328

A lady aged 45 years was examined and investigated for executive check. She was coincidentally found to have hypercalcemia. There were no significant physical illness and physical examination was unremarkable.

Investigations

- Serum Na — 138 mmol/L (Normal 137 to 144).
- Serum K — 4.1 mmol/L (Normal 3.5 to 4.9).
- Serum urea — 3.8 mmol/L (Normal 2.5 to7.5).
- Serum corrected calcium — 2.76 (Normal 2.2 to 2.6).
- Serum phosphate — 0.86 mmol/L (Normal 0.8 to 1.4).
- Serum alkaline phosphatase — 86 U/L (Normal 45 to 105).
- Plasma parathyroid hormone — 5.3 pmol/L (Normal 0.9 to 5.4).
- 24-hour urinary calcium — 0.5 mmol/24 hr (Normal 2.5 to 7.5).

QUESTIONS

a. What is your diagnosis?
b. What measure should be taken?

CASE NO. 329

A 25-year-old man was referred to outpatient department with 8 years history of recurrent chest infections. He used to take frequent antibiotic.

Investigations

* Ig G   - 6.5 g/L (Normal 6.0 to13.0).
* IgA   - 0.8 g/L (Normal 0.8 to 3.0).
* IgM   - 0.5 g/L (Normal 0.4 to 2.5).

QUESTIONS

a. What is the likely diagnosis with the above result?
b. Mention one specific treatment option which will prevent recurrent chest infection.

CASE NO. 330

A lady aged 60 years known diabetic for 3 years, well controlled with diet. She is mildly hypertensive for 2 years, well controlled with one drug. Her daughter called the GP mentioning that while the patient was going upstairs, she felt extreme weakness and fell down on the ground, but was fully conscious, no vomiting, or headache. Her GP examined her and found: pulse—80/min, regular; BP—130/80 mm Hg. Heart and lungs—normal. Reflexes—diminished in lower limbs but normal in upper limbs; plantar—normal; no sensory abnormality.

QUESTIONS

a. What is likely cause of her weakness?
b. What is the most probable drug she was getting?

CASE NO. 331

A man aged 70 years known COPD was hospitalized because of cough with hemoptysis for 10 days. He used to take different types of inhalers and steroid, salbutamol, etc. There is no significant past medical history.

On examination, the patient is emaciated, there is generalized clubbing. Heart—normal, lungs—breath sound is vesicular with prolonged expiration with plenty of ronchi on both lung fields. No organomegaly.

CXR shows opacity in the right apical region. FNAC was done. After 2 hours, the patient complains of severe respiratory distress and central chest pain.

QUESTIONS

a. Mention one immediate investigation.
b. What is the most likely diagnosis?
c. Mention two differential diagnosis.

CASE NO. 332

A lady aged 65 years, diabetic and hypertensive, well controlled with drugs, was suffering from high grade fever with severe headache and bodyache for 5 days. CBC count shows leukopenia with thrombocytopenia. She was hospitalized after bleeding gum and epistaxis. Dengue hemorrhagic was suspected. With symptomatic treatment, blood count became normal and the patient went home with request after 3 days. Again after 5 days while she came for follow-up, she mentioned that her headache is persistent and there is frequent epigastric pain and vomiting for which she was again hospitalized. With symptomatic treatment, her symptoms were not subsided and headache with vomiting were persistent. Her maid servant mentioned that 2 weeks before, she got trauma to the head while she was getting down from the car.

In her past nedical history, right mastectomy was done 8 years back with suspiscion of carcinoma of the breast, followed by chemo and radiotherapy and she was well. Total abdominal hysterectomy and cholecystectomy were done 3 years and 2 years back respectively.

Routine investigations like - CBC, Electrolytes, Creatinine, CXR, ECG, Endoscopy, USG of abdomen were normal. CT scan of head and MRI of brain were normal.

QUESTIONS

a. What is the likely cause of her headache?
b. Mention one confirmatory investigation.

CASE NO. 333

A 45-year-lady has been suffering from fever, dry cough and loss of weight for 3 months. For the last 2 months, she developed frequent hemoptysis, difficulty in hearing followed by deafness. There is no significant past medical illness. On examination- the patient looks very toxic, temperature 105 F. No lymphadenopathy or organomegaly. Heart—normal, lungs—multiple coarse crepitations with plenty of ronchi on both lungs fields. Deafness is present.

Investigations

* CXR—bilateral extensive patchy opacity consistent with tuberculosis.
* WBC—10,000/cmm; Neutrophil—80%, lympho-15%, eosinophil—5%; ESR—120 mm in 1st hour.
* MT-02mm.
* Blood and urine C/S—normal.
* CT scan shows severe sinusitis with mastoiditis.

Anti-TB was started and an ENT surgeon performed surgery with suspiscion of mastoid abscess. But her fever was persistently very high with increasing cough, respiratory distress, severe headache and also persistent deaness. Repeat CXR—persistent bilateral opacity. Other routine investigations were repeated, but no abnormality. ANA, Antids DNA were negative. Only serum ferritin was found to be moderately high.

QUESTIONS

a. What is the likely diagnosis?
b. Mention two investigations.

Chapter
2

Data Interpretation of Cardiac Catheter

(For answers: See page 447-451)

"I would live to study, and not study to live."

— Francis Bacon

Chapter

2

INTRODUCTION

Interpretation of data related to cardiac catheter is sometimes given in postgraduate examination. Before interpretation, one must know the normal pressure and also oxygen saturation in different chambers of the heart as well as great vessels. Only few common cardiac data are included in this chapter.

Normal pressures (mm Hg) in different chambers of heart and vessels

* Right atrium — 0 to 8 (mean 4).
* Right ventricle — 15 to 30 systolic (mean 24), 1 to 7 diastolic (mean 4)
* Pulmonary artery — 15 to 30 systolic (mean 22), 5 to 17 diastolic (mean 11).
* Pulmonary capillary wedge — 2 to 8 (mean 6). pressure (same left atrial pressure, same LVEDP)
* Left ventricle — Less than 140/12.

Abnormal pressure

* A pulmonary artery pressure >35 mm Hg is suggestive of pulmonary hypertension.
* A pressure drop of more 10 mm Hg across the aortic or pulmonary valve is suggestive of aortic or pulmonary stenosis respectively.
* PCWP is equal to LVEDP. When PCWP exceeds LVEDP, the diagnosis of mitral stenosis should be considered.
* Aortic regurgitation is diagnosed by a wide pulse pressure.
* Elevated and equal left and right atrial pressures, elevated and equal right and left ventricular end diastolic pressures are highly suggestive of chronic constrictive pericarditis.

Some diagnostic features in valvular lesion

* Raised right ventricular systolic pressure occurs in pulmonary hypertension, pulmonary stenosis, Eisenmenger's syndrome.
* Raised right ventricular end-diastolic pressures occurs in right ventricular failure, constrictive pericarditis, cardiomyopathy.
* Raised mean pulmonary artery pressure occurs in pulmonary hypertension, left to right shunt, mitral stenosis, left ventricular failure.
* Decreased mean pulmonary artery pressure occurs in pulmonary stenosis. (There must be a gradient greater than 20 mm Hg before stenosis is diagnosed.)
* Raised pulmonary capillary wedge pressure occurs in mitral stenosis, mitral regurgitation, left ventricular failure, aortic stenosis.
* Raised left ventricular systolic pressure occurs in systemic hypertension, aortic stenosis and non-valvular aortic stenosis including hypertrophic obstructive cardiomyopathy.
* Raised left ventricular end-diastolic pressure occurs in left ventricular failure, aortic regurgitation, cardiomyopathy.

Diagnosis of common valve lesions

1. In aortic stenosis, there is a pressure gradient between the left ventricular systolic pressure and the aortic systolic pressure.
2. In aortic regurgitation, there is a wide pulse pressure and near equalization of aortic and left ventricular end diastolic pressures.

3. In mitral stenosis, there is a difference between pulmonary capillary wedge pressure (left atrial pressure) and left ventricular diastolic pressure, which is increased by exercise.
4. If right ventricular systolic pressure is equal to aortic systolic pressure, the diagnosis may be Eisenmenger's syndrome, Fallot's tetralogy or transposition of great vessels.

NORMAL OXYGEN SATURATION

In traditional oximetry, multiple samples are taken in rapid succession from the following sites. Normal values for oxygen saturation are given:

- Right ventricle (outflow, body, inflow) - 57 to 85% (Average 71%).
- Right atrium (low, mid, high)   - 58 to 82% (Average 70%).
- Superior vena cava (low, high)   - 51 to 83% (Average 67%).
- Inferior vena cava at the level
  of diaphragm   - 54 to 90% (Average 72%).
- Pulmonary artery (main left and right) - 58 to 82% (Average 70%).
- Systemic artery   - 88 to 99% (Average 94%).

CHANGES IN DIFFERENT SHUNT ANOMALY

- If there is left-to-right shunt, pulmonary blood flow is greater than the systemic blood flow. The position of oxygen step-up indicates the position of the shunt (for example in patent ductus arteriosus, the step-up in oxygen saturation occurs between the right ventricle and pulmonary artery).
- If the shunt is from right to left, there is arterial desaturation and the position of the shunt is indicated by the left heart chamber, which is the first to show desaturation.
- If the shunt is unidirectional, its magnitude may be calculated as the difference between the pulmonary and systemic blood flow. This can be simply calculated approximately using the formula:

$$\frac{\text{Systemic arterial oxygen saturation} - \text{Mixed venous oxygen saturation}}{\text{Systemic arterial oxygen saturation} - \text{Pulmonary artery oxygen saturation.}}$$

- An accepted formula for calculating the mixed venous oxygen saturation is: 3 × SVC oxygen saturation + 1 × IVC oxygen saturation ÷ 4.

INTERPRETATION OF SOME CARDIAC CATHETER

CARDIAC CATHETER – 01

The results of cardiac catheterization in a patient of 20 years age, who presented with occasional breathlessness.

	Pressure (mm Hg)	Oxygen saturation (%)
Superior vena cava	Mean 4	74%
Inferior vena cava	Mean 2	68%
Right atrium	Mean 4	75%
Right ventricle body	40/0	81%
Right ventricle outflow tract	40/0	88%
Pulmonary artery	40/15, mean 24	88%
Left ventricle	110/2, end diastole 7	99%

QUESTIONS

a. Comment on these results.
b. Suggest the likely diagnosis.
c. Where is the commonest site of lesion?
d. Mention one physical finding.

CARDIAC CATHETER - 02

The results of cardiac catheterization of a 23-year-old lady, presented with increasing shortness of breath on exertion.

	Pressure (mm Hg)	Oxygen saturation (%)
Superior vena cava	–	66%
Inferior vena cava	–	78%
Right atrium	2 (mean)	90% (mean)
Right ventricle body	60/0	87%
Pulmonary artery	16/8 (10 mean	87%

QUESTION

Mention two diagnoses.

CARDIAC CATHETER - 03

The results of cardiac catheterization of a 3-year-old baby, with cyanosis and finger clubbing.

	Pressure (mm Hg)	Oxygen saturation (%)
Superior vena cava	–	43%
Right atrium	10	42%
Right ventricle	120/10	43%
Pulmonary artery	15/5	42%
Pulmonary capillary wedge pressure	12	98%
Left atrium	10	88%
Left ventricle	120/8	77%
Femoral artery	120/80	75%

QUESTIONS

a. What cardiac lesions may be present?
b. What two features would you expect to see in chest X-ray?
c. Mention one investigation.

CARDIAC CATHETER - 04

The results of cardiac catheterization of a 32-year-old man.

	Pressure (mm Hg)	Oxygen saturation (%)
Right atrium	0	57%
Right ventricle	120/05	55%
Left ventricle	110/70	85%
Pulmonary artery	120/70	57%
Aorta	105/60	84%

▌QUESTIONS

a. What is the diagnosis?
b. Mention one further investigation.

▌CARDIAC CATHETER - 05

The results of cardiac catheterization of a 50-year-old man investigated for systolic murmur after myocardial infarction.

	Pressure (mm Hg)	Oxygen saturation (%)
Right atrium	Mean 8	74%
Right ventricle	20/60	84%
Pulmonary artery	50/18	84%
PCWP	18	–
Left ventricle	95/18	94%
Aorta	105/60	94%

▌QUESTIONS

a. What is the diagnosis?
b. What would be the ideal management if patient remains stable?

▌CARDIAC CATHETER - 06

The results of cardiac catheterization of a 55-year-old man, who presented with dyspnea on exertion. A systolic murmur is present.

	Pressure (mm Hg)
Right atrium	Mean 3
Right ventricle	29/3
Pulmonary artery	28/14
PCWP	Mean 18
Left ventricle	190/20
Aorta	110/80

QUESTIONS

a. Mention two differential diagnoses.
b. Mention one investigation.

CARDIAC CATHETER - 07

The results of cardiac catheterization of a 26-year-old male who presented with breathlessness with moderate activity.

	Pressure (mm Hg)	Oxygen saturation (%)
Right atrium	Mean 7	79%
Right ventricle	20/6	74%
Pulmonary artery	36/17	92%
PCWP	3	–
Left ventricle	100/8	96%
Aorta	95/60	96%

QUESTIONS

a. What is the diagnosis?
b. Mention one important auscultatory finding.
c. Mention two abnormalities in above data.

CARDIAC CATHETER - 08

The results of cardiac catheterization of a 35-year-old man presented with increasing breathlessness on mild exertion.

	Pressure (mm Hg)	Oxygen saturation (%)
Right atrium	Mean 10	67%
Right ventricle	40/10	67%
Pulmonary artery	40/22	67%
PCWP	17	–
Left ventricle	160/10	98%
Aorta	110/70	98%

QUESTIONS

a. Mention three abnormalities.
b. What are the possible diagnoses?

CARDIAC CATHETER - 09

The results of cardiac catheterization of a 16-year-old tall, lean and thin boy presented with breathlessness.

	Pressure (mm Hg)	Oxygen saturation (%)
Superior vena cava	–	76%
Inferior vena cava	–	72%
Right atrium	Mean 6	74%
Right ventricle	25/6	75%
Pulmonary artery	25/18	75%
PCWP	16	–
Left ventricle	210/18	98%
Aorta	210/55	98%

QUESTIONS

a. What abnormality is seen in this data?
b. What is the cardiac diagnosis?
c. What is the underlying diagnosis?

CARDIAC CATHETER - 10

The results of cardiac catheterization of a 28-year-old male who presented with headache and intermittent claudication.

	Pressure (mm Hg)	Oxygen saturation (%)
Superior vena cava	–	75%
Inferior vena cava	–	71%
Right atrium	Mean 7	75%
Right ventricle	26/8	76%
Pulmonary artery	26/10	76%
PCWP	8	–
Left ventricle	195/5	98%
Femoral artery	155/85	96%

QUESTIONS

a. What abnormality is seen?
b. What is the diagnosis?

CARDIAC CATHETER - 11

The results of cardiac catheterization of a 22-year-old patient, known to have a heart murmur from the age of 3 months.

	Pressure (mm Hg)	Oxygen saturation (%)
Superior vena cava	–	75%
Inferior vena cava	–	71%
Right atrium	Mean 7	75%
Right ventricle	26/8	76%
Pulmonary artery	26/10	76%
PCWP	8	–
Left ventricle	195/5	98%
Aorta	120/85	96%

QUESTIONS

a. What abnormality is present here?
b. What is the diagnosis?

CARDIAC CATHETER - 12

The results of cardiac catheterization of a 33-year-old housewife, whose ECG shows left axis deviation with right bundle branch block (RBBB).

	Pressure (mm Hg)	Oxygen saturation (%)
Superior vena cava	–	69%
Inferior vena cava	–	65%
Right atrium	Mean 7	81%
Right ventricle	28/3	81%
Pulmonary artery	25/7	82%
PCWP	9	–
Left ventricle	125/9	96%
Femoral artery	120/70	96%

QUESTIONS

a. What abnormality is shown?
b. What is the diagnosis?

CARDIAC CATHETER - 13

The results of cardiac catheterization of a 45-year-old woman presented with breathlessness even on mild exertion.

	Pressure (mm Hg)
Right atrium	30/15
Right ventricle	70/15
Pulmonary artery	70/40
PCWP	35
Left ventricle	105/5
Aorta	100/70

QUESTIONS

a. Mention the diagnosis, also points in favor of the diagnosis.
b. Suggest one further investigation.

CARDIAC CATHETER - 14

The results of cardiac catheterization of a 4-year-old child with a 47 XY karyotype.

	Pressure (mm Hg)	Oxygen saturation (%)
Superior vena cava	–	66%
Inferior vena cava	–	70%
Right atrium	10	82%
Right ventricle	50/0	83%
Pulmonary artery	50/25	81%
Left atrium	10	95%
Left ventricle	95/0	96%

QUESTIONS

a. What are the diagnoses?
b. Suggest one investigation.

CARDIAC CATHETER - 15

The results of cardiac catheterization of a 35-year-old housewife presented with weakness and exertional dyspnea.

	Pressure (mm Hg)	Oxygen saturation (%)
Superior vena cava	–	68%
Inferior vena cava	–	69%
Right atrium	19	68%
Right ventricle	48/20	68%
Pulmonary artery	40/20	68%
PCWP	18	–
Left ventricle	90/20	96%
Aorta	85/65	96%

QUESTIONS

a. What is the diagnosis?
b. Suggest one investigation.

CARDIAC CATHETER - 16

The results of cardiac catheterization of a 50-year-old woman presented with exertional dyspnea.

	Pressure (mm Hg)	Oxygen saturation (%)
Superior vena cava	–	65%
Inferior vena cava	–	65%
Right atrium	6	65%
Right ventricle	24/6	67%
Pulmonary artery	24/18	67%
PCWP	16	–
Left ventricle	210/18	96%
Aorta	210/55	96%

QUESTIONS

a. What is the diagnosis?
b. Mention one auscultatory finding helpful for your diagnosis.

Family Tree (Pedigree)

(For answers: See page 453-458)

"Life is short, the art is long, opportunity fleeting, experience delusive, judgement difficult."

— Hippocrates 400 BC

"Once we have recognized that disease is naught else than the process of life under altered conditions, the concept of healing expands to imply the maintenance or re-establishment of the normal conditions of existence."

— *Rudolf Virchow*

FAMILY TREE - 01

This is a family tree (Pedigree).

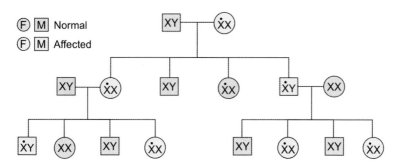

QUESTIONS

a. What is the mode of inheritance?
b. Mention one condition which follows this mode of inheritance.

FAMILY TREE - 02

This is a family tree (Pedigree).

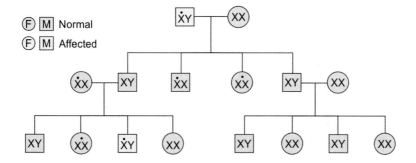

QUESTIONS

a. What is the mode of inheritance?
b. Mention five diseases which follow this mode of inheritance.

FAMILY TREE - 03

This is a family tree (Pedigree).

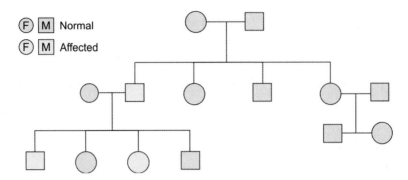

QUESTIONS

a. What is the mode of inheritance?
b. Mention five diseases which follow this mode of inheritance.

FAMILY TREE - 04

This is a family tree (Pedigree).

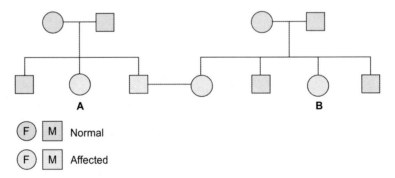

QUESTIONS

a. What is the mode of inheritance of (i) family A, and (ii) family B?
b. What is the chance of the children being affected, if both parents are affected?

FAMILY TREE - 05

This is a family tree (Pedigree) of a rare bone disease.

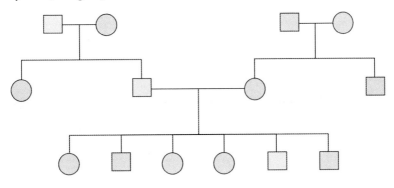

QUESTIONS

a. What is the mode of inheritance?
b. What is the chance (i) of a son (ii) of a daughter having the disease?

FAMILY TREE - 06

This is a family tree (Pedigree).

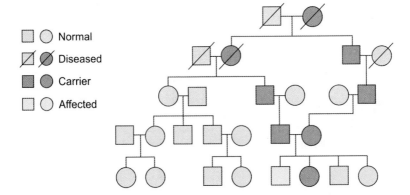

QUESTIONS

a. What is the mode of inheritance?
b. If both parents are carrier, what is the chance (i) of children being affected (ii) of children being carrier?

FAMILY TREE - 07

This is a family tree (Pedigree).

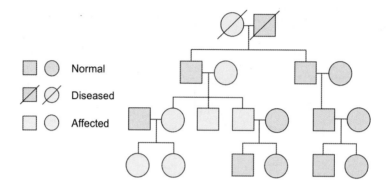

QUESTIONS

a. What is the mode of inheritance?
b. If a male is affected, what portion of his offspring will get the disease from him?
c. Mention one example of such.

FAMILY TREE - 08

This is a family tree (Pedigree).

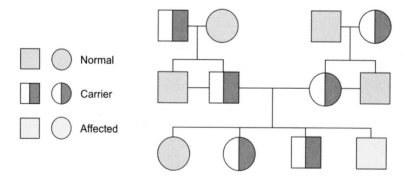

QUESTIONS

a. What is the mode of inheritance?
b. How many generations are affected?

FAMILY TREE - 09

This is a karyotype.

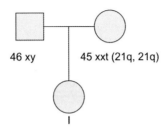

46 xy   45 xxt (21q, 21q)

QUESTIONS

a. What is the karyotype?
b. What is the chance of Down's syndrome in I?

FAMILY TREE - 10

This is a family tree (Pedigree).

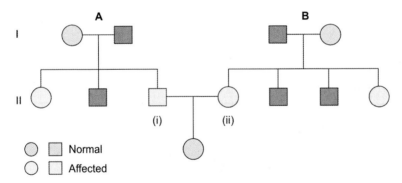

A   B

I

II

(i)   (ii)

○ □ Normal
○ □ Affected

QUESTIONS

a. What is the inheritance in II (i)?
b. What is the inheritance in II (ii)?
c. What is the chance of children to be normal if both couples are deaf?

FAMILY TREE - 11

This is a family tree (Pedigree).

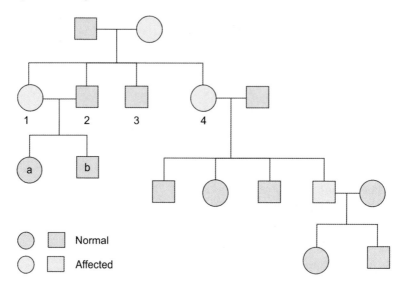

QUESTIONS

a. What is the inheritance?
b. What is the chance that individual "a" is affected?
c. What is the chance that individual "b" is affected?
d. Mention one disease.

FAMILY TREE - 12

This is a family tree of a patient with achondroplasia.

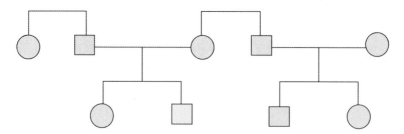

QUESTIONS

a. What is the chance of parents having another achondroplasia?
b. In the sibling who has an achondroplasia, what is the chance of getting another achondroplasia?

FAMILY TREE - 13

This is a family tree (Pedigree).

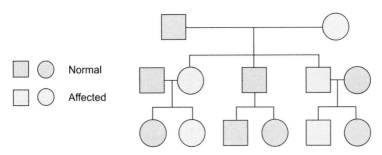

QUESTIONS

a. What is the inheritance pattern?
b. What is the chance of offspring being affected?
c. Mention five conditions of such pedigree.

FAMILY TREE - 14

This is a family tree of a patient having XXY.

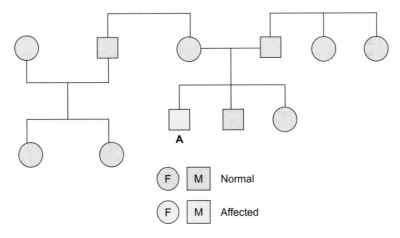

QUESTIONS

a. What disease is the patient suffering from?
b. What is the chance of parents of the affected to get another XXY?
c. What is the chance of a patient having affected child?

"Medicine is the most distinguished of all the arts, but through the ignorance of those who practice it, and of those who casually judge such practitioners, it is now of all the arts by far the least esteemed. Many are physicians by repute, very few are such in reality."

*— **Hippocrates 460–357 BC***

Chapter
4

Spirometry

(For answers: See page 459-465)

"The fruit of healing grows on the tree of understanding. Without diagnosis, there is no rational treatment. Examination comes first, then judgement, and then one can give help."

— Carl Gerhardt

"I search after truth, by which man never yet was harmed."

— Galen

SPIROMETRY

Spirometry is a method of assessing lung function by measuring the volume of air after maximal expiration following maximal inspiration. By spirometry, FEV_1 and FVC are measured. The technique involves a maximum inspiration followed by a forced expiration (as long as possible), into the spirometer. FEV_1 is expressed as a percentage of the FVC.

It is done to diagnose and differentiate obstructive airway disorders (e.g. COPD, asthma) from restrictive diseases (e.g. ILD). Spirometry can also be used to determine the severity of asthma and COPD.

By spirometry, five important measures can be detected:

1. **FEV_1 (Forced expiratory volume in 1st second):** The volume of air in the first second of forced expiration after full inspiration.
2. **FVC (Forced vital capacity):** The total volume of air expired forcibly in one breath after full inspiration.
3. **FEV_1/FVC:** The ratio of FEV_1 to FVC expressed as percentage.
4. **PEF (Peak expiratory flow):** It is the highest flow one can achieve during forceful expiration. It is used as a short-term monitoring tool at doctor's chamber and emergency room during exacerbations.
   Long-term monitoring of asthma can be done by seeing diurnal variability of PEF at patient's home by maintaining peak flow chart. This is essential for constructing self-management plan.
5. **FEF_{25-75} (Forced expiratory flow in 25 to 75 percentile):** It is the graphical measurement of average expiratory flow in between 25 to 75% of the expiration during FVC maneuver. This measurement denotes airflow condition in smaller airways of <2 mm of diameter, which are devoid of cartilages. It is especially important in smokers (with COPD and emphysema) and in children who cannot produce satisfactory FEV_1.

In spirometric tracings, three values of the above parameters are shown:

1. *Predicted values:* These are the expected normal values of a person with regard to sex, age, weight and height.
2. *Measured values:* These are the actual values achieved by a person through expiratory and inspiratory maneuvers.
3. *Percentage of predicted value:* These are measured values expressed as a percentage of predicted values.

$$\text{That is} = \frac{\text{Measured value} \times 100}{\text{Predicted value}}$$

These values are used to differentiate and classify asthma, COPD and restrictive diseases.

Peak expiratory flow rate (PEFR): Measurement of PEFR on a regular basis at home with a portable peak flow meter is especially useful for patients over 5 years of age with moderate to severe persistent asthma. The patient is asked to take a full inspiration as far as possible, then blow out forcefully into the peak flow meter. PEFR is best used to monitor progress of the disease and its treatment.

Regular measurement of PEFR on waking, in afternoon and before bed demonstrates the wide diurnal variations in airflow limitations that characterize bronchial asthma. Daily calculation of diurnal variability of PEF provides a reasonable index of asthma stability and severity. Diurnal variability in peak flow is expressed by the following formula:

$$\text{Diurnal variability} = \frac{(\text{Highest PEF} - \text{Lowest PEF}) \times 100}{\text{Highest PEF}}$$

It should be noted that, PEF physiologically falls at late night or early morning. But this fall is normally <20% of personal best result. Fall of PEF >20% in early morning is known as "morning dipping of PEF". It is characteristic of uncontrolled asthma.

Spirometry indicates presence of airway abnormality, if recordings show
- FEV_1 – <80% of predicted value.
- FVC – <80% of predicted value.
- FEV_1/FVC ratio – <75%.

Obstructive disorder shows
- FEV_1 – reduced (<80% of predicted value).
- FVC – reduced.
- FEV_1/FVC ratio – reduced (<75%).

Restrictive disorder shows
- FEV_1 – reduced (<80% of predicted value, but in proportion to FVC).
- FVC – reduced (<80% of predicted value).
- FEV/FVC ratio – normal (>75%).

Differences between restrictive and obstructive airway disease

Points	Restrictive	Obstructive
1. Both FEV_1 and FVC	Proportionately reduced	FEV_1 is markedly reduced and FVC also reduced
2. Ratio between FEV_1 and FVC	Normal	Reduced
3. RV	Reduced or normal	Increased
4. TLC	Reduced	Increased
5. Ratio between RV and TLC	Normal or slightly increased	Markedly increased

We usually do spirometry for diagnostic and monitoring purposes. For these the following tests are performed:

1. Baseline spirometry

It means spirometric assessment when patient is asymptomatic or in his best condition. It is done without reversibility test to classify asthma into intermittent and persistent (mild, moderate or severe) varieties.

2. Reversibility test

Bronchodilator reversibility test can be used to differentiate between asthma and COPD. After bronchodilatation, both >12% and >200 mL increase in FEV_1, over pre-bronchodilator levels indicates positive reversibility test, suggesting diagnosis of bronchial asthma. Negative result indicates COPD (or severe persistent asthma).

3. Bronchoprovocation test

Fall of FEV_1 >20% after inhalation of methacholine or hypertonic saline is used for diagnosis of hyper-responsiveness of airways in susceptible patients with normal spirometry. Susceptible patients are: (i) Patient with cough-variant asthma, (ii) Mild intermittent asthma, (iii) Chronic bronchitis with hyper-responsive airways.

4. Exercise challenge test

Fall of FEV_1 vor PEFR >15% from baseline value after vigorous exercise (i.e. running or climbing stairs for 6 minutes) indicates "exercise-induced asthma". The fall starts at 5 to 10 minutes after stoppage of exercise and peaks at 20 to 30 minutes and then resolves automatically. It can be reversed quickly by using bronchodilator inhalers.

■ **SPIRO – 01**

Name   ....
Sex   F
Age   39 years
Height   150 cm
Weight   60 kg
Eth. corr. 100%

Best trial report

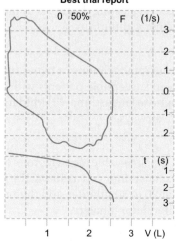

			Meas	Pred	%
Best-FVC	1		2.64	2.74	96
Best-FEV$_1$	1		1.94	2.35	83
		Repeatable FEV$_1$			
FVC	1		2.64	2.74	96
FEV$_1$	1		1.94	2.35	83
PEF	1/s		3.69	5.97	62
PIF	1/s		2.80		
FEV$_1$/FVC%	1/s		73.5	85.8	86
FEF 25-75	1/s		1.35	3.47	39
Vmax-25	1/s		3.11	5.46	57
Vmax-50	1/s		2.28	3.86	59
Vmax-75	1/s		0.33	1.71	19
FET 100%	s		2.98		

SPIRO – 02

Name	....
Sex	M
Age	35 years
Height	159 cm
Weight	46 kg
Eth. corr.	100%

Best trial report

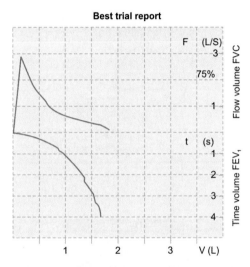

		Meas	Pred	%
Best-FVC	1	1.90	3.91	49
Best-FEV$_1$	1	1.16	3.33	35
Repeatable FEV$_1$				
FVC	1	1.90	3.91	49
FEV$_1$	1	1.11	3.33	33
PEF	1/s	2.97	8.41	35
FEV$_1$/FVC%	1/s	58.4	85.2	69
FEF 25-75	1/s	0.58	4.28	14
Vmax-25	1/s	1.38	7.20	19
Vmax-50	1/s	0.66	4.59	14
Vmax-75	1/s	0.31	1.90	16
FET 100%	s	4.00		

SPIRO – 03

Name   ....
Sex   F
Age   39 years
Height   150 cm
Weight   60 kg
Eth. corr.   100%

Best trial report

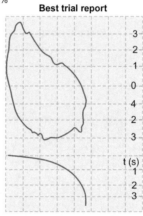

		Meas	Pred	%
Best-FVC	1	2.35	2.74	86
Best-FEV$_1$	1	1.87	2.35	80
Repeatable FVC and FEV$_1$				
FVC	1	2.35	2.74	86
FEV$_1$	1	1.95	2.35	79
PEF	1/s	3.51	5.97	60
PIF	1/s	3.13		
FEV$_1$/FVC%		78.7	85.8	92
FEF 25-75	1/s	1.65	3.47	48
Vmax-25	1/s	3.91	5.46	55
Vmax-50	1/s	2.7	3.86	54
Vmax-75	1/s	0.99	1.71	57
FET 100%	s	3.50		

SPIRO – 04

Name   ....
Sex   F
Age   60 years
Height   150 cm
Weight   35 kg
Eth. corr.   100%

Best trial report

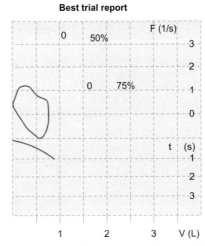

		Meas	Pred	%
Best-FVC	1	0.79	2.19	36
Best-FEV$_1$	1	0.79	1.82	43
Repeatable FVC and FEV$_1$				
FVC	1	0.79	2.19	36
FEV$_1$	1	0.79	1.82	43
PEF	1/s	1.25	5.34	23
PIF	1/s	0.92		
FEV$_1$/FVC%	1/s	100.0	83.1	120
FEF 25-75	1/s	0.89	2.75	32
Vmax-25	1/s	1.20	4.93	24
Vmax-50	1/s	1.06	3.33	32
Vmax-75	1/s	0.62	1.18	53
FET 100%	s	0.90		

SPIRO – 05

Name   ....
Sex   M
Age   25 years
Height   167 cm
Weight   64 kg
Eth. corr. 100%

Best trial report

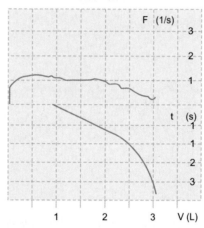

		Meas	Pred	%
Best-FVC	1	3.22	4.63	70
Best-FEV$_1$	1	1.78	3.97	45
Repeatable FVC				
FVC	1	3.10	4.63	67
FEV$_1$	1	1.28	3.97	45
PEF	1/s	1.16	9.33	12
FEV$_1$/FVC%	1/s	57.4	85.7	67
FEF 25-75	1/s	0.89	4.87	18
Vmax-25	1/s	1.97	7.92	14
Vmax-50	1/s	0.93	5.20	18
Vmax-75	1/s	0.88	2.37	29
FET 100%	s	4.78		

SPIRO – 06

Name   ....
Sex   M
Age   25 years
Height   170 cm
Weight   60 kg
Eth. corr.   100%

Best trial report

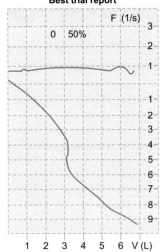

		Meas	Pred	%
Best-FVC	1	6.98	4.20	45
Best-FEV$_1$	1	1.35	4.10	45
FVC	1	6.98	4.80	45
FEV$_1$	1	1.34	4.10	33
PEF	1/s	1.76	9.51	19
FEV$_1$/FVC%	1/s	19.2	85.4	22
FEF 25-75	1/s	0.54	4.92	11
Vmax-25	1/s	0.83	8.09	10
Vmax-50	1/s	0.71	5.32	13
Vmax-75	1/s	1.02	2.44	42
FET 100%	s	9.28		

SPIRO – 07

Name   ....
Sex   F
Age   72 years
Height   153 cm
Weight   61 kg
Eth. corr. 100%

Best trial report

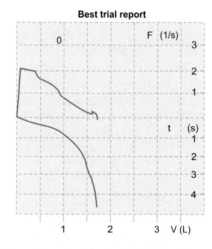

		Meas	Pred	%
Best-FVC	1	1.18	2.01	90
Best-FEV$_1$	1	1.18	1.64	72
Repeatable FEV$_1$				
FVC	1	1.80	2.01	90
FEV$_1$	1	1.18	1.64	72
PEF	1/s	2.13	5.15	41
FEV$_1$/FVC%	1/s	65.6	81.6	80
FEF 25-75	1/s	0.77	2.38	32
Vmax-25	1/s	1.70	4.73	36
Vmax-50	1/s	0.94	3.11	30
Vmax-75	1/s	0.30	0.91	33
FET 100%	s	4.98		

SPIRO – 08

Name	....
Sex	M
Age	48 years
Height	167 cm
Weight	53 kg
Eth. corr.	100%

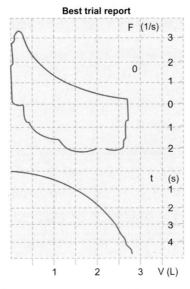

Best trial report

		Meas	Pred	%
Best-FVC	1	2.80	4.03	69
Best-FEV$_1$	1	1.49	3.30	45
FVC	1	2.80	4.03	69
FEV$_1$	1	1.49	3.30	45
PEF	1/s	1.37	8.34	40
PEF	1/s	2.16		
FEV$_1$/FVC%	1/s	53.2	81.9	65
FEF 25-75	1/s	0.76	3.88	20
Vmax-25	1/s	1.77	7.26	24
Vmax-50	1/s	0.83	4.49	18
Vmax-75	1/s	0.42	1.77	24
FET 100%	s	4.72		

SPIRO – 09

Name	....
Sex	M
Age	70 years
Height	157 cm
Weight	42 kg
Eth. corr.	100%

Best trial report

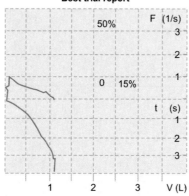

		Meas	Pred	%
Best-FVC	L	1.11	2.88	39
Best-FEV$_1$	L	0.55	2.23	25
....				
FVC	L	1.11	2.88	39
FEV$_1$	L	0.55	2.23	25
PEF	L/s	0.88	6.78	13
PIF	L/s	0.29		
FEV$_1$/FVC%	L/s	49.5	77.4	64
FEF 25-75	L/s	0.37	2.74	14
Vmax-25	L/s	0.55	6.07	9
Vmax-50	L/s	0.36	3.43	10
Vmax-75	L/s	0.28	0.94	30
FET 100%	L/s	3.84		

SPIRO – 10

Name   ....
Sex   F
Age   22 years
Height   150 cm
Weight   48 kg
Eth. corr.   100%

Best trial report

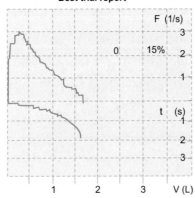

		Meas	Pred	%
Best-FVC	L	1.66	3.18	52
Best-FEV$_1$	L	1.39	2.77	50
FVC	L	1.66	3.18	52
FEV$_1$	L	1.39	2.77	50
PEF	L/s	2.91	6.48	45
PIF	L/s	0.40		
FEV$_1$/FVC%	L/s	83.7	87.1	96
FEF 25-75	L/s	1.34	4.4	33
Vmax-25	L/s	2.61	5.88	45
Vmax-50	L/s	1.57	4.28	37
Vmax-75	L/s	0.67	2.13	31
FET 100%	L/s	1.90		

SPIRO – 11

Name   ....
Sex   M
Age   25 years
Height   168 cm
Weight   80 kg
Eth. corr.   100%

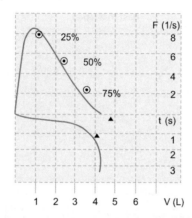

		Meas	Pred	%
Best-FVC	L	4.15	4.69	88
Best-FEV$_1$	L	3.73	4.01	93
....				
FVC	L	4.15	4.69	88
FEV$_1$	L	3.70	4.01	92
PEF	1/s	8.44	9.39	90
FEV$_1$/FVC%	1/s	89.2	85.5	104
FEF$_{25-75}$	1/s	4.81	4.88	99

SPIRO – 12

Name   ....
Sex   M
Age   40 years
Weight   66 kg

		Pred	PRE	% (Pre/perd)
VC MAX	[L]	4.42	4.01	90.8
FVC	[L]	4.24	3.80	89.6
FEV$_1$	[L]	3.53	3.69	104.5
FEV$_1$ % VC MAX	[96]	80.01	92.04	115.0
FEV$_1$ % FVC	[%]		97.18	
FEF 25	[L/s]	7.49	6.48	86.5
FEF 50	[L/s]	4.74	5.62	118.7
FEF 75	[L/s]	1.98	2.63	132.7
FEV6	[L]		3.80	
PIF	[L/s]		4.76	
FE T	[s]		1.19	
VC IN	[L]	4.42	4.01	90.8
FEV$_1$ % FVC	[%]		97.18	

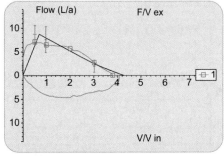

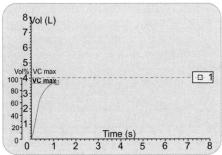

SPIRO – 13

Name   ....
Age   40 years
Sex   Male
Weight   74 kg

		Pred	Pre	% (Pre/Pred)
VC MAX	[L]	4.36	3.47	79.7
FVC	[L]	4.18	3.18	76.1
FEV$_1$	[L]	3.49	2.16	61.9
FEV$_1$ % VC MAX	[%]	80.01	62.25	77.8
FEV$_1$ % FVC	[%]		67.84	
FEF 25	[L/s]	7.43	2.52	33.8
FEF 50	[L/s]	4.70	1.74	36.9
FEF 75	[L/s]	1.95	0.25	12.9
FEV$_6$	[L]		3.01	
PIF	[L/s]		3.97	
FET	[s]		12.76	
VC IN	[L]	4.36	3.47	79.7
FEV$_1$ % FVC	[%]		67.84	

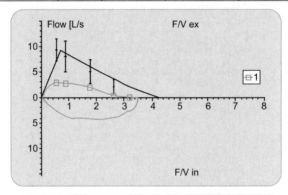

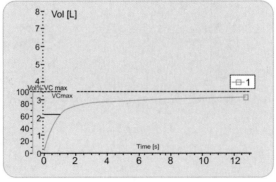

SPIRO – 14

Name   ....
Age   40 years
Sex   Female
Weight 50 kg

		Pred	Pre	% (PRE/Pred)
VC MAX	[L]	2.86	2.67	93.6
FVC	[L]	2.89	2.65	91.7
FEV₁	[L]	2.48	1.77	71.2
FEV₁ % VC MAX	[%]	81.50	66.13	81.1
FEV₁ % FVC[$]	[%]		66.70	
FEF 25	[L/s]	5.56	2.56	46.0
FEF 50	[L/s]	3.93	1.44	36.7
FEF 75	[L/s]	1.73	0.34	19.7
FEV₁	[L]		2.49	
PIF	[L/s]		2.57	
FET	[s]		9.79	
VC IN	[L]	2.86	2.67	93.6
FEV₁ % FVC	[%]		66.70	

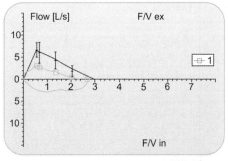

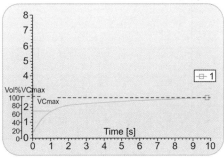

SPIRO – 15

Name   ....
Age   25 years
Sex   Female
Weight 40 kg

		Pred	PRE	% (PRE/Pred)
VC MAX	[L]	3.11	2.50	80.3
FVC	[L]	3.15	2.38	75.6
FEV$_1$	[L]	2.74	1.96	71.6
FEV, % VC MAX	[%]	84.35	78.57	93.1
FEV, % FVC	[%]		82.36	
FEF 25	[L/S]	5.84	2.93	50.2
FEF 50	[L/s]	4.23	2.10	49.6
FEF 75	[L/s]	2.07	0.96	46.3
FEV$_6$	[L]		2.38	
PIF	[L/s]		2.49	
PE T	[s]		2.88	
VC IN	[L]	3.11	2.50	80.3
FEV$_1$ % FVC	[%]		82.36	

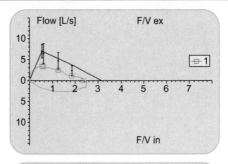

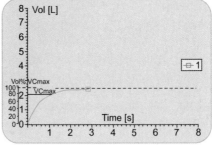

SPIRO – 16

Name ....
Age 60 years
Sex Female
Weight 48 kg

		Pred	PRE	% (PRE/Pred)
VC MAX	[L]	3.25	1.19	36.7
FVC	[L]	3.14	0.94	29.9
FEV1	[L]	2.52	0.59	23.4
FEV$_1$ % VC Max	[%]	76.41	49.58	64.9
FEV$_1$ % FVC	[%]		62.94	
FEF 25	[L/s]	6.36	0.62	9.7
FEF 50	[L/s]	3.74	0.23	6.3
FEF 75	[L/s]	1.20	0.14	11.7
FEV6	[L]		0.94	
PIF	[L/s]		1.02	
FE T	[s]		4.00	
VC IN	[L]	3.25	1.19	36.7
FEV1 % FVC	[%]		62.94	

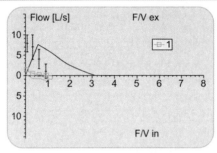

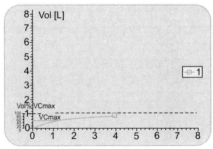

SPIRO – 17

Name ....
Age 42 years
Sex Male
Weight 69 kg

		Pred	PRE	% (PRE/Pred)
FVC	[L]	4.24	3.17	74.8
FEV1	[L]	3.52	2.64	75.2
FEV1/FVC	[%]		83.33	
PEF	[L/s]	8.66	5.31	61.3
FEF 25	[L/s]	7.48	5.31	70.9
FEF 50	[L/s]	4.72	3.59	76.1
FEF 75	[L/s]	1.95	0.88	45.2
MMEF 75125	[LS]	4.15	2.50	60.2

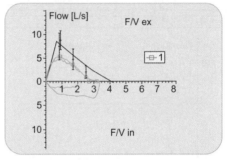

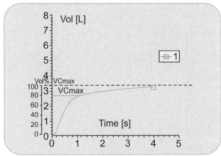

SPIRO – 18

Name   ....
Age   44 years
Sex   Male
Weight   65 kg

		Pred	PRE	% (PRE/Pred)
FVC	[L]	4.25	3.18	79.0
FEV$_1$	[L]	3.50	3.13	89.5
FEV$_1$ % FVC	[%]		98.44	
PEF	[L/s]	8.63	4.07	47.1
FEF 25	[L/s]	7.48	4.07	54.4
FEF 50	[L/s]	4.69	3.03	64.5
FEF 75	[L/s]	1.93	0.66	34.3
MMEF 75/25	[LS]	4.09	2.69	65.9

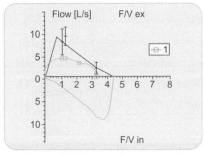

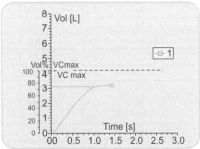

SPIRO – 19

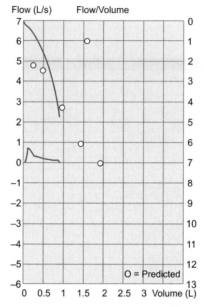

Comment

Par (BTPS)	Pred	Best	PRE	% Pred
FVC	1.90	0.93	0.93	49.0
FEV$_1$	1.59	0.41	0.38	23.9
FEV$_1$/FVC	84.0	53.2	40.9	48.7
PEF	4.80	0.72	0.71	14.8
PEF25	4.54	0.42	0.32	7.0
PEF50	2.74	0.26	0.21	7.7
FEF75	0.96	0.19	0.14	14.5
FEF25-75	2.09	0.27	0.20	9.6
FET	4.72	4.72		
ELA	59			

SPIRO – 20

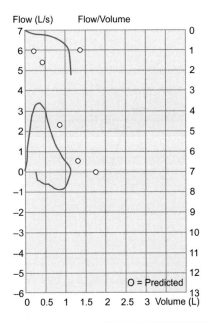

Par (BTPS)	Pred	Best	PRE	% Pred
FVC	1.77	1.28	1.21	68.3
FEV$_1$	1.37	1.22	1.12	81.8
FEV$_1$%	78.7	95.3	92.6	117.7
PEF	5.92	3.75	3.41	57.6
FEF25	5.36	3.54	3.37	62.8
FEF50	2.28	2.87	2.07	90.8
FEF75	0.57	0.97	0.71	123.6
FEF25-75	1.70	2.23	1.66	97.8
FET		2.20	2.20	
FIVC	1.77	1.25	0.91	51.4
FIV$_1$	1.37	1.25	0.78	57.0
FIV$_1$%	78.7	100.0	85.7	108.9
PIF	5.92	1.88	0.92	15.5
ELA	76		85	111.8

SPIRO – 21

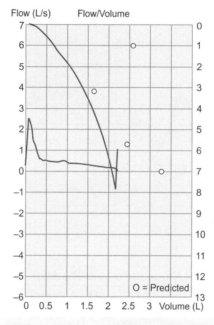

Par (BTPS)	Pred	Best	PRE	% Pred
FVC	3.27	2.27	2.27	69.3
FEV₁	2.59	0.66	0.66	25.5
FEV₁/FVC%	79.4	29.1	29.1	36.6
PEF	7.85	2.57	2.57	32.7
FEF25	7.19	0.41	0.41	5.7
FEF50	3.77	0.31	0.31	8.2
FEF75	1.29	0.17	0.17	13.1
FEF25-75	2.99	0.31	0.31	10.4
FET		6.00	6.00	
ELA	69			

SPIRO – 22

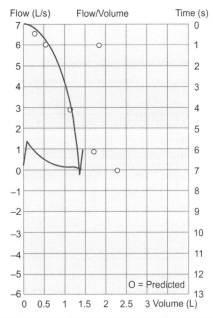

Par (BTPS)	Pred	Best	PRE	% Pred
FVC	2.28	1.48	1.48	65.0
FEV$_1$	1.82	0.80	0.64	35.1
FEV$_1$%	79.9	70.8	43.2	54.1
PEF	6.58	2.32	1.65	25.1
FEF25	6.01	1.27	0.64	10.6
FEF50	2.89	0.74	0.24	8.3
FEF75	0.92	0.38	0.10	10.9
FEF25-75	2.27	0.61	0.22	9.7
FET	6.00	6.00		
ELA		65		

SPIRO - 23(A)

Name   ....
Age   44 years
Sex   Male
Weight   65 kg

See next spirometry for reversibility

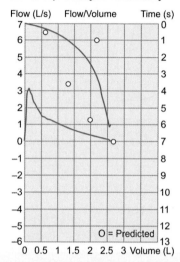

Par (BTPS)	Pred	Best	PRE	% Pred
FVC	2.67	2.73	2.66	99.8
FEV₁	2.20	1.34	1.32	59.9
FEV₁%	81.4	49.6	49.6	60.9
PEF	7.11	3.21	3.15	44.3
FEF25	6.54	1.34	1.31	20.0
FEF50	3.44	0.77	0.77	22.4
FEF75	1.27	0.29	0.29	22.9
FEF25-75	2.82	0.68	0.68	24.2
FET		6.00	6.00	
FIVC	2.67	1.54	1.54	57.8
FIV₁	2.20	1.54	1.54	69.9
FIV₁%	81.4	100.0	100.0	122.8
ELA	50		84	168.0

SPIRO - 23(B)

Reversibility test of same patient

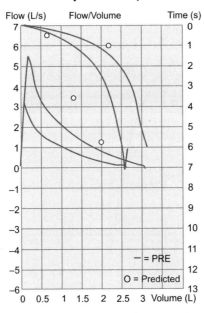

Par (BTPS)	Pred	Best	%PRE	Pred	Post	% Pred	% Pre
FVC	2.67	2.73	2.73	102.4	3.20	120.1	+17.2
FEV$_1$	2.20	1.34	1.34	60.8	1.93	87.6	+44.4
FEV$_1$%	81.4	49.6	49.1	60.3	60.3	74.0	+22.8
PEF	7.11	3.21	3.21	45.2	5.50	77.4	+71.3
FEF25	6.54	1.34	1.34	20.5	2.31	35.3	+72.4
FEF50	3.44	0.77	0.66	19.2	1.26	36.7	+90.9
FEF75	1.27	0.29	0.25	19.8	0.41	32.4	+64.0
FEF25-75	2.82	0.68	0.63	22.4	1.03	36.6	+63.5
FET		6.00	6.00		6.00		
FIVC	2.67	1.54			1.91	71.7	
FIV$_1$	2.20	1.54			1.91	86.7	
ELA	50		83	166.0			

SPIRO - 24(A)

Name   ....
Age   36 years
Sex   Male
Weight   105 kg

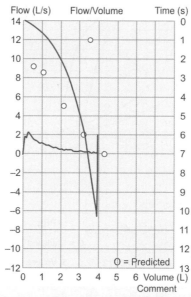

Par (BTPS)	Pred	Best	% PRE	% Pred
FVC	4.28	4.01	4.01	93.8
FEV$_1$	3.54	1.32	1.32	37.3
FEV$_1$%	82.9	32.9	32.9	39.7
PEF	9.20	2.25	2.25	24.5
FEF25	8.52	1.04	1.04	12.2
FEF50	5.11	0.53	0.53	10.4
FEF25	2.11	0.27	0.27	12.8
FEF25-75	4.31	0.48	0.48	11.1
FET	6.00	6.00		
ELA	36			

SPIRO - 24(B)

Name ....
Age   36 years
Sex   Male
Weight   105 kg

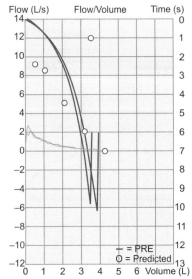

Par (BTPS)	Pred	Best	Pre	% Pred	Post	% Pred	% Pre
FVC	4.28	4.01	4.01	93.8	3.68	86.1	−8.2
FEV₁	3.54	1.32	1.32	37.3	1.32	37.3	
FEV₁%	82.9	32.9	32.9	39.7	35.9	43.3	+9.1
PEF	9.20	2.25	2.25	24.5	2.70	29.4	+20.0
FEF25	8.52	1.04	1.04	12.2	1.10	12.9	+5.8
FEF50	5.11	0.53	0.53	10.4	0.49	9.6	−7.5
FEF25	2.11	0.27	0.27	12.8	0.23	10.9	−14.8
FEF25-75	4.31	0.48	0.48	11.1	0.47	10.9	−2.1
FET		6.00	6.00		6.00		
ELA	36						

SPIRO – 25

Name	....
Sex	M
Age	55 years
Height	150 cm
Weight	65 kg
Eth. corr.	100%

Name	....
Quantity	400
Sex	M
Age	55 years
Height	169 cm
Weight	65 kg
Eth. corr.	100%

Before bronchodilator

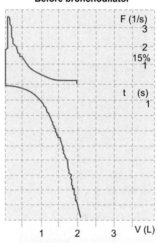

After bronchodilator

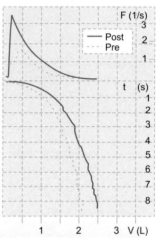

		Meas	Pred	%
Best-FVC	1	2.00	3.96	51
Best-FEV$_1$	1	1.01	3.18	32
Repeatable FVC and FEV$_1$				
....				
FVC	1	2.00	3.96	51
FEV$_1$	1	0.94	3.18	30
PEF	1/s	3.50	8.16	43
FEV$_1$/FVC%	1/s	47.0	80.3	59
FEF 25-75	1/s	0.28	3.61	8
Vmax-25	1/s	1.18	7.16	16
Vmax-50	1/s	0.37	4.35	9
Vmax-75	1/s	0.16	1.64	10
FET 100%	s	8.64		

		Meas	Pred	%
Best-FVC	1	2.41	2.00	121
Best-FEV$_1$	1	1.23	1.01	122
....				
FVC	1	2.41	2.00	121
FEV$_1$	1	1.23	1.01	122
PEF	1/s	3.74	1.69	221
FEV$_1$/FVC%	1/s	51.0	51.5	101
FEF25-75	1/s	0.64	0.33	194
Vmax-25	1/s	2.01	1.42	142
Vmax-50	1/s	0.79	0.47	168
Vmax-75	1/s	0.30	0.15	200
FET 100%	s			

SPIRO - 26(A)

Name ....
Age   65 years
Sex   Male
Weight 58 kg

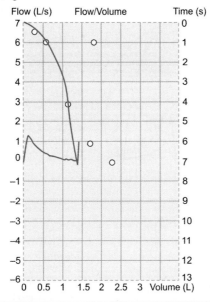

Par (BTPS)	Pred	Best	% PRE	% Pred
FVC	2.28	1.48	1.48	65.0
FEV$_1$	1.28	0.80	0.64	35.1
FEV$_1$%	79.9	70.8	43.2	54.1
PEF	6.58	2.32	1.65	25.1
FEF25	6.01	1.27	0.64	10.6
FEF50	2.89	0.74	0.24	8.3
FEF75	0.92	0.38	0.10	10.9
FEF25-75	2.27	0.61	0.22	9.7
FET		6.00	6.00	
ELA	65			

SPIRO - 26(B)

Name ....
Age 65 years
Sex Male
Weight 58 kg

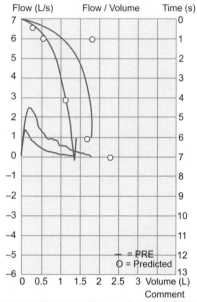

Par (BTPS)	Pred	Best	PRE	% Pred	POST	% Pred	% PRE
FVC	2.28	1.48	1.48	65.0	1.90	83.5	+28.4
FEV$_1$	1.28	0.80	0.64	35.1	1.12	61.5	+75.0
FEV$_1$%	79.9	70.8	43.2	54.1	58.9	73.8	+36.3
PEF	6.58	2.32	1.65	25.1	2.51	38.1	+52.1
FEF25	6.01	1.27	0.64	10.6	1.31	21.8	+104.7
FEF50	2.89	0.74	0.24	8.3	0.57	19.7	+137.5
FEF75	0.92	0.38	0.10	10.9	0.24	26.1	+140.0
FEF25-75	2.27	0.61	0.24	9.7	0.57	25.1	+159.1
FET		6.00	6.00		6.00		
ELA	65						

Chapter
5

Pictures of Multiple Diseases

(For answers: See page 467-486)

"You see but you do not observe."

— Sir Arthur Conan Doyle

"I search after truth, by which man never yet was harmed."

— Galen

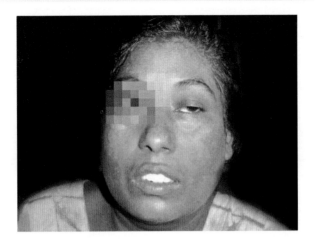

PICTURE - 01

a. What is the likely diagnosis?
b. Suggest one alternative diagnosis.
c. Mention one physical finding in this case.

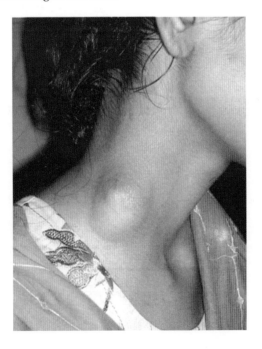

PICTURE - 02

a. What is the finding?
b. What is the diagnosis?
c. How to confirm the diagnosis?

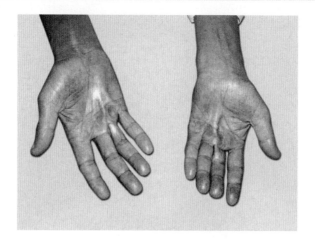

PICTURE - 03

a. Mention two findings.
b. Suggest the likely diagnosis.

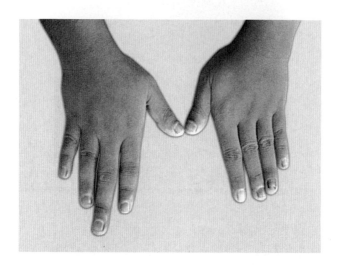

PICTURE - 04

a. What is the finding?
b. What is the diagnosis?

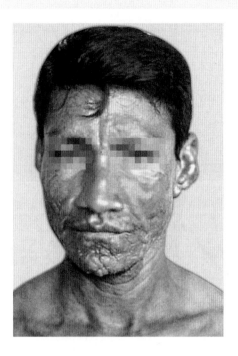

PICTURE - 05

a. What is the appearance?
b. What is the diagnosis?
c. Mention one alternative diagnosis.

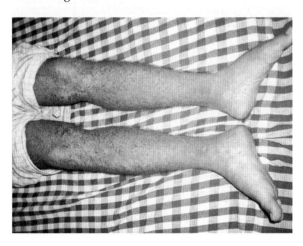

PICTURE - 06

a. This patient is suffering from fever for 5 days. What is the finding?
b. What is the likely diagnosis?

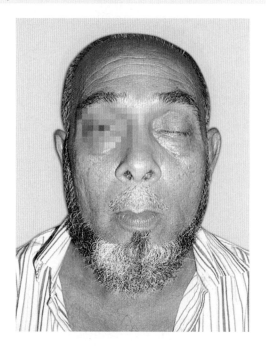

PICTURE - 07

a. This patient is complaining of severe weakness for few months. Mention two findings.
b. What is the most likely diagnosis?

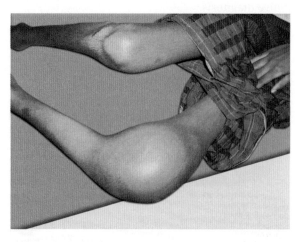

PICTURE - 08

a. This patient of 16 years presented with gradual painful hard swelling in left knee with weight loss. What is the diagnosis?
b. Mention one investigation to confirm the diagnosis.

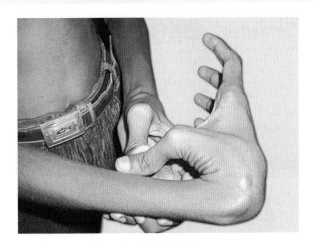

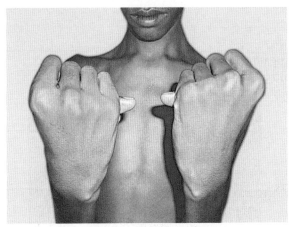

PICTURES - 09 AND 10

a. What is shown in the picture "9"?
b. What is the sign in the picture "10"?
c. What is the diagnosis?

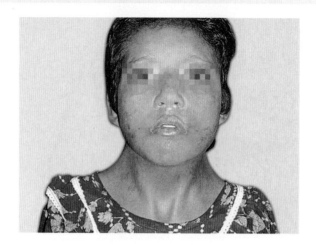

PICTURE - 11

  a. What is the diagnosis?
  b. Mention one investigation to confirm the diagnosis.
  c. What is the common presentation in this case?

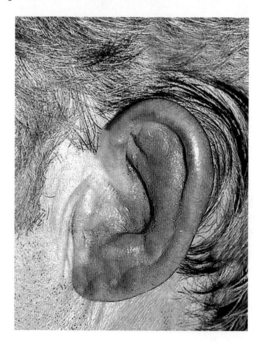

PICTURE - 12

  a. This patient presented with recurrent attack of this symptom. What is the diagnosis?
  b. How to confirm the diagnosis?

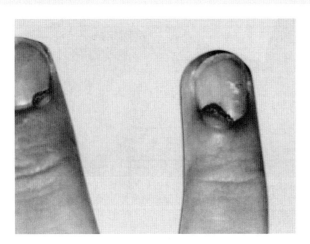

PICTURE - 13

a. What is the lesion?
b. What is the diagnosis?
c. Write one common presentation.

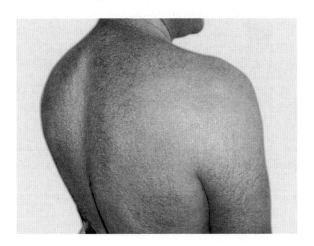

PICTURE - 14

a. What is the finding in this asymptomatic patient?
b. What history do you like to take in this patient?

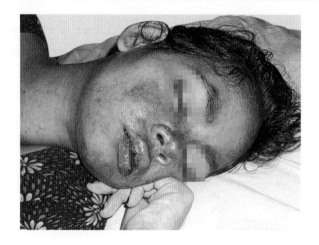

PICTURE - 15

Suggest three differential diagnoses.

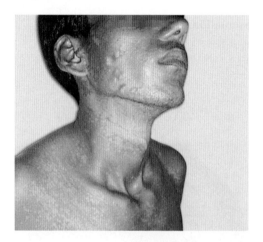

PICTURE - 16

This patient was suffering from fever 1 year back. What is the diagnosis?

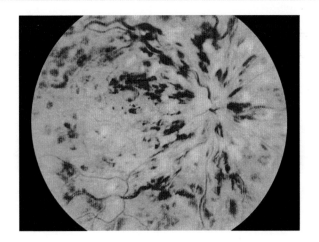

PICTURE - 17

a. What is the diagnosis?
b. Mention two common causes.

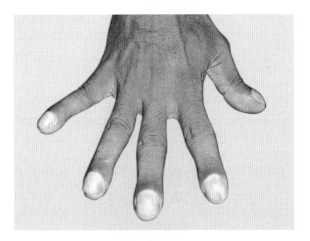

PICTURE - 18

a. What is the appearance of nails?
b. The patient has bilateral coarse end inspiratory crepitations. What is the likely cause?

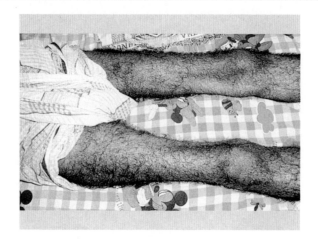

PICTURE - 19

a. What is the finding?
b. What is the diagnosis?
c. Patient is 20 years old. What may be the likely cause?

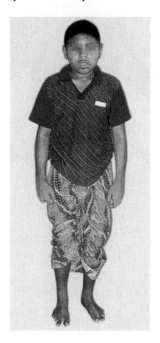

PICTURE - 20

a. This patient presented with recurrent seizure. His serum calcium is low. What is the diagnosis?
b. Mention two physical findings.

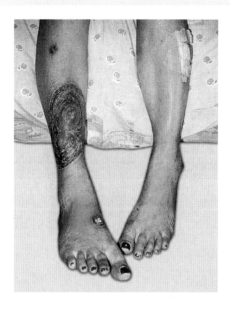

PICTURE - 21

What is the diagnosis?

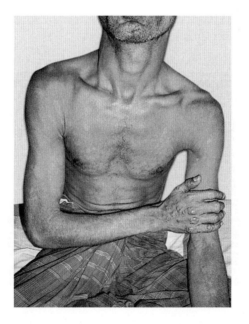

PICTURE - 22

a. What are the findings?
b. What is the diagnosis?
c. What physical examination do you want to see?

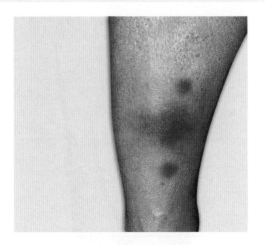

PICTURE - 23

a. This patient presents with polyarthritis and cough. What is the finding?
b. Mention two differential diagnoses.

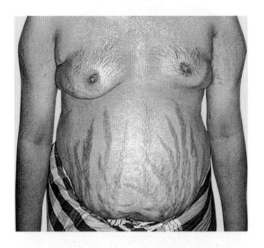

PICTURE - 24

a. Mention two findings.
b. What is the commonest cause of this disease?

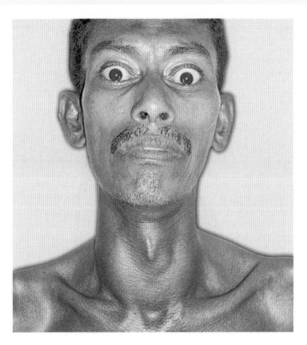

PICTURE - 25

a. Mention two findings in this patient.
b. What is the diagnosis?
c. Mention one physical finding to be seen for your diagnosis.

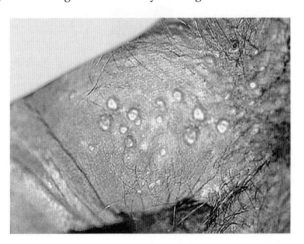

PICTURE - 26

a. What is the diagnosis?
b. Mention one underlying disease, which is associated with it.
c. How to treat?

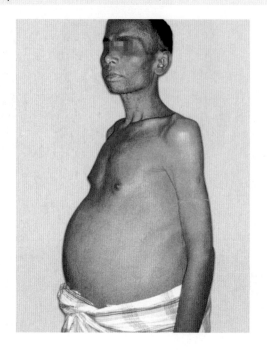

PICTURE - 27

a. What four findings can you see in this patient?
b. What is the diagnosis?

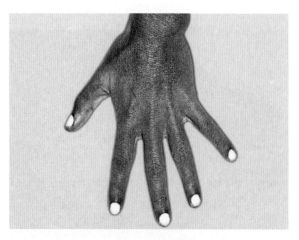

PICTURE - 28

a. What is the finding?
b. What does it indicate?

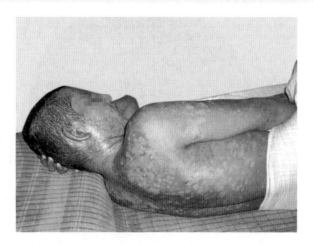

PICTURE - 29

a. Patient is highly toxic. What is the diagnosis?

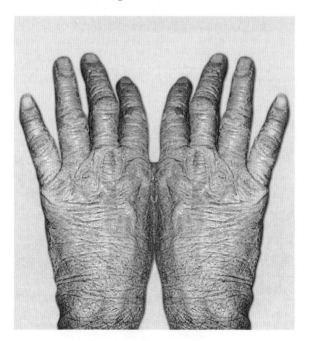

PICTURE - 30

a. What is the diagnosis?
b. Suggest one underlying cause.

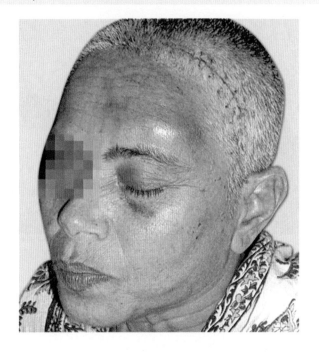

PICTURE - 31

a. What are the findings?
b. What is the diagnosis?
c. What is the underlying cause?

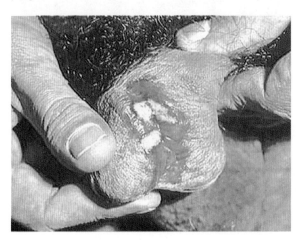

PICTURE - 32

a. What is the diagnosis?
b. What is the differential diagnosis?

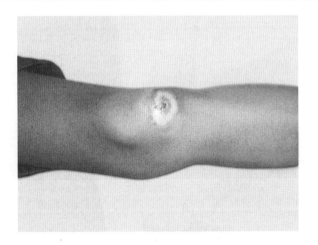

PICTURE - 33

a. What is the diagnosis of this sheep farmer?
b. What is the causative organism?

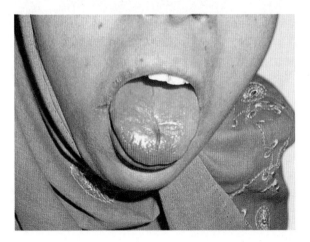

PICTURE - 34

a. What are the findings?
b. What is the cause?

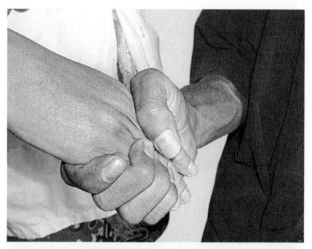

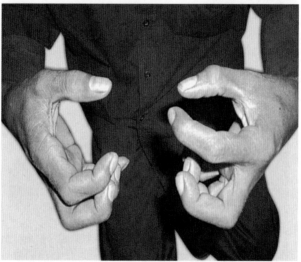

▌PICTURES - 35 AND 36

a. What sign is shown here?
b. What is the diagnosis?

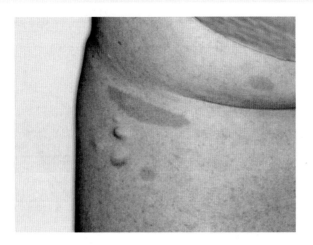

PICTURE - 37

a. What are the findings?
b. What is the diagnosis?

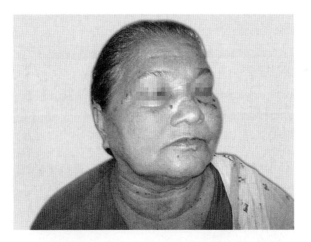

PICTURE - 38

a. What are the findings?
b. Mention two differential diagnoses.

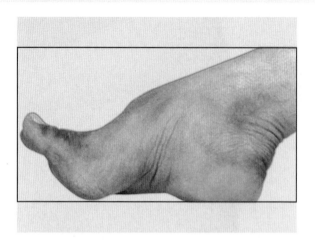

PICTURE - 39

a. What is the finding?
b. What is the common cause?

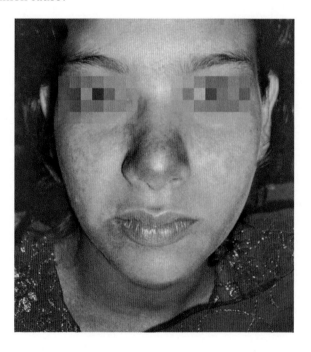

PICTURE - 40

a. What is the finding?
b. What is the diagnosis?

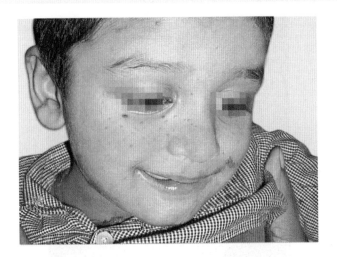

PICTURE - 41

a. This patient presented with epilepsy. What is the finding?
b. What is the diagnosis?
c. Mention two other physical findings.

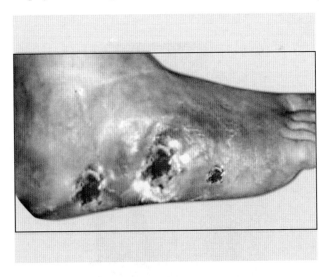

PICTURE - 42

a. What are the findings?
b. Mention one single investigation.
c. What is the likely diagnosis?

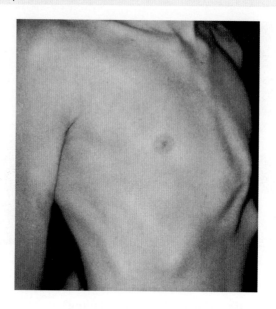

PICTURE - 43

a. What is the finding?
b. What are the causes?

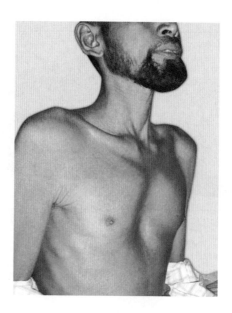

PICTURE - 44

a. What is the finding?
b. What are the causes?

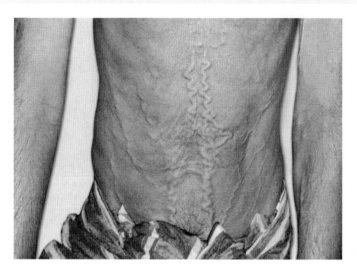

PICTURE - 45

a. Mention one physical finding to be seen.
b. Mention two differential diagnosis in this case.

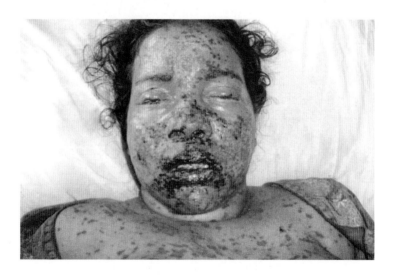

PICTURE - 46

a. What is the diagnosis?
b. Mention the name of three drugs responsible for this.

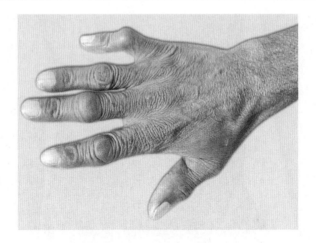

PICTURE - 47

a. What is the finding?
b. What is the diagnosis?

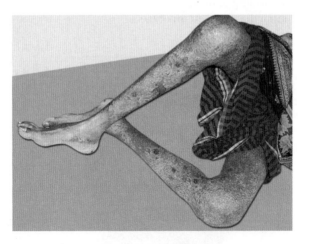

PICTURE - 48

a. What is the finding?
b. What is the diagnosis?

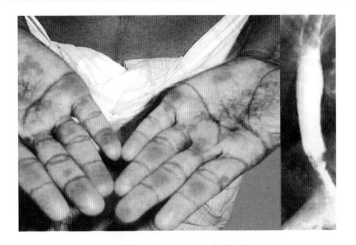

PICTURE - 49

a. What are the findings of hands and X-ray of same patient?
b. What is the diagnosis?

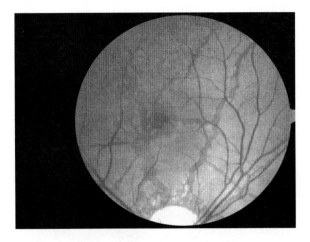

PICTURE - 50

a. What is the finding?
b. What are the causes?

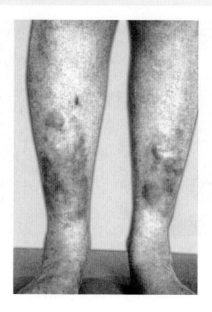

▊ PICTURE - 51

a. What is the finding?
b. What is the diagnosis?

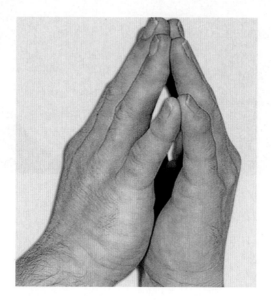

▊ PICTURE - 52

a. This patient is diabetic. What is the likely diagnosis?
b. What is the cause?

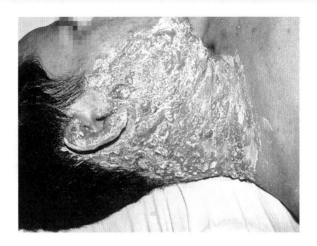

PICTURE - 53

a. What is the likely diagnosis?
b. Mention four complications.

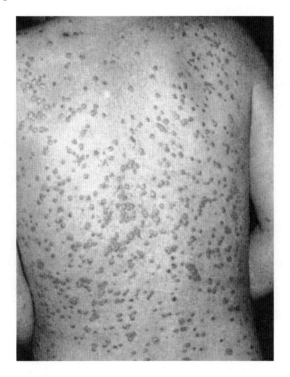

PICTURE - 54

a. What is the diagnosis?

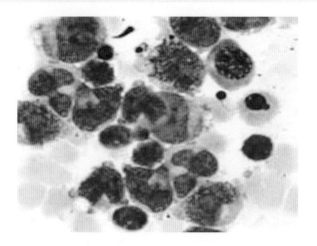

PICTURE - 55

a. This patient presents with severe anemia, multiple purpuric spots and fever. His prothrombin time and APTT are prolonged. What is the diagnosis with this film?
b. What is the likely cause of his blood picture?

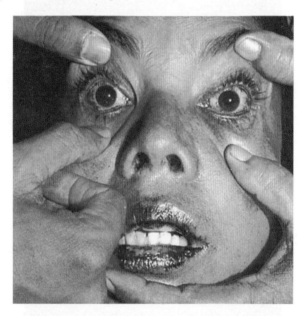

PICTURE - 56

a. This patient also has genital ulcer. What is the likely diagnosis?

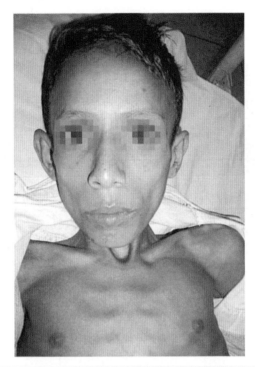

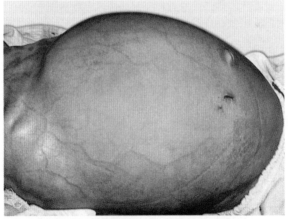

PICTURES - 57 AND 58

a. This young patient presents with rapid development of upper abdominal pain, tender hepatomegaly and huge ascites. Six months back, there is history of DVT. What is your diagnosis?
b. Mention two investigations.

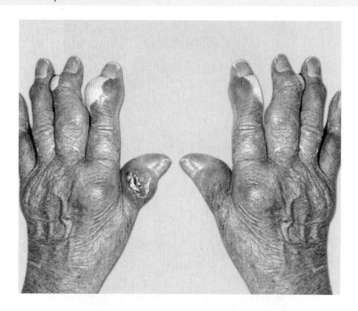

PICTURE - 59

a. What is the diagnosis?
b. How to confirm the diagnosis?

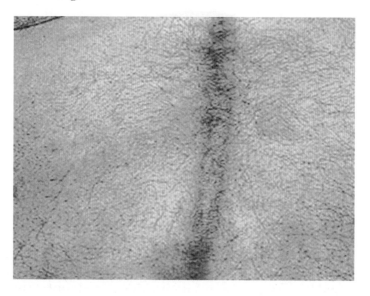

PICTURE - 60

a. This patient had abdominal surgery few weeks back. What is the finding?
b. What is the diagnosis?

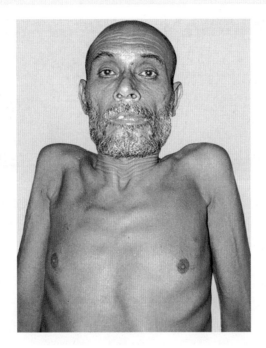

PICTURE - 61

a. What are the findings?
b. The patient presented with pale stool with itching. What is the most likely cause?
c. Suggest one investigation.

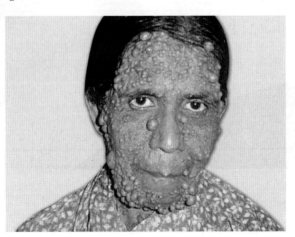

PICTURE - 62

a. What is the diagnosis?
b. Mention one dangerous complication.

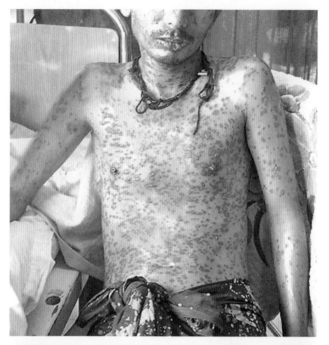

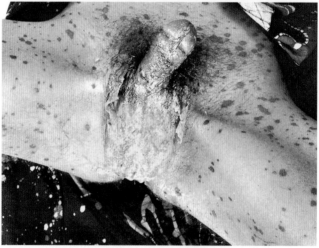

PICTURES - 63 AND 64

a. This patient was suffering from epilepsy. This has developed following antiepileptic drug. What is the diagnosis?
b. What is the cause?

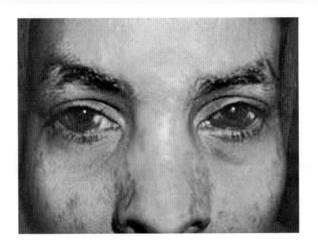

PICTURE - 65

a. This patient is suffering from high-grade fever for 5 days. What is the diagnosis?
b. Mention one single investigation to be done immediately.

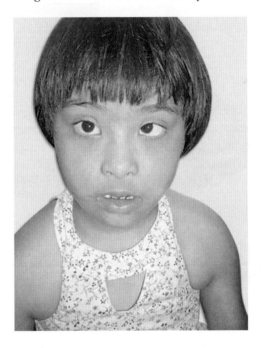

PICTURE - 66

a. What is the diagnosis?
b. What are the causes?

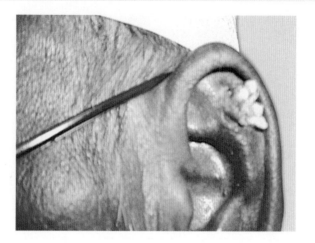

PICTURE - 67

a. What is the diagnosis?

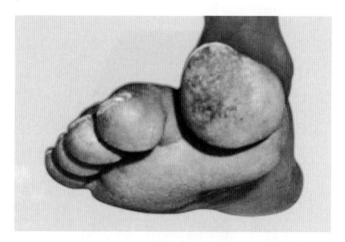

PICTURE - 68

a. What single history would you ask to this young patient?
b. What is the diagnosis?

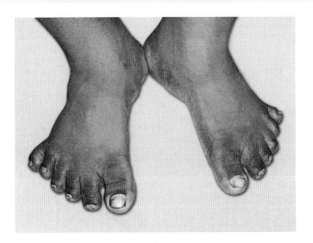

PICTURE - 69

a. What is the finding?
b. What is the underlying diagnosis?

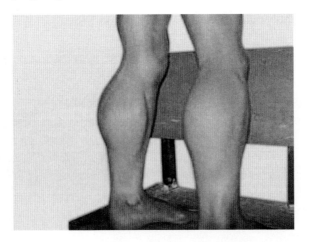

PICTURE - 70

a. What is the finding in this 8 years old boy?
b. Mention one typical physical finding.
c. What is the diagnosis?

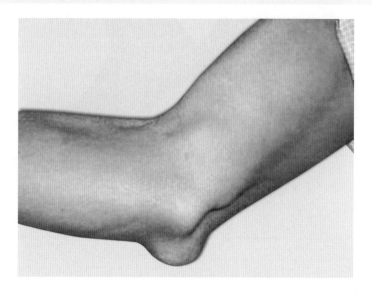

PICTURE - 71

Mention three differential diagnoses.

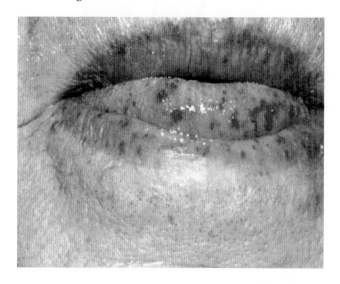

PICTURE - 72

a. What is the diagnosis?
b. Mention one common presentation.

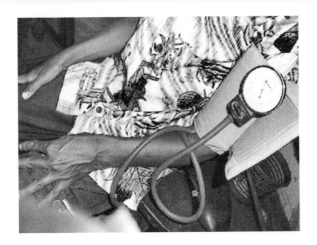

PICTURE - 73

a. What is shown here?
b. What sign is this?
c. What is the underlying pathology?

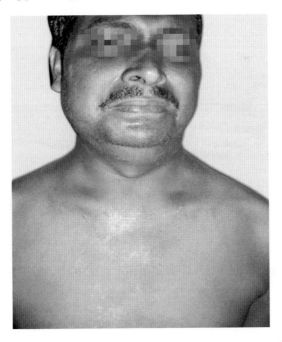

PICTURE - 74

a. What is the finding?
b. What is the diagnosis?

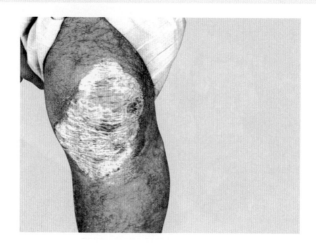

PICTURE - 75

What is the diagnosis?

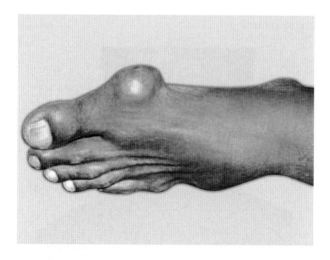

PICTURE - 76

a. This patient has been suffering from long-standing arthritis. What is the diagnosis?
b. What is this sign?

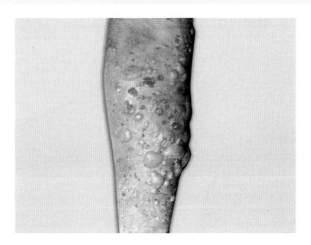

PICTURE - 77

a. What are the findings?
b. Mention three differential diagnoses.

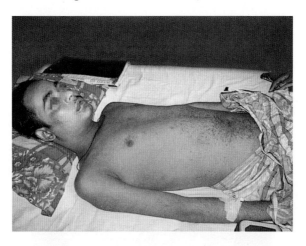

PICTURE - 78

a. This patient was diagnosed as a case of non-hodgkin lymphoma (NHL). After six cycles of chemotherapy, this is the picture of the patient. What may be the cause?

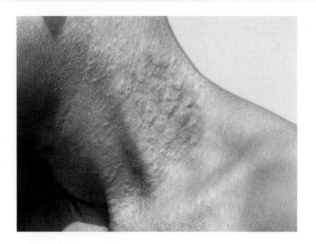

PICTURE - 79

a. What is the finding?
b. What is the diagnosis?

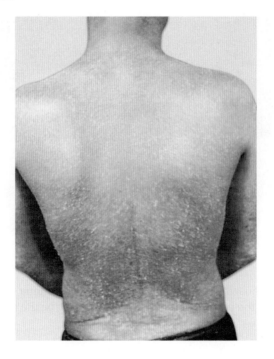

PICTURE - 80

a. What is the finding?

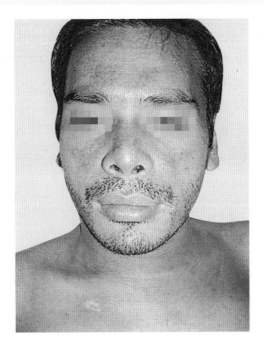

PICTURE - 81

a. What is the finding?
b. Mention five systemic diseases causing this.

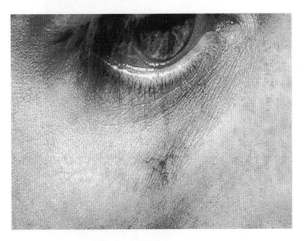

PICTURE - 82

a. What is the diagnosis?
b. What is the likely cause?

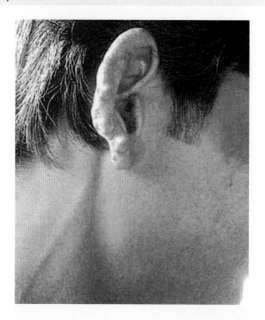

PICTURE - 83

a. What are the findings?
b. What is the diagnosis?

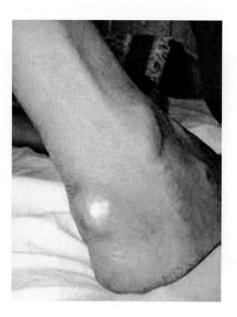

PICTURE - 84

a. What is the most likely diagnosis?
b. Mention one single investigation.
c. Mention four differential diagnoses.

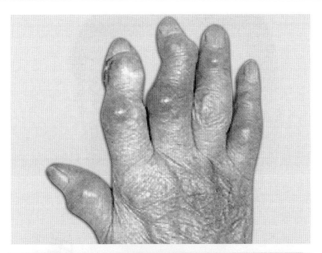

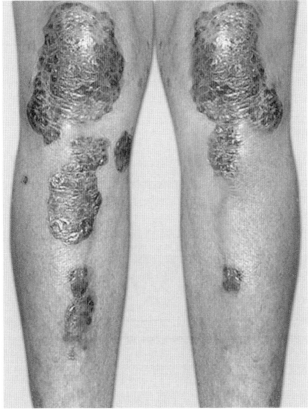

PICTURES - 85 AND 86

What metabolic abnormality is present in such patient?

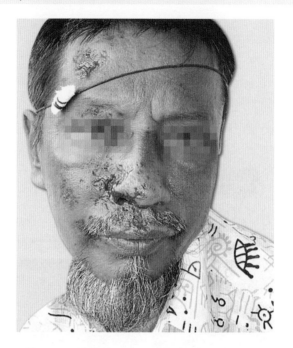

PICTURE - 87

What is the diagnosis?

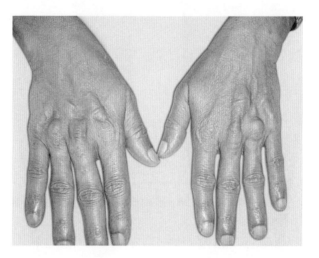

PICTURE - 88

a. What is the diagnosis in this asymptomatic patient?
b. What investigation do you want to do?

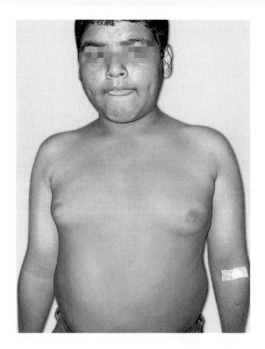

PICTURE - 89

a. What is the finding?
b. What are the causes relevant to the patient?

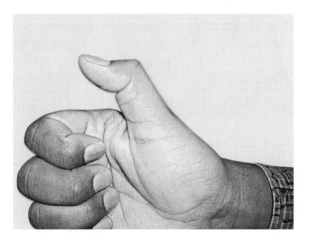

PICTURE - 90

a. What is the finding?
b. What is the diagnosis?

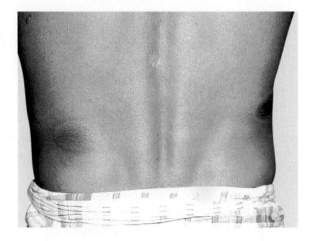

PICTURE - 91

a. What is the finding?

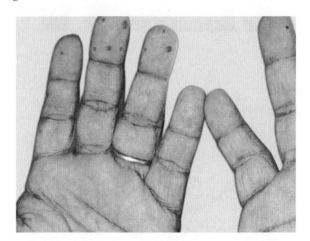

PICTURE - 92

a. Patient is suffering from fever for 15 days. What is the finding?
b. What is the diagnosis?
c. Mention one investigation.

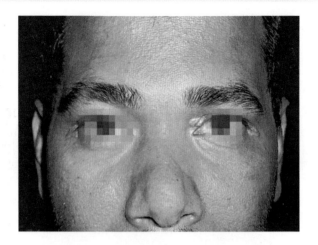

PICTURE - 93

a. What is the finding?
b. What is the diagnosis?

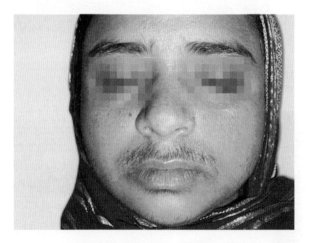

PICTURE - 94

a. This patient presented with complaints of deepening of voice and shrinking of breasts. She also noticed increased incidence of acne recently. What is the diagnosis?
b. What are the causes?

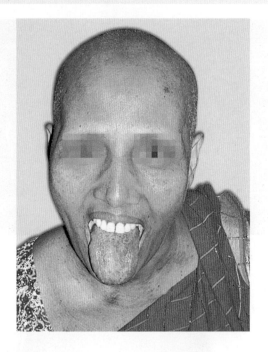

▌PICTURE - 95

a. What is the finding?
b. What are the causes?

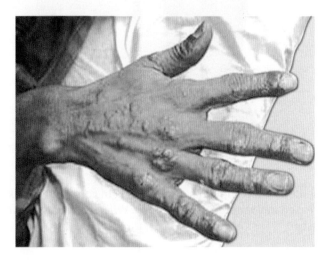

▌PICTURE - 96

a. What is the finding?
b. What is the diagnosis?

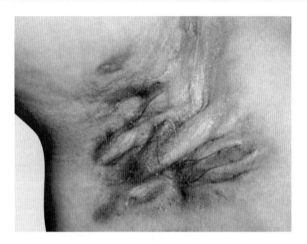

PICTURE - 97

a. There is occasional discharge from right axilla. What is the diagnosis?
b. How to treat such cases?

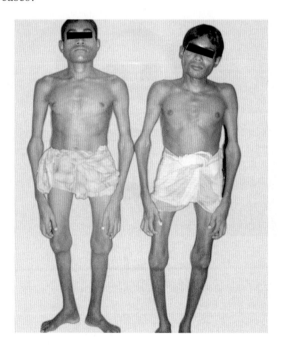

PICTURE - 98

a. Both of these brothers (aged 30 and 33 years) are suffering since childhood. Mention one question you would like to ask them.
b. What is the possible diagnosis?

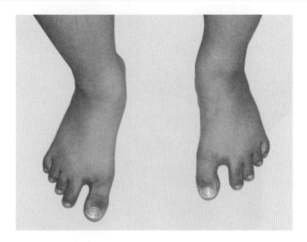

PICTURE - 99

a. What is the finding?
b. What is the diagnosis?

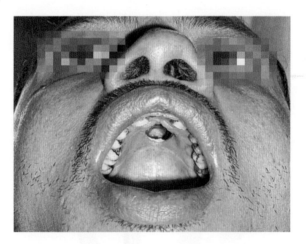

PICTURE - 100

a. What is the diagnosis?
b. Mention three causes.

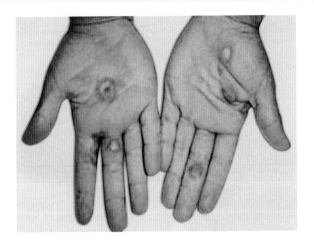

PICTURE - 101

a. What is the finding?
b. What is the diagnosis?

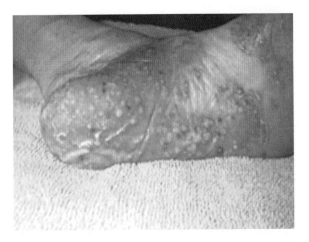

PICTURE - 102

a. What is the likely diagnosis?
b. Suggest one alternative diagnosis.

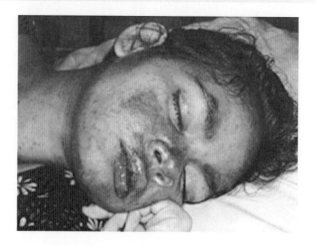

PICTURE - 103

a. What is the finding?
b. What is the diagnosis?
c. How to confirm the diagnosis?

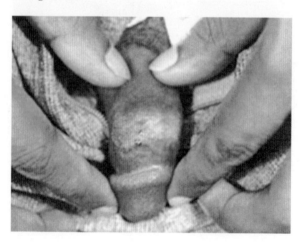

PICTURE - 104

a. What is the finding?
b. What is your diagnosis?

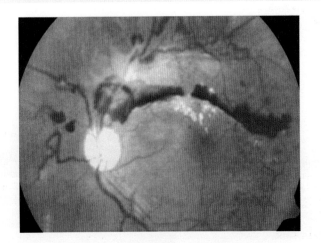

PICTURE - 105

a. What is the finding?
b. What is your diagnosis?

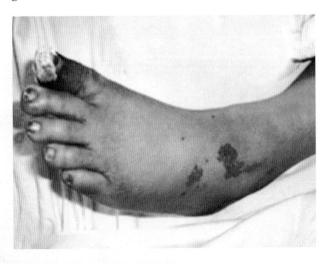

PICTURE - 106

a. What is the finding?
b. What is your diagnosis?

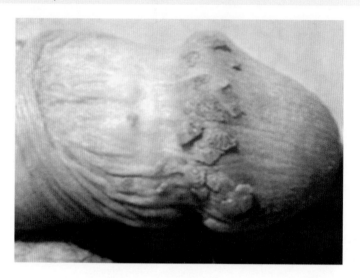

PICTURE - 107

a. What is your diagnosis?

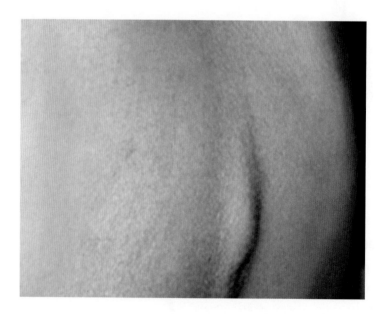

PICTURE - 108

a. What is the finding?
b. What is your diagnosis?

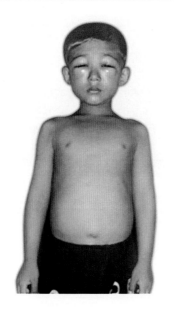

PICTURE - 109

a. What is the finding?
b. What is your diagnosis?

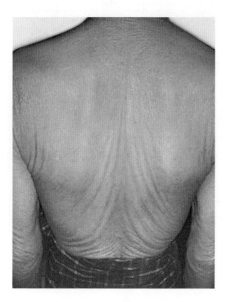

PICTURE - 110

a. What is the finding?
b. What is your diagnosis?

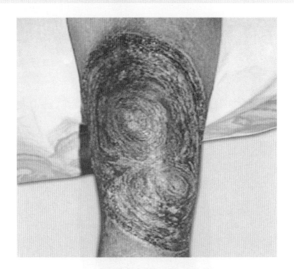

PICTURE - 111

a. What is the finding?
b. What is your diagnosis?

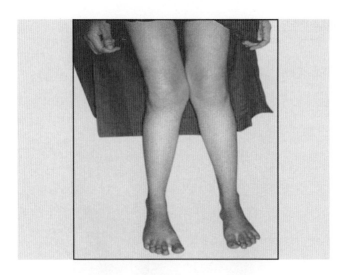

PICTURE - 112

a. What is the finding?
b. What is your diagnosis?

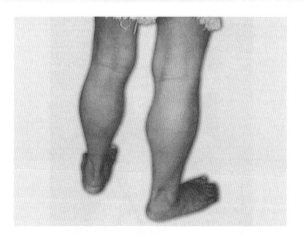

PICTURE - 113

a. What is the finding?
b. What is your diagnosis?

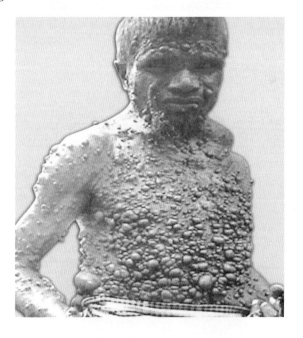

PICTURE - 114

a. What is the finding?
b. What is your diagnosis?

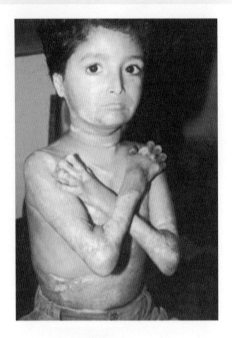

PICTURE - 115

a. What is the finding?
b. What is your diagnosis?

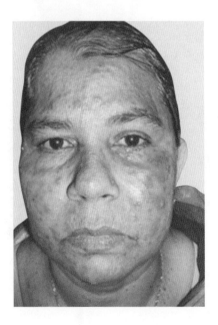

PICTURE - 116

a. What is the finding?
b. What is your diagnosis?

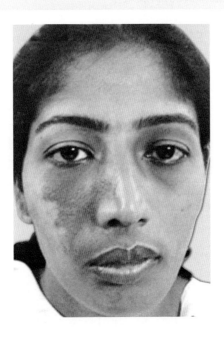

PICTURE - 117

a. What is the finding?
b. What is your diagnosis?

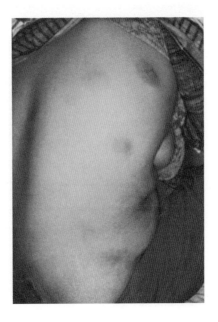

PICTURE - 118

a. What is the finding of this patient with fever for 10 days?
b. What is your diagnosis?

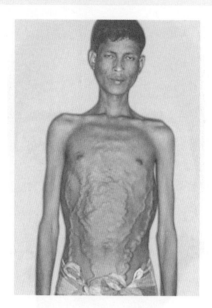

PICTURE - 119

a. What is the finding?
b. What is your diagnosis?

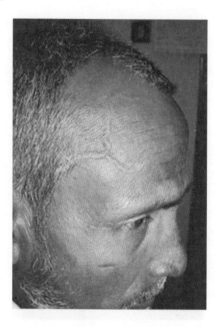

PICTURE - 120

a. What is the finding?
b. What is your diagnosis?

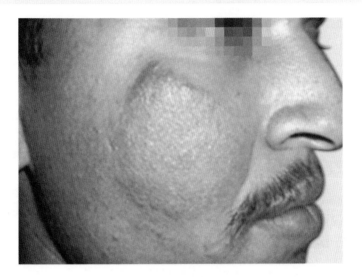

PICTURE - 121

a. What is the finding?
b. What is your diagnosis?

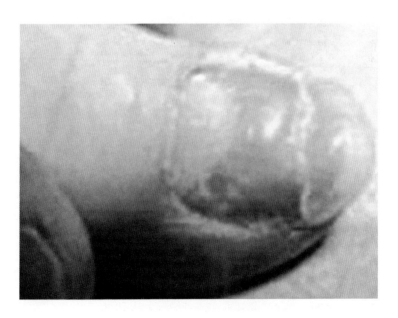

PICTURE - 122

a. What is the finding?
b. Mention three causes.

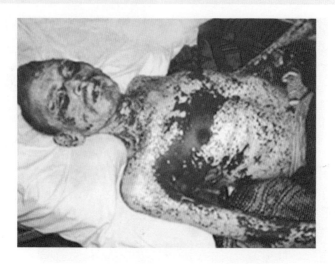

PICTURE - 123

a. What is your diagnosis?

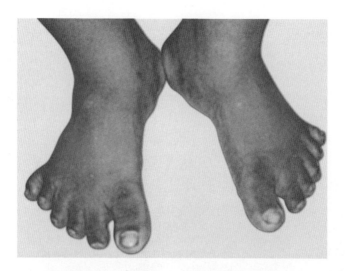

PICTURE - 124

a. What is the finding?
b. What is your diagnosis?

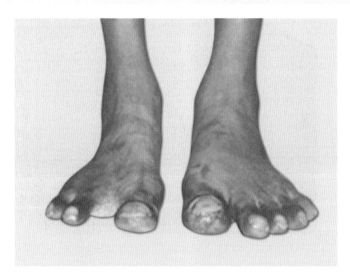

PICTURE - 125

a. What is the finding?
b. What is your diagnosis?

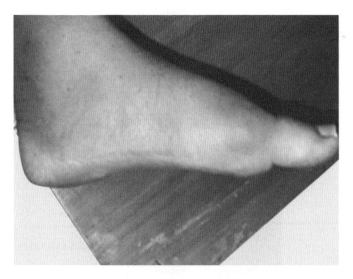

PICTURE - 126

a. What is the finding?
b. What is your diagnosis?

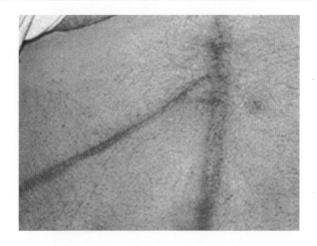

▌PICTURE - 127

a. What is the finding?
b. What is your diagnosis?

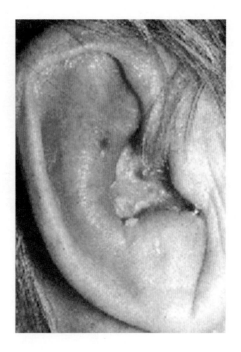

▌PICTURE - 128

a. What neurological may be present with this picture?
b. What is the underlying diagnosis ?

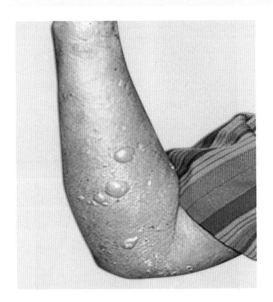

PICTURE - 129

a. What is the finding?
b. What is your diagnosis?

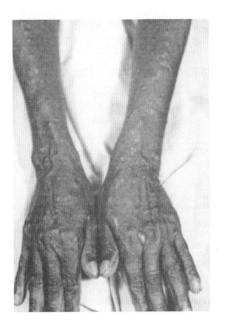

PICTURE - 130

a. What is the finding?
b. What is your diagnosis?

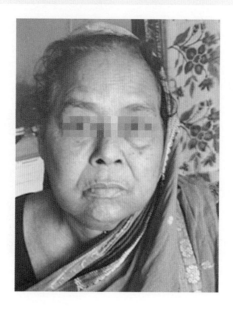

PICTURE - 131

a. What is your diagnosis?

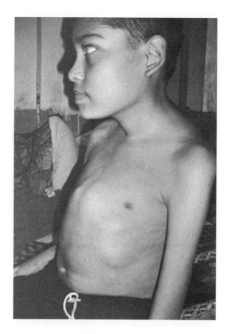

PICTURE - 132

a. What is the finding?
b. Mention two causes

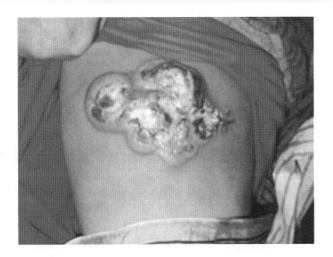

PICTURE - 133

a. What is the finding?
b. What is your diagnosis?

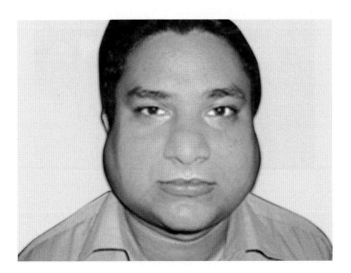

PICTURE - 134

a. What is your diagnosis?
b. Mention two causes.

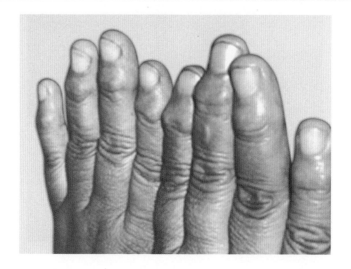

PICTURE - 135

a. What is the finding?
b. What is your diagnosis?

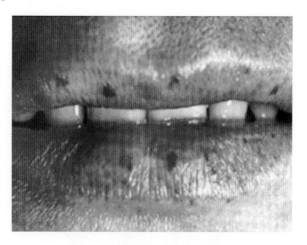

PICTURE - 136

a. What is the finding?
b. What is your diagnosis?

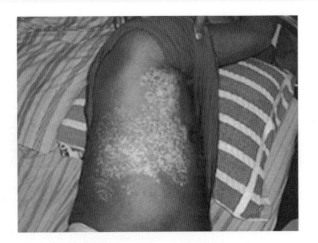

PICTURE - 137

a. What is the finding?
b. What is your diagnosis?

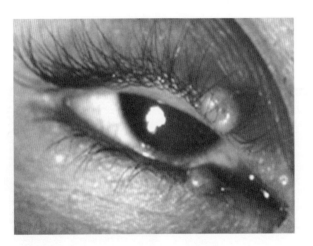

PICTURE - 138

a. What is your diagnosis?

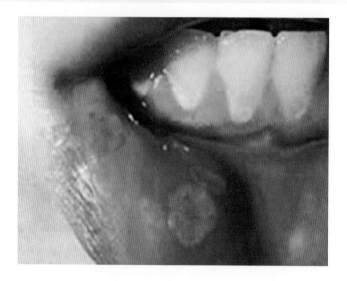

▌PICTURE - 139

a. What is the finding?
b. What is your diagnosis?

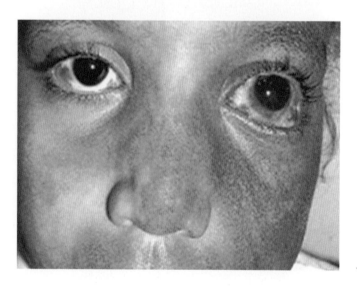

▌PICTURE - 140

a. What is the finding?
b. What is your diagnosis?

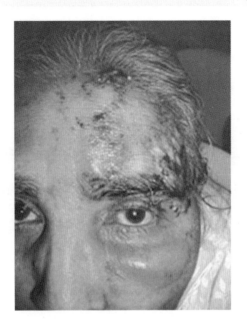

PICTURE - 141

a. What is the finding?
b. What is your diagnosis?

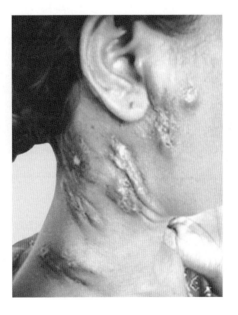

PICTURE - 142

a. What is the finding?
b. What is your diagnosis?

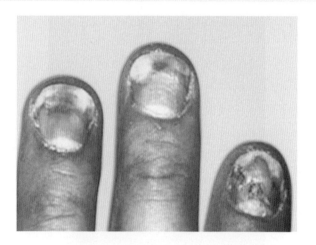

PICTURE - 143

What is your diagnosis?

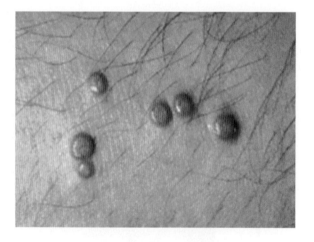

PICTURE - 144

What is your diagnosis?

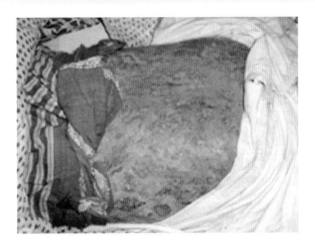

PICTURE - 145

a. What is the finding?
b. What is your diagnosis?

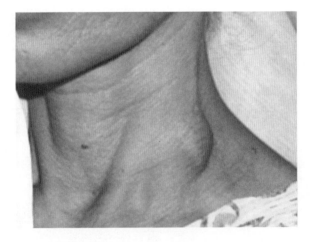

PICTURE - 146

a. What is the finding?
b. What is your diagnosis?

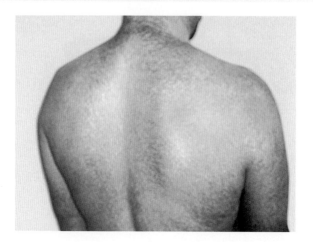

PICTURE - 147

a. What is the finding?
b. What is your diagnosis?

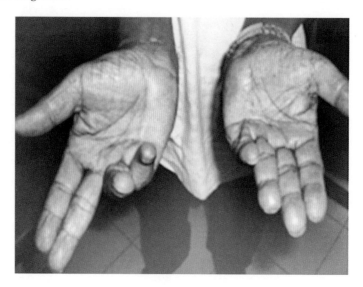

PICTURE - 148

a. What is the finding?
b. What is your diagnosis?

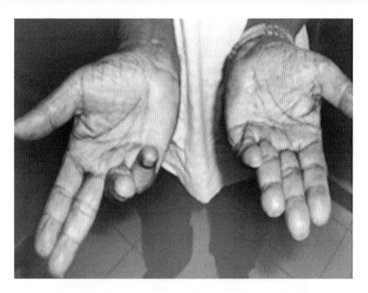

PICTURE - 149

a. What is the finding?
b. What is your diagnosis?

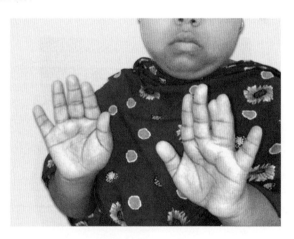

PICTURE - 150

a. What is the finding?
b. What is your diagnosis?

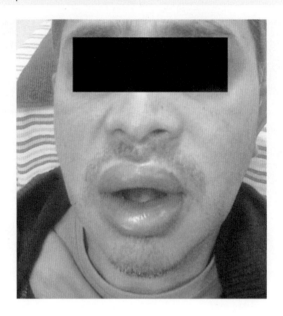

PICTURE - 151

a. What is the finding?
b. What is your diagnosis?

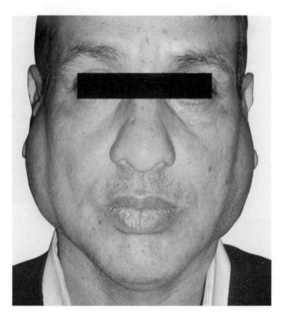

PICTURE - 152

a. What is the finding?
b. What is your diagnosis?

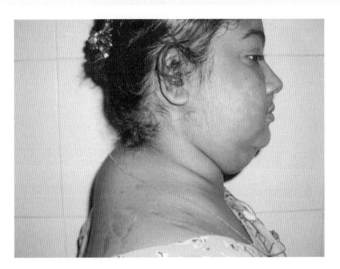

PICTURE - 153

a. What is the finding?
b. What is your diagnosis?

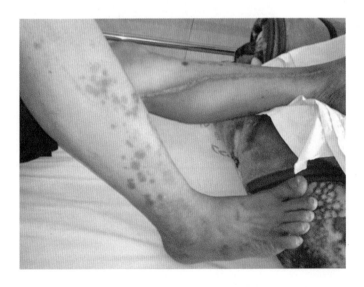

PICTURE - 154

This is the leg of a diabetic patient
a. What is the finding?
b. What is your diagnosis?

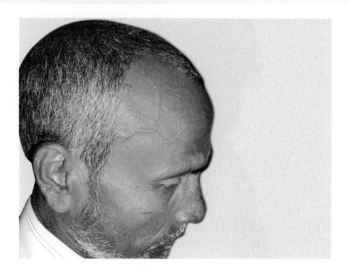

PICTURE - 155

a. What is the finding?
b. What is your diagnosis?

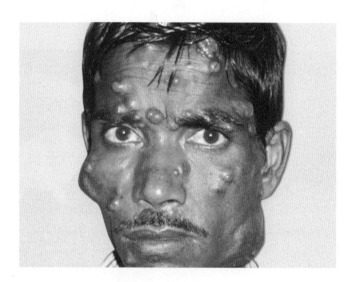

PICTURE - 156

a. What is the finding?
b. Mention three differential diagnosis

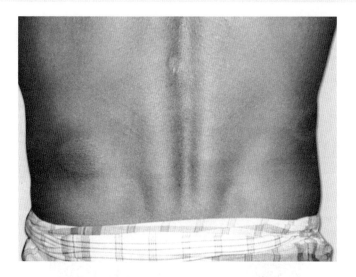

PICTURE - 157

a. What is the finding?
b. What history will be taken ?

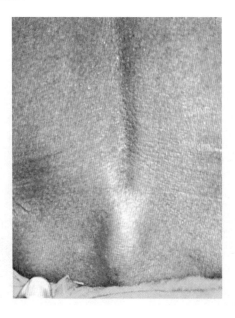

PICTURE - 158

a. What is the finding?
b. What is your diagnosis?

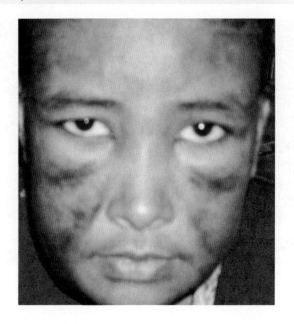

PICTURE - 159

   a. What are the finding?

   b. What is your diagnosis?

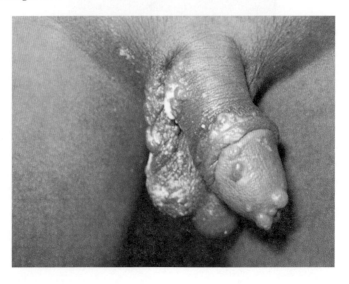

PICTURE - 160

   a. What is the finding?

   b. What is your diagnosis?

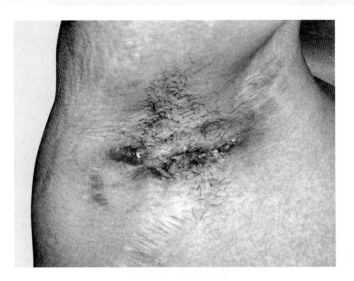

PICTURE - 161

a. What is your diagnosis?

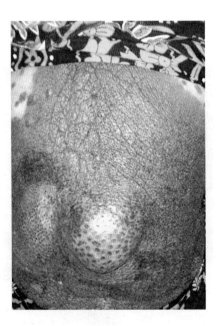

PICTURE - 162

a. What is the finding?
b. What is your diagnosis?

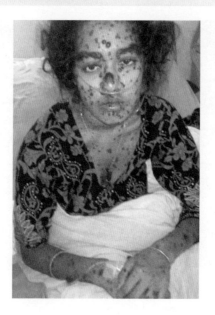

PICTURE - 163

a. What is the finding?
b. What is your diagnosis?

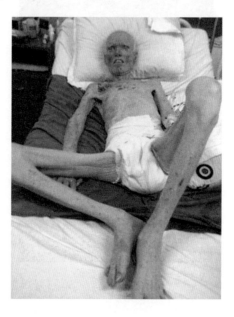

PICTURE - 164

a. What is the finding?
b. What is your diagnosis?

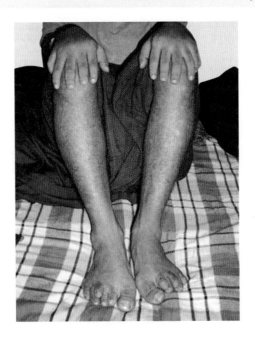

PICTURE - 165

a. What is the finding?
b. What is your diagnosis?

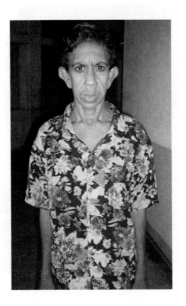

PICTURE - 166

This is the photograph of 14 years old.
a. What is your diagnosis?

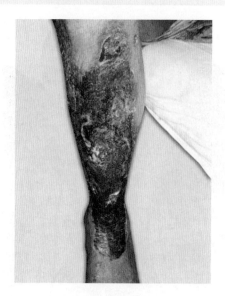

PICTURE - 167

a. What is the finding?
b. What is your diagnosis?
c. Mention two important causes.

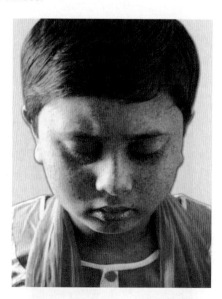

PICTURE - 168

This 7 years old girl cannot go outside the room:
a. What is the finding?
b. What is your diagnosis?

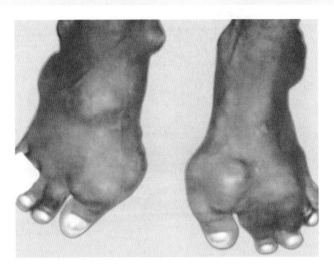

PICTURE - 169

a. What is the finding?
b. What is your diagnosis?

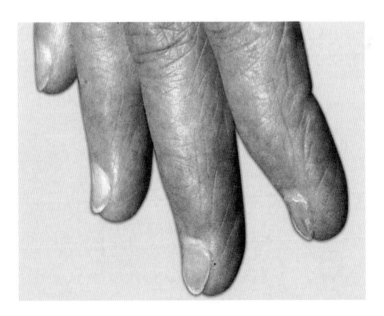

PICTURE - 170

a. What is the finding?
b. What is your diagnosis?

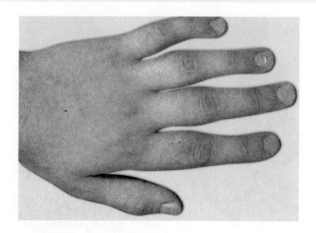

PICTURE - 171

a. What is the finding?
b. What is your diagnosis?

Answers

Case History and Data Interpretation

"To all students of medicine who listen, look, touch and reflect: may they hear, see, feel and comprehend."

— John B

CASE NO. 001

a. Sideroblastic anemia with hemosiderosis.
b. Bone marrow study to see ring sideroblast.
c. Avoid iron.

Note: Blood picture is dimorphic (microcytic and normocytic) with severe anemia, high iron, ferritin and TIBC, which are highly suggestive of sideroblastic anemia.

Sideroblastic anemias are a group of disorders, in which dimorphic blood picture is associated with marked dyserythropoiesis and abnormal iron granules in the cytoplasm of erythroblast, called ring sideroblast (seen by Prussian blue staining).

Types of sideroblastic anemia:
a. Hereditary.
b. Acquired, which may be (i) Primary and (ii) Secondary.

Primary sideroblastic anemia is one of the types of myelodysplastic syndrome, a refractory anemia with ring sideroblast.

Secondary sideroblastic anemia may be due to (i) Drugs and chemicals (INH, cycloserine, alcohol, chloramphenicol, lead), (ii) Hematological disease (myelofibrosis, polycythemia rubra vera, myeloma, Hodgkin's lymphoma, hemolytic anemia, leukemia), (iii) Inflammatory disease (rheumatoid arthritis, SLE), (iv) Others (carcinoma, myxedema, malabsorption).

Treatment: Primary cause should be treated. Offending drug should be stopped. In some cases, high dose pyridoxine, 200 mg daily may be helpful. Folic acid should be given.

CASE NO. 002

a. HELLP syndrome (HELP syndrome).
b. Reticulocyte count, viral screen (hepatitis A, B, E).
c. Termination of pregnancy (or delivery of the baby).

Note: HELLP syndrome stands—**H** for hemolysis, **EL** for elevated liver enzyme, **LP** for low platelet in a patient with preeclampsia. HELLP syndrome is a variant of preeclampsia, affects 1 per 1000 pregnancies, common in multiparous women. It is common in multipara, perinatal mortality is 10 to 60% and maternal mortality is 1.5 to 5%. In 15% cases, BP may be normal and proteinuria may be absent. HELLP syndrome usually occurs in last trimester of pregnancy or within first week of delivery. Liver disease is associated with hypertension, proteinuria and fluid retention. Serum transaminases are high and the condition can be complicated by hepatic infarction and rupture. Differential diagnoses are HUS (hemolytic uremic syndrome), TTP (thrombotic thrombocytopenic purpura) and fatty liver. However, in TTP and HUS, no hypertension or no proteinuria. In fatty liver, transaminase are very high and clotting screen is usually abnormal.

Treatment of HELLP syndrome: Prompt delivery is indicated for any of the following—1. Pregnancies ≥34 weeks of gestation. 2. Nonreassuring tests of fetal status (e.g. biophysical profile, fetal heart rate testing. 3. Maternal disease: multiorgan dysfunction, DIC, liver infarction or hemorrhage, renal failure, or abruptio placenta.

In <34 weeks, intravenous steroid (Dexamethasone) may be given. Other therapy—(i) Control of hypertension, (ii) Platelet and blood transfusion may be necessary, (iii) If convulsion, magnesium sulfate intravenously, (iv) Sometimes in severe renal failure, dialysis may be necessary.

Maternal complications—DIC, abruptio placentae, acute renal failure, pulmonary edema, subcapsular liver hematoma, retinal detachment.

Fetus/neonate complications—Prematurity, intrauterine growth restriction and sequelae of abruptio placenta, perinatal mortality. Maternal HELLP does not affect fetal/neonatal liver function.

CASE NO. 003

a. Insulinoma.
b. Factitious intake of insulin.
c. Retroperitoneal fibrosarcoma, mesothelioma.
d. Serum glucose with simultaneous insulin and C-peptide, USG or CT scans of pancreas, 72 hours fasting with measurement of glucose, insulin and C-peptide.

Note: Her symptoms are due to recurrent hypoglycemia secondary to recurrent insulin secretion. Weight gain is due to frequent intake of food for hypoglycemia. Insulinoma is the commonest cause of nondiabetic fasting hypoglycemia. It is the insulin-secreting tumor of beta cell of pancreas, small <5 mm and occurs in any part of pancreas. 90% are benign and slow growing, 10% may be malignant. Common in middle age. Symptoms of hypoglycaemia occur during fasting and relieve by taking food. The patient frequently takes food and gains weight. Whipple's triad is use for clinical diagnosis—1. Symptoms are associated with fasting or exercise 2. Hypoglycemia is confirmed during these episodes 3. Glucose relieves these symptoms. A 4th criteria is inappropriately high insulin during hypoglycemia.

There are more synthesis of pro-insulin, insulin and high C-peptide. It may be confused with self-induced insulin intake. In such a case, there is high serum insulin, but C-peptide is absent or low.

Insulinoma is detected by CT, MRI or endoscopic or laparoscopic USG.

Retroperitoneal fibrosarcoma and mesothelioma can cause hypoglycemia due to secretion of insulin-like substance (insulin-like growth factor-2).

Treatment: Resection, if possible. Diazoxide may be use. Symptoms may remit with octreotide or lanreotide (somatostatin analog). Verapamil or Phenytoin also can be used. It reduces insulin secretion from the tumor.

CASE NO. 004

a. Bartter's syndrome.
b. The 24 hours urine potassium, serum renin and aldosterone (others—24 hours urinary calcium, which is high).
c. Diuretic abuse, laxative abuse.

Note: This young patient has hypokalemia, metabolic alkalosis and normal blood pressure. Differential diagnoses are diuretic abuse, laxative abuse, self-induced vomiting, etc. All are absent in the history, only remaining is Bartter's syndrome. This disease is characterized by hypokalemia, metabolic alkalosis, normal blood pressure, high renin and high aldosterone, hypercalciuria, occasionally hypomagnesemia. Primary defect is impairment of sodium and chloride reabsorption in the ascending limb of Henle's loop. Urinary calcium is >40 mmol/L. Prostaglandin levels are also high. It may be associated with short stature and mental retardation.

Diagnosis: Low serum potassium (<3 mmol) and high 24 hours urine potassium (>20 mmol) plus high renin and high aldosterone. Biopsy of the kidney shows hyperplasia of juxtaglomerular cells (prominent interstitial cells and interstitial fibrosis may be present).

Treatment: Potassium, spironolactone, ACE inhibitor in some cases. Indomethacin, interfere with tubular prostaglandin production may be helpful. Magnesium supplement may be necessary, if hypomagnesemia.

(Two other syndromes—(i) **Liddle's syndrome**—characterized by hypokalemia, metabolic alkalosis, high blood pressure, low renin and low aldosterone, (ii) **Gitelman's syndrome**—variant of Bartter's syndrome characterized by hypokalemia, metabolic alkalosis, normal blood pressure, high renin and high aldosterone, hypocalciuria, hypomagnesemia).

CASE NO. 005

a. Acute intermittent porphyria.
b. Urine for Ehrlich's aldehyde test, urine for α-aminolevulinic acid (ALA-increased), PBG (increase).
   Others—urine for porphobilinogen. Assay of red cells for the enzyme PBG deaminase (very low).

Note: Recurrent abdominal pain, hypertension and also psychiatric problem with low sodium is highly suggestive of acute intermittent porphyria. AIP, inherited as autosomal dominant, is characterized by recurrent abdominal pain, neurological and psychiatric problem. There may be peripheral neuropathy (usually motor), respiratory failure, ophthalmoplegia, optic atrophy, constipation, psychiatric problem such as anxiety, depression and frank psychosis. Epileptic convulsion, hypertension and tachycardia may occur. Respiratory muscle paralysis may be life-threatening, may require assisted ventilation.

Common in female, usually after 30 years. Primary defect is deficiency of porphobilinogen deaminase in the heme biosynthetic pathway. Precipitating factors—barbiturate, oral pills, griseofulvin, sulfonamide, alcohol, even fasting.

When urine is kept for long time, it turns red brown or dark red color (Portwine). Bedside test is Ehrlich's aldehyde test in which reagent is added to urine, which shows pink color due to presence of porphobilinogen (which persists after addition of chloroform). Pink color may be due to urobilinogen, which disappears after addition of chloroform. Sodium may be low due to syndrome of inappropriate antidiuretic hormone (SIADH).

Treatment: No specific treatment. Acute attack is treated by administration of large quantities of glucose 500 g/day (it reduces ALA synthetase activity). If no response in 48 hours, intravenous infusion of heme (hematin or hem-arginate) is helpful. Hypertension and tachycardia are treated with β-blocker. Avoid precipitating factors. High carbohydrate and fluid intake should be maintained. Cyclical attack in woman may respond to suppression of menstrual cycle by GnRH analog.

CASE NO. 006

a. Fitz-Hugh-Curtis syndrome (Chlamydia or gonococcal perihepatitis).
b. Acute cholecystitis, liver abscess.
c. USG of HBS, X-ray chest, endocervical swab for microscopy and culture, urine for routine and culture.

Note: History of urethritis, vaginitis followed hepatitis is highly suggestive of Fitz-Hugh-Curtis syndrome. It is caused by *Chlamydia* or *Gonococcus* infection, which tracks up the right paracolic gutter to cause perihepatitis, secondarily from endocervical or urethral infection. It is characterized by fever, pain in the right hypochondrium with radiation to right shoulder, tender hepatomegaly, hepatic rub, small right pleural effusion, etc. (*Chlamydia* infection may be asymptomatic in 80% cases).

Investigations: Endocervical swab for microscopy and special culture, direct fluorescent antibody for *Chlamydia*, ELISA, PCR may be done.

Treatment: Tetracycline or doxycycline or erythromycin or azithromycin are used for *Chlamydia* infection.

CASE NO. 007

a. Sarcoidosis, SLE, lymphoma, disseminated tuberculosis.
b. Sarcoidosis.
c. Full blood count and ESR, X-ray chest, MT, ANA and anti-ds DNA, FNAC or biopsy from lymph node.

Note: Fever, arthritis or arthralgia, skin rash (erythema nodosum) and bilateral hilar lymphadenopathy in chest X-ray is highly suggestive of sarcoidosis. It is a multisystem granulomatous disorder of unknown cause characterized by presence of non-caseating granuloma in different organs. More in female than male, also common in black people. Usual features are fever, polyarthritis or arthralgia, erythema nodosum. X-ray shows bilateral hilar lymphadenopathy.

Other features: Dry cough, breathlessness, lupus pernio, plaque, skin rash, uveitis, bilateral parotid involvement, cardiomyopathy, arrhythmia, hepatosplenomegaly, etc. Neurological features are cranial nerve palsy, aseptic meningitis, seizure, psychosis, multiple sclerosis type syndromes (neurosarcoid).

Investigations: CBC (low lymphocyte), high calcium, high ACE (related to activity), chest X-ray (BHL), MT (usually negative), biopsy of involved tissue (lymph node, lung). Lung function test—restrictive with impaired gas exchange.

Bronchoscopy: Cobble stone appearance of mucosa, bronchial lavage shows increased CD4: CD8 T cell ratio. CT scan of chest may be done.

Biopsy shows non-caseating granuloma consisting of epithelioid cells, lymphocytes around it and multinucleated giant cells.

Two syndromes in sarcoidosis are (i) **Heerfordt's or Waldenstrom's syndrome**—fever, uveitis, parotid enlargement and seventh nerve palsy, (ii) **Lofgren's syndrome**—erythema nodosum, iritis and bilateral hilar lymphadenopathy.

The patient with sarcoidosis may have lacrimal and parotid gland enlargement, called Mikulicz syndrome, characterized by xerostomia and gritty eyes.

CASE NO. 008

a. Berger's IgA nephropathy.
b. Serum IgA, immune complex estimation, kidney biopsy.
c. Henoch Schonlein purpura.

Note: Young patient with history of sore throat followed by hematuria with urinary abnormality indicates Berger's nephropathy. It is a type of immune-complex mediated focal and segmental proliferative glomerulonephritis with mesangial deposition of IgA. In some cases, IgG, IgM, C_3 may be deposited in mesangium. Common in children and young males, 20 to 35 years of age. Most patients are asymptomatic, presents with recurrent microscopic or even gross hematuria. It may follow a viral respiratory or GIT infection. Hematuria is universal, proteinuria is usual and hypertension is common, 5% may develop nephrotic syndrome. In some cases, progressive loss of renal function, leading to end stage renal failure (20%) in 20 years.

Kidney biopsy shows focal proliferative glomerulonephritis. Immune deposits are present diffusely in mesangium of all glomeruli and contain usually IgA.

Treatment: Episodic attack resolves spontaneously. Patient with proteinuria over 1 to 3 g/day, mild glomerular change and good renal function should be treated with steroid. In progressive renal disease, prednisolone plus cyclophosphamide for 3 months, then prednisolone plus azathioprine. Combination of ACE inhibitor and ARB should be given to all cases. Tonsillectomy may be helpful, if recurrent tonsillitis.

CASE NO. 009

a. Thyrotoxic crisis.
b. FT_3, FT_4 and TSH.

Note: Clue for the diagnosis is goiter with loss of weight, loose motion, palpitation which are due to thyrotoxicosis. Consolidation has precipitated thyrotoxic crisis. It is characterized by life-threatening increase in severity of the signs and symptoms of thyrotoxicosis (also called thyroid storm). There is high fever, restlessness, agitation, irritability, nausea, vomiting, diarrhea, abdominal pain, confusion, delirium and coma. Precipitated by infection, stress, and surgery in unprepared patient and following radio-iodine therapy (due to radiation thyroiditis).

Treatment: (i) Better in ICU, (ii) carbimazole 15 mg 8 hourly or propylthiouracil 150 mg 6 hourly, (iii) propranolol 80 mg 6 hourly, (iv) IV-normal saline and glucose, (v) antibiotic, (vi) steroid-dexamethasone (2 mg 6 hourly), (vii) Na-iopodate (radiographic contrast)—500 mg daily orally rapidly effective, reduces release of thyroid hormone and also reduces conversion of T_4 to T_3. Mortality rate in thyrotoxic crisis is 10%.

CASE NO. 010

a. Hyperosmolar non-ketotic diabetic coma with UTI.
b. RBS, urine for ketone bodies, serum osmolality, urine for C/S.
c. IV 1/2 strength saline (0.45%), soluble insulin (preferably with insulin pump, 2 to 6 units hourly). When osmolality is normal, 0.9% normal saline should be given.

Note: Glycosuria, high sodium, hyperchloremic acidosis are the clue for the diagnosis of hyperosmolar non-ketotic diabetic coma (HNDC). It may be the first presentation in diabetes mellitus. Common in elderly, NIDDM, characterized by very high blood glucose (>50 mmol/L) and high plasma osmolality. No ketosis, because insulin deficiency is partial and low insulin is present, which is sufficient to prevent ketone body formation, but insufficient to control hyperglycemia. Hyperchloremic mild acidosis may be present due to starvation, increased lactic acid and retention of inorganic acid. Precipitating factors are large amount of sweet drink, infection, steroid, thiazide, myocardial infarction, etc. Plasma sodium is usually high (may be false low due to pseudohyponatremia). There may be high BUN, urea, creatinine and serum osmolality may be very high. Mortality rate may be up to 40%. Osmolality is calculated by $= 2 \times Na + 2 \times K + plasma \ glucose + plasma \ urea$ (all in mmol/L).

Normal 280 to 300 mOsm/kg. Consciousness is depressed, if it is > 340 mOsm.

Other treatments: NG tube feeding, catheter if needed, antibiotic if infection, correction of electrolytes, low dose heparin (as thrombosis is common).

Differences between diabetic ketoacidosis and HNDC

Points	DKA	HNDC
1. Age	Young, may be any age	Elderly, >40 years
2. Precipitating factor	Insulin deficiency	Partial insulin deficiency
3. Breath	Acetone present	Absent
4. Kussmaul's breathing	Present	Absent
5. Sodium	Low	High
6. Bicarbonate	Low	Normal
7. Ketonuria	Present	Absent
8. Osmolality	Normal	High
9. Mortality	5 to 10%	30 to 40%

Differences between diabetic ketoacidosis and lactic acidosis

Points	DKA	Lactic acidosis
1. Precipitating factor	Insulin deficiency, infection, no biguanide	Biguanide
2. Dehydration	Present	Absent
3. Breath	Acetone	Absent
4. Ketonuria	Present	Absent or mild
5. Serum lactate	Normal	High >5 mmol/L
6. Mortality	5 to 10%	>50%

CASE NO. 011

a. Bilateral occipital cortex (cortical blindness).
b. Basilar artery occlusion by mural thrombus from left ventricle.
c. MRI of brain.
d. Poor.
e. Murmur is due to mitral regurgitation or VSD.

Note: Sudden blindness with normal pupil and normal papillary reaction to light indicates cortical blindness. Thromboembolism may occur following myocardial infarction. Widespread bilateral cortical damage causes cortical blindness (Anton's syndrome). Causes are infarction, trauma, tumor. The patient cannot see and lacks insight into the degree of blindness and may even deny it. Pupillary response is normal. In myocardial infarction, rupture of the papillary muscles causes mitral regurgitation and rupture of interventricular septum causes VSD.

CASE NO. 012

a. Any skin rash with the onset of fever, which disappears with fall of temperature (Salmon rash).
b. Adult Still's disease.

c. Lymphoma, SLE (others—septicemia, disseminated tuberculosis).

d. Serum ferritin (very high), ANA, anti-ds DNA, FNAC of lymph node.

Note: High fever, polyarthritis, pleurisy, hepatosplenomegaly, lymphadenopathy are consistent with adult Still's disease. It may be confused with SLE, lymphoma, disseminated tuberculosis. ANA is negative and also high CRP is against SLE. Lymphoma is another possibility, but very high fever, seronegative arthritis, leukocytosis, etc. are against lymphoma.

Adult Still's disease is a clinical condition of unknown cause, characterized by high fever, seronegative arthritis, skin rash and polyserositis. It is usually diagnosed by exclusion of other diseases. Common in young adult, 16 to 35 years of age, rare after 60 years.

Diagnostic criteria of adult Still's disease are:

A. Each of the four (i) fever, >39°C, (ii) arthralgia/arthritis lasting 2 weeks or longer, (iii) Evanescent rash (iv) RA and ANA-negative.

B. Plus two of (i) Leukocytosis >15,000/cmm, (ii) evanescent macular/maculopapular rash, Salmon colored, nonpruritic, (iii) serositis (pleurisy, pericarditis), (iv) hepatomegaly, (v) splenomegaly, (vi) lymphadenopathy.

Another criteria (Yamaguchi criteria)

❖ Major criteria—(i) Arthralgia >2 weeks (ii) Fever >39°, intermittent ≥ 1 week (iii) Typical rash (iv) WBC >10 000 (>80% granulocytes).

❖ Minor—(i) Sore throat (ii) Lymphadenopathy and/or splenomegaly, (iii) LFT abnormal, (iv) ANA and RF—negative.

Diagnosis—five criteria at least two major.

Lymph node biopsy shows reactive hyperplasia.

Treatment: NSAID, high dose steroid, disease-modifying drugs (Methotrexate). If no response, biologic agent (e.g. TNF alpha, etanercept, infliximab).

CASE NO. 013

a. Late onset congenital adrenal hyperplasia (CAH).

b. Polycystic ovarian syndrome (PCOS).

c. Dexamethasone suppression test.

d. Steroid (prednisolone or dexamethasone).

e. Serum 17-hydroxyprogesterone (high), urine for pregnanetriol (high).

Note: Differential diagnosis of hirsutism is congenital adrenal hyperplasia, polycystic ovarian syndrome (PCOS), androgen-secreting adrenal tumor, Cushing's syndrome, arrhenoblastoma. Serum 17-hydroxyprogesterone is high in 21 α-hydroxylase deficiency. In late onset CAH, this may be normal and if it is high after synacthen test, is highly suggestive of late onset CAH (which is due to mild enzyme defect).

After dexamethasone suppression test, there is fall of 17-hydroxyprogesterone and other androgens in CAH, but in PCOS and other androgen-secreting tumor of ovary or adrenal cortex, these do not fall after dexamethasone suppression test.

Hirsutism is present in late onset congenital adrenal hyperplasia. Also, the patient is tall, there is precocious sexual development. In children with CAH, there may be salt loss, adrenal crisis, increased pigmentation and ambiguous genitalia.

In 95% cases, CAH is due to 21 β-hydroxylase deficiency.

Rarely, 11 β-hydroxylase deficiency or 17 β-hydroxylase deficiency may be present. Both are associated with hypertension. There is less synthesis of cortisol, aldosterone and increased synthesis of 17-hydroxyprogesterone, testosterone, other androgen such as dehydro-epiandrosterone, androstenedione, increased ACTH and 24 hours urinary pregnanetriol.

Treatment: Steroid in high dose at night and low dose in morning. Late onset CAH may not require steroid. Hirsutism should be treated with anti-androgen.

CASE NO. 014

a. Meningococcal septicemia with DIC.
b. Dengue hemorrhagic fever.
c. Prothrombin time, APTT, serum FDP.
d. Blood culture and sensitivity.
e. LP and CSF study.

Note: High fever, multiple purpuric rash with DIC are highly suggestive of meningococcal septicemia, caused by *Neisseria meningitidis*. Septicemia due to other cause may be also responsible. Full blood count, blood culture, LP and CSF study are necessary. Meningococcal meningitis and septicemia are caused by *Neisseria meningitidis*, a gram-negative *Diplococcus*. Septicemia may be associated with multiple petechial hemorrhage, also conjunctival hemorrhage. In CSF, pressure is high, color is purulent, high neutrophil, high protein and low glucose. Gram staining, culture and sensitivity are also necessary. Complications of meningococcal septicemia—DIC, peripheral gangrene following vascular occlusion, Waterhouse-Friderichsen syndrome, renal failure, meningitis, shock, arthritis (septic or reactive), pericarditis may occur. Skin rash in 70% (by *N. meningitidis*).

After sending blood for C/S, treatment should be started immediately. Usually, benzyl penicillin in high dose plus cephalosporin or aminoglycoside should be given intravenously.

Lumbar puncture (LP) is mandatory, provided there is no contraindication.

Leukocytosis is not a feature of dengue hemorrhagic fever (usually leukopenia).

CASE NO. 015

a. Spontaneous bacterial peritonitis (SBP).
b. Aspiration of ascitic fluid for cytology, biochemistry and C/S.
c. Liver transplantation.

Note: In a chronic liver disease (CLD) patient with ascites, if fever develops, SBP is the most likely diagnosis. Spontaneous bacterial peritonitis means infection of the ascitic fluid in a patient with cirrhosis of liver, in the absence of primary source of infection. SBP may develop in 8% cases of ascites with cirrhosis (may be as high as 20 to 30%), usually by single organism (monomicrobial).

It is due to migration of enteric bacteria through gut wall by hematogenous route or mesenteric lymphatics, commonly caused by *E coli*. Other organisms are *Klebsiella*, *Haemophilus*, *Enterococcus*, other enteric gram-negative organism, rarely *Pneumococcus*, *Streptococcus*. Anaerobic bacteria are not usually associated with SBP.

Features of spontaneous bacterial peritonitis:
a. Fever, abdominal pain, rebound tenderness, increasing ascites not responding to diuretic, absent bowel sound. Features of hepatic encephalopathy and fever may occur (in 1/3rd cases).

b. Abdominal symptoms may be mild or absent (in 1/3rd cases) and in this patient, portal-systemic encephalopathy (PSE) and fever are main features.
c. Ascitic fluid shows (i) cloudy (exudative—high protein and low sugar), (ii) neutrophil in fluid >250 or WBC >500/cmm.

Treatment: Broad spectrum antibiotic (cefotaxime or ceftazidime) plus metronidazole IV. Recurrence is common (70%) within one year, which may be prevented by norfloxacin 400 mg daily or ciprofloxacin 250 mg daily. Mortality is 10 to 15%. SBP is an indication for referral to liver transplant center.

CASE NO. 016

a. Avascular necrosis of head of femur with lupus gut (with UTI with lupus nephritis).
b. Avascular necrosis of head of femur.
c. MRI of hip joint.

Note: Any patient who is getting steroid for long time, if complains of severe backache with difficulty in walking, avascular necrosis should be excluded. In SLE, avascular necrosis may be due to prolonged use of steroid and also due to vasculitis. MRI is the most sensitive test to diagnose early. X-ray may be normal in early case.

Limping gait is a recognized complication of SLE. Severe acute abdominal pain, nausea, vomiting, diarrhea, etc. may occur in SLE due to vasculitis (called lupus gut).

CASE NO. 017

a. Fat embolism in brain.
b. CT scan/MRI of brain, urine for fat cells.

Note: Fat embolism may occur after bony fracture, more common with closed than open fracture. It is usually caused by trauma to the long bone or pelvis, orthopedic procedures, sometimes parenteral lipid infusion, recent corticosteroid therapy, burns, liposuction, sickle cell crisis. Fat embolism is characterized by hypoxemia, petechial rash over the upper part of the body, neurological abnormality, within 24 to 72 hours of injury. Retinal hemorrhage with intra-arterial fat globules may be seen with fundoscope. Fat cells can be detected in urine or sputum. Treatment is supportive, such as maintenance of oxygenation, hydration, prophylaxis against thrombosis, nutrition, etc.

CASE NO. 018

a. Postpartum cardiomyopathy.
b. Echocardiography, serum electrolytes.

Note: If any patient after delivery develops respiratory distress or pulmonary edema or features of heart failure, postpartum cardiomyopathy is the likely diagnosis. Differential diagnosis is pulmonary embolism. Postpartum cardiomyopathy is characterized by dilatation of the heart with biventricular failure, usually in the last trimester or within 6 months of delivery. It is a type of dilated cardiomyopathy. Cause is unknown. Immune and viral causes are postulated. Other factors are advanced age, multiple pregnancy, multiparity and hypertension in pregnancy. Commonly occurs immediately after or in the month before delivery (peripartum).

It occurs usually in multipara, age above 30 years. The patient usually presents with heart failure, dyspnea, orthopnea, cough with frothy sputum, weakness, pain in abdomen, swelling of leg, etc. Atrial fibrillation or other arrhythmia may occur.

Diagnostic criteria are (four criteria):
i. Presentation in last month of pregnancy or within 5 months of delivery.
ii. Absence of an obvious cause for heart failure.
iii. Previously normal cardiac status.
iv. Echocardiographic evidence of systolic left ventricular dysfunction.

Treatment: Symptomatic for heart failure (diuretics, ACE inhibitor, digoxin). β-blocker may be helpful in some cases. Inotropic agent may be given. More than half cases have a complete or near complete recovery over several months. Immunosuppressive therapy has doubtful value. Mortality rate is 10 to 20%.

The patient should avoid subsequent pregnancy, due to risk of relapse. However, if the heart size is normal in the first episode following heart failure, subsequent pregnancy is tolerated in some cases. If heart size remains enlarged, further pregnancy causes refractory chronic heart failure.

CASE NO. 019

a. Primary hyperparathyroidism.
b. Serum Ca, PO_4 and alkaline phosphatase, parathormone assay, hydrocortisone suppression test, X-ray of hand (to see subperiosteal erosion in the medial side of phalanges) and X-ray of skull (to see pepper pot), USG or CT scan of neck (other test—thallium/technetium subtraction scan of thyroid and parathyroid).
c. Plenty of fluid (infusion of normal saline 4 to 6 liters daily) for hypercalcemia.

Note: This patient presents with the features of hypercalcemia and nephrocalcinosis, suggestive of hyperparathyroidism. It may be primary (due to adenoma, hyperplasia or carcinoma of parathyroid), secondary (chronic renal failure, malabsorption, rickets or osteomalacia) or tertiary (autonomous from secondary). Most symptoms are due to hypercalcemia. There may be band keratopathy (corneal calcification), nephrocalcinosis, pancreatitis, peptic ulcer, pseudogout, spontaneous fracture, and osteoporosis. X-ray of skull shows pepper pot and loss of lamina dura. X-ray of hand shows resorption of terminal phalanges.

Treatment: For primary hyperparathyroidism, total parathyroidectomy followed by transplantation of a small amount of parathyroid in the forearm muscles. After surgery, calcium may fall rapidly and tetany may occur. Hypocalcemia may persist for several months. So, it is necessary to continue vitamin D supplement. In mild and asymptomatic case, follow-up. Surgery is also required for tertiary hyperparathyroidism. Treatment of secondary causes should be done.

CASE NO. 020

a. Cerebral lupus erythematosus with autoimmune hemolytic anemia with renal lupus.
b. ANA, anti-ds DNA, antiphospholipid antibody, MRI of brain.

Note: Young female with long time fever, arthritis or arthralgia, eye problem, etc. with low platelet, SLE should be considered. In SLE, cerebral involvement may occur in up to 15%

of cases. The patient may present only with psychiatric manifestations, such as behavior abnormality, irritability, confusion, hallucination, obsessional or paranoid or frank organic psychosis. Epilepsy or convulsion, stroke, peripheral neuropathy, chorea, transverse myelitis may also occur. CSF will show features of aseptic lymphocytic meningitis. Antiphospholipid or anticardiolipin antibody is present in 30 to 40%. ANA is positive in 90%, anti-dsDNA is positive in up to 60%. CRP is usually normal, high if secondary infection. Complement, mainly C_3 is low.

Treatment: High dose prednisolone or methylprednisolone plus pulse cyclophosphamide intravenously.

CASE NO. 021

a. Cerebral abscess.
b. Full blood count (leukocytosis), CT scan or MRI of brain, blood for culture and sensitivity.

Note: Infection in ear with fever and cerebral features are highly suggestive of brain abscess. It may occur as a complication from ear infection. Other causes include infection in nose, paranasal sinus and tooth, head injury, penetrating trauma, septicemia, HIV infection, immunocompromised case, Fallot's tetralogy, etc. Organisms are *Streptococcus anginosus, Bacteroids, Staphylococcus,* and fungus. Mixed infections are common. Multiple abscesses are common in HIV. CT scan will show ring-like shadow in the brain.

Treatment: Broad spectrum antibiotic, metronidazole (in anaerobic). Surgery may be necessary, if drug fails. Mortality 25%. Epilepsy may occur in survivor.

CASE NO. 022

a. Neuroleptic malignant syndrome.
b. ANA and anti-ds DNA (to exclude SLE), serum ferritin (to exclude adult Still's disease).
c. Serum CPK (raised).

Note: If unexplained high fever develops in a psychiatric patient who is on antipsychotic drug, neuroleptic malignant syndrome is the likely diagnosis. It is rare, but serious complication of any neuroleptic drug therapy, such as phenothiazine, butyrophenones (commonly haloperidol), irrespective of dose. It occurs in 0.2% of cases, usually after days or weeks of neuroleptic drug therapy. May be precipitated after abrupt withdrawal of antiparkinsonian drug. It is characterized by high fever, stiffness of body, fluctuating consciousness, autonomic dysfunction (tachycardia, labile BP, pallor). There may be leukocytosis and abnormal liver function tests. High CPK (due to myonecrosis) is highly suggestive of the diagnosis. Sometimes, metabolic acidosis, respiratory failure, cardiac failure, rhabdomyolysis and even renal failure may occur. Mortality is 20% in untreated cases and 5% in treated cases.

Treatment: (i) Stop the offending drug (ii) dopamine receptor agonist—bromocriptine, (iii) antispastic agent—dantrolene IV may be helpful and (iv) supportive therapy (hydration, reduction of temperature).

CASE NO. 023

a. Obstructive airway disease.
b. Pulmonary emphysema.
c. X-ray chest, HRCT scan of chest.

Note: Ratio of FEV_1: FVC is low, which indicates obstructive airway disease. Low ratio, reduced transfer factor of CO and high residual volume is highly suggestive of emphysema. HRCT scan is the most sensitive noninvasive investigation for diagnosis of emphysema. It is diagnosed by histological examination (not done usually).

Other causes of low transfer factor are pulmonary fibrosis, severe ventilation/perfusion mismatch, pulmonary edema, lobectomy, severe anemia.

CASE NO. 024

a. Henoch Schonlein purpura.
b. Serum IgA, skin biopsy.
c. Renal biopsy.

Note: Combination of abdominal pain, bloody diarrhea, arthritis and purpura or skin rash in a young patient is highly suggestive of Henoch Schonlein purpura. This is a small vessel vasculitis, common in boys of 5 to 15 years, but may occur in any age. It is characterized by purpura or petechial rash (in buttock and ankles), polyarthritis (in big joints), glomerulonephritis and gastrointestinal symptoms (pain and bleeding). If occurs in older children and adults, GN is more prominent. Acute abdominal pain may be due to intussusception. It usually follows upper respiratory infection. There is vasculitis, bowel is edematous and inflamed causing bleeding and obstruction. 30 to 70% have renal involvement with hematuria and proteinuria. Renal disease is usually mild, but nephrotic syndrome and ARF may occur. Only 1% develops end stage renal failure.

Diagnosis is usually clinical. Serum IgA is high in 50% cases. Skin biopsy may show leukocytoclastic vasculitis with IgA deposition. Kidney biopsy shows IgA deposition within and around the blood vessels. There may be focal and segmental proliferative GN.

Treatment: Usually self-limiting. Steroid is indicated, if there is GIT and joint symptoms. If renal involvement, pulse IV steroid (methylprednisolone) and immunosuppressive therapy. Prognosis is good in children, relatively worse in adults.

Adverse factors in adults are—presentation with hypertension, abnormal renal function and proteinuria >1.5 g/day.

CASE NO. 025

a. Gilbert's syndrome.
b. 48 hours 400 kcal restriction test, IV 50 mg nicotine (there is rise of bilirubin).
c. Reassurance, therapeutic trial with phenobarbitone 60 mg TDS. Avoid prolong fasting.
Note: In any young patient with recurrent jaundice, Gilbert's syndrome is the commonest cause. This syndrome is a type of unconjugated nonhemolytic hyperbilirubinemia. It occurs in 2 to 7% of normal individual, some cases may be inherited as autosomal dominant.

Most patients remain asymptomatic, diagnosis may be done as an incidental finding during routine examination. Jaundice is usually mild, occurs intermittently during infection or prolonged fasting. All other liver biochemistry is normal and no signs of liver disease. It is due to defect in the uptake of bilirubin by the liver and also there is deficiency of UDP glucuronyl transferase activity, the enzyme that conjugates bilirubin with glucuronic acid. Usually, no hemolysis, bilirubin in urine is absent, urobilinogen in urine is present. Liver biopsy—normal (may show increased centrilobular lipofuscin).

Treatment: Reassurance, avoid fasting.

Other causes of nonhemolytic hyperbilirubinemia are Crigler-Najjar syndrome (type 1 and 2), Dubin Johnson syndrome (liver is black due to increased deposition of lipofuscin and melanin), Rotor syndrome.

CASE NO. 026

a. Rhabdomyolysis with acute renal failure.
b. Urine for ammonium sulfate test, spectroscopic examination of urine to detect myoglobin.
c. Hemodialysis.

Note: Muscle injury due to any cause followed by acute renal failure is highly suggestive of rhabdomyolysis. In this case, clue to the diagnosis of rhabdomyolysis are history of multiple injury, followed by severe renal failure. Acute muscle destruction is called rhabdomyolysis, associated with high myoglobinemia and myoglobinuria. Myoglobin is highly toxic to the renal tubules and precipitates renal failure. Urine is red, but no RBC. Myoglobinuria gives a false positive dipstick result for blood (hemoglobin), which can be distinguished by the ammonium sulfate test. This test gives a colored precipitate with hemoglobinuria and colored supernatant with myoglobinuria.

Rhabdomyolysis is associated with high AST, CPK, creatinine, potassium, phosphate and uric acid. There is low calcium, because free calcium becomes bound by myoglobin.

Treatment: Supportive, such as adequate hydration, alkalinization of urine to reduce precipitation of myoglobin in the renal tubules. Dialysis, if renal failure. Nonsymptomatic hypocalcemia does not require treatment. Loop diuretics should be avoided, as they result in an acidic urinary pH.

Causes of rhabdomyolysis—trauma (crush injury), severe exercise, convulsion or epilepsy, electrocution, hypothermia, heat stroke, alcoholism, polymyositis, neuroleptic malignant syndrome, burn, septicemia, infection (influenzae, Legionnaire's disease), ecstasy or amphetamine abuse. Rhabdomyolysis is one of the important causes of acute renal failure.

CASE NO. 027

a. Giant cell arteritis (GCA).
b. Temporal artery biopsy.
c. High dose prednisolone to prevent blindness.

Note: In any elderly patient with unilateral headache associated with unexplained fever, arthritis, etc. with very high ESR, always think of giant cell arteritis or temporal arteritis. GCA is an inflammatory granulomatous arteritis of unknown cause involving the large arteries, predominantly affecting temporal and ophthalmic artery. Common in female (F: M = 4:1), 60 to 75 years of age, rare < 50 years.

Headache is invariable, mostly on temporal and occipital region. There is local tenderness; temporal artery is thick, hard, tortuous and tender. Jaw claudication, worse on eating, pain in the face, jaw and mouth (due to involvement of facial, maxillary and trigeminal branch of external carotid artery), TIA, visual disturbance, even blindness may occur. It is one of the important causes of PUO in elderly. Simple test is very high ESR and high CRP. ANA and ANCA are negative.

Temporal artery biopsy shows (i) Intimal hypertrophy, (ii) Inflammation of intima and subintima, (iii) Breaking up or fragmentation of internal elastic lamina, (iv) Infiltration of lymphocyte, plasma cells and giant cells in internal elastic lamina with necrosis of arterial media.

Biopsy from the affected site should be taken before starting or within 7 days of starting steroid. Whole length of the artery (>1 cm) should be taken, because the lesion is patchy or skip. Biopsy is negative in 30% cases, due to typical patchy nature of inflammation. Negative does not exclude the diagnosis.

Treatment: Prednisolone 60 to 100 mg/day for 1 to 2 months, then taper slowly (with the guide of ESR and CRP). To be continued for long time, 75% settle in 12 to 36 months. 25% may require low dose steroid for years. In some cases, steroid may be needed for lifelong. ESR and CRP are done, which are the markers of disease activity. Relapse may occur in 30% cases. May be difficult to taper the dose, then methotrexate or azathioprine may be added.

CASE NO. 028

a. Intestinal malabsorption.
b. Celiac disease.
c. Endoscopic small bowel (Jejunal) biopsy, serum antiendomysial antibody detection.
d. Dermatitis herpetiformis.
e. Howel-Jolly body, target cells.
f. Avoid gluten-containing diet.

Note: Blood picture is dimorphic (both macrocytic and microcytic), due to deficiency of both iron, folic acid and rarely B_{12}. Diarrhea, weight loss, abdominal discomfort, all are suggestive of intestinal malabsorption, associated with itchy vascular rash, which is due to dermatitis herpetiformis. All the features are suggestive of celiac disease.

Celiac disease is characterized by mucosal destruction of proximal small bowel due to hypersensitivity to gliadin fraction of gluten protein. There is atrophy of villi, crypt hypertrophy, infiltration of plasma cells and lymphocytes in lamina propria.

Antiendomysial antibody (Sensitive in 85 to 95%, specific in 99%) and tissue transglutaminase antibody (Anti-tTG) may be present in the serum. Antiendomysial antibodies are IgA antibodies, which may not be detected in patient with low IgA antibody level. Since celiac disease may be associated with IgA deficiency, it is important to analyze in coexisting IgA deficiency. Antireticulin antibody may be present which is very sensitive, but less specific. Antigliadin antibody is also less sensitive (not used).

Complications: Hyposplenism, gastric or small bowel T cell lymphoma, esophageal squamous carcinoma and small bowel carcinoma, ulcerative jejunoileitis may occur. Dermatitis herpetiformis may be associated with celiac disease. Target cells, Howel-Jolly body are due to hyposplenism.

Treatment: Avoid gluten-free diet (wheat, rye, barley, oat). Iron, folic acid, calcium, magesium should be given.

CASE NO. 029

a. Toxic shock syndrome.
b. Blood for C/S, high endocervical swab for C/S.
c. History of using tampons.
d. DIC.

Note: If menstruating female presents with burning micturition, multiple skin rash and high fever, likely diagnosis is toxic shock syndrome. It is characterized by local infection in genital tract by *Staph. aureus* producing exotoxin, which causes high fever, shock, diffuse macular rash, desquamation of palms and soles, widespread damage of multiple organs. TSS toxin 1 is responsible in 75% cases. Local source of infection usually from tampons used during menstruation. Blood culture is usually negative. DIC may occur.

Diagnosis is done by five criteria (i) Temperature >39°C, (ii) Widespread erythematous macular rash, (iii) BP systolic <90 mm Hg or postural diastolic drop, (iv) Source of localized TSST producing infection, (v) Evidence of toxic action on three systems—diarrhea or vomiting, myalgia or high CPK, drowsiness or confusion, high urea or creatinine, low platelet (<1,00,000).

Treatment: Management of shock, inotropic support, broad spectrum antibiotics (e.g. clindamycin, vancomycin, linezolid and flucloxacillin). High dose steroid and immunoglobulin IV may be given. Mortality—10%.

CASE NO. 030

a. Tricyclic antidepressant poisoning (TCA).
b. ECG, arterial blood gas analysis.
c. Gastric lavage, cardiac monitoring.

Note: Clue of the diagnosis is history of taking drugs, unconsciousness, dilated pupil, tachycardia are all suggestive of anticholinergic side effects of tricyclic antidepressant drug. TCA poisoning is characterized by drowsiness, confusion, delirium, hallucination, agitation, myoclonic fit, convulsion and coma. Pupil dilated, loss of accommodation. Reflex- exaggerated, hypertonia or spasticity. Plantar–extensor, divergent strabismus, retention of urine may occur. ECG–sinus tachycardia, QRS is prolonged, P is small, arrhythmia (SVT, VT).

There may be metabolic acidosis, respiratory failure. Most patients recover in 48 hours. However, in some cases, there may be persistent agitation, confusion, hallucination, rapid jerky movement which may last for several days.

Treatment: (i) Gastric lavage, if >250 mg tablet is taken. TCA cause delay gastric emptying, so lavage can be given up to 12 hours of poisoning, and activated charcoal may be given if the patient presents within 1 hour. (ii) Protection of airways and oxygen is given. (iii) Intravenous fluid. (iv) Cardiac monitor— if ECG shows prolong QRS (> 0.16 sec), arrhythmia may develop. (v) If epileptic seizure, IV lorazepam or diazepam should be given. (vi) For acidosis, sodium bicarbonate (50 cc of 8.4%) should be given. Lipid emulsion therapy in severe intractable poisoning may be tried. No role of forced diuresis or hemodialysis.

CASE NO. 031

a. Lactic acidosis due to metformin.
b. Serum lactate level, urine for ketone body, blood for pH.
c. IV isotonic (1.26%) sodium bicarbonate (high dose), IV soluble insulin and glucose.
d. Diabetic ketoacidosis, renal failure, renal tubular acidosis, salicylate poisoning.

Note: Clue for the diagnosis is diabetic patient on metformin, with severe metabolic acidosis and high anion gap. In lactic acidosis, there is high anion gap without hyperglycemia or ketosis. Mortality is >50%. Sodium dichloroacetate may be given to lower lactate.

Lactic acidosis may be of two types:

1. *Type A*—due to tissue hypoxia. It may occur in shock, severe anemia, cyanide or carbon monoxide poisoning, respiratory failure.
2. *Type B*—due to impaired hepatic metabolism. It may occur in diabetes mellitus, hepatic failure, drug (biguanide, salicylate), toxin (methanol, ethanol), hematological malignancy, severe infection.

Anion gap is calculated by = $(Na + K) - (Cl + HCO_3)$ in mmol/L. Normal value = 8 to 14 mmol/L.

Metabolic acidosis with high anion gap may occur in (i) diabetic ketoacidosis, (ii) renal failure, (iii) lactic acidosis, (iv) salicylate poisoning.

Metabolic acidosis with normal anion gap may occur in (i) renal tubular acidosis, (ii) diarrhea, (iii) ureterosigmoidostomy, (iv) acetazolamide therapy, (v) ammonium chloride ingestion.

❖ Normal cation in blood—Na^+, K, Ca, Mg.
❖ Normal anions in blood—Cl, HCO_3, albumin, sulfate, lactate, phosphate.

CASE NO. 032

a. Primary sclerosing cholangitis.
b. Ultrasonography of hepatobiliary system, ERCP or MRCP.
c. Liver transplantation.

Note: In long-standing inflammatory bowel disease, when there is biochemical evidence of cholestasis, one should exclude primary sclerosing cholangitis. 75% of primary sclerosing cholangitis is due to inflammatory bowel disease, commonly ulcerative colitis. The frequency of primary sclerosing cholangitis is inversely proportional to the severity of ulcerative colitis. About 3 to 10% cases of ulcerative colitis may cause primary sclerosing cholangitis, less in Crohn's disease. Other liver disorders in inflammatory bowel disease are fatty liver, pericholangitis, sclerosing cholangitis, cholangiocarcinoma, cirrhosis of liver, granuloma, abscess, gallstone, etc. P-ANCA is positive in 60 to 80%.

Patient with primary sclerosing cholangitis may be asymptomatic, but may present with advance liver disease. Fatigue, pain in right hypochondrium and pruritus are common complaints. Diagnosis is confirmed by ERCP that shows multiple stricture and dilatations in the intrahepatic biliary ducts. MRCP is another investigation of choice. Antibiotic prophylaxis before instrumentation of biliary tree is mandatory to prevent bacterial cholangitis.

Treatment: Supportive—Cholestyramine for pruritus, ursodeoxycholic acid, fat-soluble vitamins supplementation. Immunosuppressive such as prednisolone, azathioprine, cyclosporine, tacrolimus, MTX. Anti-TNF agent such as etanercept and infliximab may be given. Biliary stenting may improve biochemistry and symptoms. Orthotopic liver transplantation is the definitive treatment.

CASE NO. 033

a. Tuberculous peritonitis.
b. MT, chest X-ray, ascitic fluid analysis (cytology, biochemistry, AFB, PCR), laparoscopy and peritoneal biopsy.
c. SLE, lymphoma.

Note: Unexplained ascites, weight loss, diffuse abdominal pain, fever; bowel abnormality may be associated with intestinal TB with peritoneal involvement. It may be secondary to pulmonary TB. Ascitic fluid is straw-colored, exudative (high protein and low glucose, high lymphocyte and high ADA. AFB and PCR may be positive. Laparoscopy may show tubercle which is taken for biopsy.

Treatment: Anti-Koch's therapy, continued for one year. Steroid may be added.

CASE NO. 034

a. Pancytopenia.
b. Aplastic anemia, hypersplenism, megaloblastic anemia, aleukemic leukemia.
c. Pernicious anemia.
d. Bone marrow study, serum B_{12}, Schilling test, endoscopy and biopsy.
e. Due to immature red cells.

Note: Anemia with high MCV, pancytopenia and presence of vitiligo is the clue for the diagnosis of pernicious anemia. It is due to absence of intrinsic factor secondary to gastric atrophy resulting in deficiency of vitamin B_{12}. Parietal cell antibodies are present in 90% cases, intrinsic factor antibody present in 60%. Common in elderly above 60 years, more in females and blood group A.

There may be peripheral neuropathy, subacute combined degeneration, optic atrophy, dementia. Carcinoma of stomach in 1 to 3%.

In PBF, macrocytosis with hypersegmented neutrophil may be present. Bone marrow shows megaloblastic changes, reduction of precursor of granulocyte, megakaryocyte. There may be increased iron, bilirubin and LDH.

Pernicious anemia may be associated with vitiligo, Hashimoto's thyroiditis, Graves' disease, Addison's disease, alopecia areata, PBC, chronic active hepatitis, primary ovarian failure.

Treatment: Injection vitamin B_{12} 1000 µg IM, 6 doses, 2 to 3 days apart, and then 1000 µg IM every 3 months for lifelong. Following therapy, hypokalemia and also iron deficiency may occur.

Oral B_{12}, usually 2 mg/day may be given. 1 to 2% is absorbed by diffusion without intrinsic factor. Sublingual B_{12} may be effective.

CASE NO. 035

a. Wernicke's encephalopathy.
b. Injection vitamin B_1 250 mg IM/IV BD or TDS for 48 to 72 hours. Correction of dehydration and electrolyte imbalance. Add other B-complex.
c. Prothrombin time, serum vitamin B_1, CT scan of brain, endoscopy.

Note: In alcoholic, with repeated vomiting associated with confusion, drowsiness with eye abnormality, Wernicke's encephalopathy should be suspected. It is the acute cerebral manifestation of vitamin B_1 deficiency, commonly in long-standing heavy drinking and inadequate diet. Occurs after repeated vomiting, alcoholism, prolonged starvation or diarrhea.

Lesion may be in (i) Brainstem causing ophthalmoplegia, nystagmus and ataxia, (ii) Superior vermis of cerebellum causing ataxia, (iii) Dorsomedial nucleus in thalamus and adjacent area of gray matter, causing amnesia.

Common features are (I) **Cognitive change**—acute confusion, disorientation, drowsiness or altered consciousness. (II) **Eye change**—bilateral symmetrical ophthalmoplegia, bilateral or unilateral paralysis of lateral conjugate gaze, horizontal or vertical nystagmus, abnormal pupillary reflex. Rarely, ptosis, meiosis and unreactive pupil—(III) **Gait ataxia**—broad based gait, cerebellar sign and vestibular **paralysis.** When associated with memory disturbance and confabulation, it is called Korsakoff's psychosis. Loss of recent memory is common, but past memory may be normal. Confabulation means falsification of memory with clear consciousness. The patient makes new stories unrelated to truth.

Diagnosis is clinical. CT scan is normal and CSF also normal, but slight rise of protein may occur.

Treatment: Injection B_1, 500 mg IV over 30 min. TDS 2 days, then 500 mg IV or IM daily for 5 days. Then oral B_1 100 mg TDS and other B complex vitamins. If promptly treated, it is reversible. If not treated promptly, lesion may be irreversible.

CASE NO. 036

a. Paraneoplastic syndrome.
b. X-ray chest, CPK, EMG, CT or MRI of brain, muscle biopsy.
c. Treatment of primary cause.

Note: Bizzare neurological presentation, especially in elderly, is highly suggestive of para-neoplastic syndrome. This is characterized by multiple signs and symptoms associated with malignancy unrelated to metastasis. Actual mechanism unknown, causes vary according to the type of malignancy. Probable causes are (i) secretion of tumor product usually polypeptide, (ii) autoimmunity—cross reaction between tumor antigen and normal tissue antigen, (iii) release of cytokines (TNF α), (iv) myelitis—commonly in cervical cord.

Features: Varies with primary cause. Some are (i) Neurological—neuropathy, cerebellar degeneration, motor neuron disease, myasthenic myopathic syndrome (Lambert-Eaton syndrome), GBS, (ii) Musculoskeletal—polymyositis or dermatomyositis, clubbing, hyper-trophic osteoarthropathy, (iii) Endocrine SIADH, ectopic ACTH syndrome, hypercalcemia. (iv) Cachexia. Most are associated with carcinoma of lung (small cell), ovary, breast, pancreas, prostate, nasopharyngeal and lymphoma. Paraneoplastic syndrome may precede the clinical presentation of primary carcinoma in 50% cases.

Investigations: X-ray chest or other organ, USG of abdomen, CT/MRI, EMG, CPK, biopsy of muscles. Other investigation according to suspicion of cause.

CASE NO. 037

a. Polycythemia rubra vera (PRV).
b. Measurement of red cell mass (increased).
c. Venesection.

Note: This patient has high hemoglobin and RBC, also high PCV, which suggests polycythemia. There is nothing in the history to suggest secondary causes. High WBC and platelet count associated with splenomegaly are all in favor of polycythemia rubra vera. Differential diagnosis of high hemoglobin and high PCV are polycythemia rubra vera, pseudopolycythemia and also secondary polycythemia. In case of pseudopolycythemia, hemoglobin and PCV are high, but red cell volume is normal (which is high in PRV).

Polycythemia rubra vera (PRV) is characterized by increased hemoglobin, RBC, hematocrit, WBC and platelet. Neutrophil leukocytosis in 70%, basophil and platelet in 50%. Also increased LAP (leukocyte alkaline phosphatase), vitamin B_{12} and uric acid (may cause gout). Bone marrow shows hypercellular with increased megakaryocyte. Abnormal karyotype may be found in bone marrow.

In vitro, culture of marrow demonstrate autonomous growth in the absence of other growth factor.

In secondary polycythemia, only RBC is increased but WBC, platelet and plasma volume are normal. Also, red cell mass is normal.

Complications: AML, thromboembolism (cerebral, coronary), hypertension, gout, peptic ulcer, myelofibrosis.

Polycythemia may be (i) relative due to reduced plasma volume (e.g. dehydration, diuretic) or (ii) true.

True polycythemia may be primary (PRV) or secondary, which may be due to (i) high altitude, cyanotic heart disease, COPD, smoking, (ii) inappropriate and excess erythropoietin secretion (renal cyst, renal cell carcinoma, cerebellar hemangioblastoma, hepatoma, uterine fibroma).

CASE NO. 038

a. Psoriatic arthritis.
b. Skin biopsy from the lesion, HLA B_{27}.
c. Methotrexate.

Note: In any patient with skin lesion and ankylosing spondylitis, one should suspect psoriatic arthritis. 7% cases of psoriasis develop arthritis.

Types of arthritis in psoriasis. Five types—(i) Asymmetrical inflammatory oligoarthritis (of hands and foot)—40%. (ii) Symmetrical seronegative polyarthritis (like rheumatoid)—25% (no rheumatoid nodule and involvement of PIP, DIP, MCP joints, nail changes help to diagnose. 50% develop arthritis mutilans). (iii) Sacroilitis or spondylitis—15%. More in male, psoriatic lesion before arthritis and nail changes are usually present. (iv) Predominant DIP joint arthritis—15% (typical), nail dystrophy is invariable. (v) Arthritis mutilans—5%. Skin lesions with nail changes are usually present. Methotrexate, sulfasalazine azathioprine, leflunamide are helpful both in skin lesion and arthritis. In persistent peripheral arthritis, sulfasalazine, methotrexate or azathioprine may be helpful, but not in axial disease. Retinoid acitretin may be helpful in arthritis and skin lesion.

Other causes of arthritis and skin lesion are Reiter's syndrome, inflammatory bowel disease (there may be erythema nodosum, pyoderma gangrenosum), Behcet's syndrome, SLE, dermatomyositis, lyme disease.

CASE NO. 039

a. Blastic crisis, AML.
b. Splenic infarction.
c. Bone marrow study.

Note: Blastic crisis can be suspected when there is rapid deterioration, increasing splenomegaly and blood picture shows increase of blast cells, basophils. Blastic crisis may occur in chronic granulocytic leukemia (CGL). Commonly there is AML in 70% and ALL in 30%. It is very severe, may be refractory to treatment with bad prognosis. Treatment response is relatively better in lymphoblastic than in myeloblastic.

CASE NO. 040

a. Pernicious anemia, folate deficiency, carcinoma of stomach.
b. Endoscopy and biopsy, bone marrow study.
c. Hypothyroidism, chronic liver disease and alcoholism.

Note: Features of anemia with high MCV are suggestive of macrocytic anemia, due to deficiency of B_{12} or folic acid. Macrocytic anemia may also occur in hypothyroidism, chronic liver disease, alcoholism, etc. Bone marrow study is normoblastic in these cases. Thyroid function and liver function tests should be done. Oral B_{12} may not be effective in deficiency of intrinsic factor in the stomach. Associated folate deficiency should be considered also.

CASE NO. 041

a. Iron deficiency anemia, β thalassemia minor, sideroblastic anemia.
b. Hb-electrophoresis and serum ferritin.

Note: Here, blood picture is microcytic hypochromic, which may occur in iron deficiency anemia, β thalassemia, sideroblastic anemia and anemia of chronic disorders. Before giving iron therapy, other conditions should be excluded. In β thalassemia, there is defect in globin synthesis. In other cases, there is defect in heme synthesis.

CASE NO. 042

a. Euthyroid state.
b. FT_3 and FT_4.
c. Pregnancy, oral contraceptive pill, estrogen therapy, acute intermittent porphyria.

Note: In this case, patient's symptoms are due to pregnancy. Thyroid gland may be normally enlarged in pregnancy. So, her total T_3 and T_4 are high, but TSH is normal, which is common in pregnancy.

Any causes of high TBG will also cause high T_3 and T_4, but FT_3 and FT_4 will be normal. Alternately, any cause of low TBG will also cause low T_3 and T_4.

Causes of high TBG: Congenital or hereditary, pregnancy, drug (estrogen, clofibrate, phenothiazine), oral contraceptive pills, acute intermittent porphyria, acute viral hepatitis. Also in hypothyroidism.

Causes of low TBG: Hereditary, malnutrition, nephrotic syndrome, liver failure, drugs (sulfonylurea, salicylate, phenytoin, phenylbutazone, anabolic steroid, androgen, corticosteroid), active acromegaly. Also in hyperthyroidism.

CASE NO. 043

a. Pseudohyponatremia.
b. Repeat the test after ether extraction of lipid.

Note: In this case, there is high cholesterol and triglyceride, but the patient has no symptoms, which is the clue for the diagnosis. Pseudohyponatremia may occur in hyperlipidemia or paraproteinemia. Normally, sodium ions are distributed in aqueous phase of plasma, but in these conditions, volume of distribution of sodium ions is lower than the volume of the sample. Ether extract of lipid would give the real result. Also, in true hyponatremia, the patient would have more symptoms and also would be more ill.

CASE NO. 044

a. Acute pancreatitis, dissecting aneurysm, rupture of esophagus.
b. X-ray chest, ultrasonogram of hepatobiliary system with pancreas, serum amylase, endoscopy.

Note: Esophageal rupture or perforation may occur following severe violent vomiting or retching, sometimes following alcohol ingestion. It may be associated with subcutaneous emphysema, left-sided pleural effusion or hydropneumothorax. This is called Boerhaave's syndrome. The patient presents with severe chest pain and shock as esophagogastric contents enter into the mediastinum and thoracic cavity. Diagnosed radiologically by barium swallow with water-soluble contrast. Careful endoscopy or CT scan may be done.

Treatment: Surgery. Mortality is very high, if treatment is delayed.
    In dissecting aneurysm, there may be unequal pulse, aortic regurgitation, widening of mediastinal shadow in plain X-ray chest. Transesophageal echocardiogram is confirmatory.

CASE NO. 045

a. Addison's disease with renal tuberculosis.
b. Serum morning and midnight cortisol, synacthen test, urine for AFB and mycobacterial C/S (MT may be done).
c. Pigmentation, blood pressure in standing and lying.

Note: In any patient with weakness, hypotension, associated with low sodium and high potassium, is highly suggestive of Addison's disease. Long continued fever with weight loss, night sweating, etc. may be due to tuberculosis.
    Addison's disease is the primary adrenocortical insufficiency, due to destruction of adrenal gland, resulting in deficiency in glucocorticoid and mineralocorticoid. There is asthenia or weakness, hypotension and pigmentation. Supine BP may be normal, but marked drop of systolic pressure on standing may occur. Low serum cortisol and high ACTH is highly suggestive of Addison's disease. Causes are autoimmune (80%), tuberculosis. Rarely, hemochromatosis, sarcoidosis, secondary deposit, amyloidosis. Short synacthen test is helpful for diagnosis.
    Serum cortisol may be normal or inappropriately low. To find out causes, adrenal autoantibody, plain X-ray abdomen (to see adrenal calcification in TB), MT, USG or CT scan of adrenal should be done.

Treatment: Hydrocortisone 15 mg in the morning and 5 mg in afternoon (1800 hour). Mineralocorticoid may be necessary (9α fluorohydrocortisone, 0.05 to 0.1 mg daily). Steroid card should be maintained. Anti-TB, if suspected.

CASE NO. 046

a. Non-cirrhotic portal hypertension.
b. Doppler study of portal vein, venography of portal vein, liver biopsy to exclude cirrhosis.
c. Splenectomy.

Note: Huge spleen, ascites, normal liver but esophageal varices are highly suggestive of noncirrhotic portal hypertension. In this case, the patient presents with features of portal hypertension and variceal bleeding without cirrhosis or hepatocellular damage, no stigmata of CLD and liver function tests are normal.

Causes: Unknown, but arsenic, vinyl chloride and other toxic agents have been implicated. The liver disease usually does not progress and the prognosis is relatively good.

CASE NO. 047

a. Pregnancy with renal glycosuria.
b. Reduction of renal threshold.

Note: Patient's symptoms are due to hypoglycemia, following insulin therapy. Antidiabetic therapy should not be started on the basis of urine examination, as there may be renal glycosuria. Reduced renal threshold may be associated with glycosuria, which is common in pregnancy. Also, increased sensitivity to insulin occurs in pregnancy, especially in the first trimester.

CASE NO. 048

a. Pickwickian syndrome.
b. Hypothyroidism, sleep apnea syndrome.
c. Secondary polycythemia.
d. Type II respiratory failure due to alveolar hypoventilation.

Note: In any patient with obesity, sleep disturbance or sleep apnea with polycythemia, the likely diagnosis is Pickwickian syndrome. It is also called obesity-hypoventilation syndrome. Gross obesity is associated with respiratory failure. In most cases, $PaCO_2$ is normal, but may be high. Airway obstruction may be present, more in smokers. There is reduced respiratory drive. Serum leptin is high. Complications such as pulmonary hypertension and cor pulmonale may occur in Pickwickian syndrome.

Treatment: Weight reduction, smoking should be stopped. Progesterone may be given (which increases respiratory drive).

CASE NO. 049

a. Sick euthyroid syndrome.
b. Repeat FT_3, FT_4 and TSH after cure of pneumonia.
c. Obesity.

Note: This type of thyroid function may be confused with secondary hypothyroidism. He was always in good health and MRI is normal that indicates normal pituitary. So, the abnormal thyroid function is likely due to sick euthyroid syndrome. In any extrathyroidal illness (acute myocardial infarction, pneumonia, CVD), there may be abnormal thyroid function tests, even the patient is euthyroid, called sick euthyroid syndrome.

In other illness, thyroid functions are affected in several ways (i) Reduced concentration of binding protein and their affinity for thyroid hormones, (ii) Decreased peripheral conversion of T_4 to T_3, occasionally more rT_3 (inactive reverse T_3), (iii) Reduced hypothalamic-pituitary TSH production. So, the patient with any systemic illness may have low both total and free T_3 and T_4. Also, TSH is low or normal. Level usually mildly below normal and thought to be mediated by interleukins (IL-1 and IL-6). The tests should be repeated after recovery of the systemic disease, usually after 6 weeks.

So, biochemical thyroid function should not be done in patient with acute nonthyroidal illness, unless there is good evidence of thyroid disease (such as goiter, exophthalmos) or previous history of thyroid disease.

CASE NO. 050

a. Factitious hyperthyroidism.
b. Serum thyroglobulin (low or absent), $T_4{:}T_3 = 70{:}1$.

Note: Factitious hyperthyroidism due to self-intake of thyroxine may occur in anxious or psychologically upset patient. Clues for the diagnosis are high thyroid hormones, but low radio-iodine uptake. Thyroglobulin level is zero or low and high ratio of $T_4{:}T_3 = 70{:}1$ (typically, in conventional thyrotoxicosis, the ratio is 30:1). Combination of negligible radio-iodine uptake, high $T_4{:}T_3$ ratio and low or undetectable thyroglobulin is diagnostic.

Causes of high T_3 and T_4, but low radio-iodine uptake are found in subacute thyroiditis, postpartum thyroiditis, iodine-induced hyperthyroidism and factitious hyperthyroidism.

CASE NO. 051

a. Malignant hypertension.
b. Secondary aldosteronism.
c. Chronic renal failure.
d. Fundoscopy to see papilledema.
e. Burr cell.

Note: Malignant hypertension (also called accelerated hypertension) is characterized by high blood pressure, mainly the diastolic >120 mm Hg, with rapidly progressive end organ damage such as retinopathy (grades 3 and 4), renal dysfunction (proteinuria, renal failure) and/or hypertensive encephalopathy. Acute LVF may occur. There is fibrinoid necrosis in retinal arteries and arterioles. Unless treated, death may occur due to LVF, renal failure, stroke, aortic dissection. There is high risk of cerebral edema, hemorrhage and encephalopathy. Change in renal artery circulation leads to progressive renal failure, proteinuria and hematuria.

Treatment: Complete bed rest, sublingual nifedipine and oral antihypertensive (atenolol or amlodipine). Blood pressure should be reduced slowly over 24 to 48 hours. If BP is rapidly reduced, there may be cerebral, renal, retinal or myocardial infarction. IV furosemide may be used. In emergency, IV labetalol or glycerin nitrate or Na-nitroprusside or IM hydralazine may be used. Without treatment, 1 year survival is less than 20%. Renal function may be permanently lost in 20%.

CASE NO. 052

a. Hypothyroidism with pernicious anemia.
b. TSH, serum vitamin B_{12} assay, bone marrow study.
c. Pericardial effusion, anemic heart failure.

Note: Typical features, cardiomegaly and low voltage tracing is highly suggestive of hypothyroidism. This may be associated with any autoimmune disease blood picture shows pancytopenia which may be due to megaloblastic anemia. In pernicious anemia, there may be pancytopenia. Bone marrow study will show megaloblastic changes. Upper GIT endoscopy should be done to see gastric atrophy. Schilling test may be done.

CASE NO. 053

a. Taking the drug irregularly, insufficient dose, took thyroxine just before the test (occasionally, if antithyroid antibody is present, may interfere with the assay of thyroid hormones).
b. Hypothyroidism still present.
c. Thyroxine dose should be increased.

Note: In this case, the patient is still hypothyroid. High T_4 with high TSH indicates that the patient took thyroxine before the test and still hypothyroid. Presence of antithyroid antibody may also give abnormal result. For follow-up, in a case with hypothyroidism, only TSH estimation is sufficient.

CASE NO. 054

a. Polymyositis.
b. Heliotrope rash, proximal myopathy.
c. CPK, EMG, muscle biopsy.

Note: The patient has muscular weakness with pain and difficulty in deglutition, which are suggestive of polymyositis. Differential diagnosis is polymyalgia rheumatica. Both the diseases may present with muscular weakness, polyarthritis and tender muscles. However, high muscle enzyme and positive RA test, ANA and anti Jo-1 are characteristics of polymyositis.

Polymyositis is a connective tissue disease of unknown cause, characterized by nonsuppurative inflammation and necrosis of skeletal muscles. When it is associated with skin rash, it is called dermatomyositis. Cause—unknown, HLA B_8/DR_3, virus (coxsackie, rubella, influenza) are implicated. Common in female (3:1), 4th or 5th decade, may be associated with malignancy (10%), commonly oat cell carcinoma of bronchus. Heliotrope rash is pathognomonic. May cause renal failure due to myoglobinuria. Pharyngeal, laryngeal and respiratory muscles involvement may lead to dysphagia, dysphonia and respiratory failure. ILD in 30% cases, strongly associated with antisynthetase (e.g. Jo-1) antibody.

RA test, ANA may be positive. Anti Jo-1 may be positive in 30% cases.

CPK is typically high. EMG shows (i) Spontaneous fibrillation (at rest), (ii) Small amplitude, short duration, polyphasic action potential (after voluntary activity), (iii) Spontaneous bizarre, high potency salvos of repetitive discharge (on mechanical stimulation of nerve).

Muscle biopsy shows focal necrosis, regeneration and inflammatory cells infiltration. MRI may be used to detect abnormal muscles.

Diagnostic criteria: (1) Typical clinical history, (2) Increased muscle enzyme (CPK), (3) EMG findings (4) Muscle biopsy.

CASE NO. 055

a. Chronic granulocytic leukemia with chronic liver disease with portal hypertension.
b. USG of HBS, endoscopy, bone marrow study.
c. Blood transfusion, endoscopy with banding or sclerotherapy.

Note: This patient's presentation is likely to due to rupture of esophageal varices. There is huge splenomegaly with high WBC count, consistent with the diagnosis of chronic granulocytic leukemia. In CGL, the patient may be asymptomatic in 25% cases. There may be huge splenomegaly, anemia, repeated infection, bleeding manifestations, etc. Bone marrow is hypercellular with increased myeloid precursors. Philadelphia chromosome is positive in 95% cases. Philadelphia chromosome is negative in older male, which is associated with poor response to therapy, with median survival of <1 year. Blastic crisis may occur, which may be myeloid (70%), or lymphoblastic (30%). Myelofibrosis may occur. CGL may be associated with low LAP score, high uric acid, high vitamin B$_{12}$ and high LDH.

Treatment: Imatinib is the drug of choice, response in 95% cases.

CASE NO. 056

a. Nephrogenic diabetes insipidus with hypothyroidism due to lithium.
b. Water depletion.
c. Plasma and urine osmolality, serum ADH, serum lithium.

Note: Patient with polyuria, but normal blood glucose, diabetes mellitus is excluded. Other differential diagnoses of polyuria are cranial diabetes insipidus, nephrogenic diabetes insipidus and compulsive water drinking. The patient was on lithium. Likely diagnosis is nephrogenic diabetes insipidus, due to lithium. In this condition, plasma osmolality is high, but urine osmolality is low, which is not affected by desmopressin. In cranial diabetes insipidus, where plasma osmolality is high and urine osmolality is low, that increases following desmopressin therapy, toxicity of lithium may occur early, as therapeutic window is narrow. 95% is excreted in glomerulus, followed by tubular reabsorption in competition with sodium. During sodium depletion, more lithium is absorbed and in sodium excess, more lithium is lost. Toxicity is increased during diarrhea, vomiting, sweating, etc. Lithium level >2.0 mmol/L is associated with toxicity. Lithium may cause NDI, hypothyroidism, hyperglycemia, hyperparathyroidism, neurological complications (dysarthria, nystagmus, coarse tremor, seizure, hyperreflexia), renal failure and even collapse.

Treatment: The drug should be stopped, replacement of water and salt. Hemodialysis, if lithium level >3.5 mmol/L.

CASE NO. 057

a. Hypokalemic hyperchloremic metabolic acidosis.
b. Distal renal tubular acidosis.
c. pH of overnight urine, blood pH, ammonium chloride load test, plain X-ray abdomen (to see nephrocalcinosis).
d. Osteomalacia.

Note: Biochemical abnormality is hypokalemic, hyperchloremic acidosis, also low calcium and phosphate. These are consistent with renal tubular acidosis. It is characterized by severe metabolic acidosis associated with failure to acidify urine either due to defect in excretion of hydrogen ion by distal tubule or due to failure of absorption of bicarbonate by proximal tubule. There is failure of acidification of urine despite severe metabolic acidosis.

RTA is of 4 types:

Type-1: Distal tubular acidosis—common. There is acidosis, hypokalemia and inability to lower urine pH<5.3, despite severe acidosis. Causes are congenital (AD, AR or sex linked), autoimmune disease (Sjogren's syndrome, chronic active hepatitis, primary biliary cirrhosis, SLE), drugs (amphotericin B, lithium, NSAID, lead), amyloidosis, cryoglobulinemia, obstructive uropathy, renal transplant rejection.

Treatment: Sodium bicarbonate, potassium supplement and treatment of underlying cause.

Type-2: Proximal tubular acidosis—common in children. Causes are congenital (AD), cystinosis, Wilson's disease, tyrosinemia, glycogen storage disease type 1, multiple myeloma, hyperparathyroidism, drugs (degraded tetracycline, carbonic anhydrase inhibitor).

Treatment: Sodium bicarbonate in high dose, potassium supplement and treatment of underlying cause.

In PTA, there is proximal tubular defect resulting in aminoaciduria, glycosuria, phosphaturia, called Fanconi syndrome.

Type-3: Combined proximal and distal tubular acidosis (rare).

Type-4: Also called hyporeninemic hypoaldosteronism.

Patient with distal RTA may present at any age. In children, the patient presents with failure to thrive. Adult patient presents with renal colic, muscular weakness due to hypokalemia, osteomalacia, etc. Patient with proximal RTA presents with features of acidosis, polydipsia, polyuria, hypokalemic myopathy and rickets or osteomalacia. Diagnosis is suspected in any patient with hyperchloremic acidosis and can be confirmed by early morning urinary pH >5.5. In patient in whom the diagnosis is suspected, but no acidosis is present, an acid load test using ammonium chloride is done.

CASE NO. 058

a. Parasagittal meningioma.
b. Normal pressure hydrocephalus.
c. CT scan of brain, MRI.

Note: The patient has spastic paraplegia, but no sensory loss, more likely cause here is cerebral. It may be due to parasagittal meningioma (Falx meningioma), thrombosis of superior longitudinal sinus, thrombosis of unimpaired anterior cerebral artery, trauma. In childhood, commonest cause is cerebral palsy. No sensory loss, which indicates no spinal cord compression. Treatment—neurosurgery.

CASE NO. 059

a. Nephrotic syndrome due to rheumatoid arthritis.
b. Amyloidosis.
c. Renal biopsy or rectal biopsy.

Note: In long-standing rheumatoid arthritis, if nephrotic syndrome develop, amyloidosis is the likely diagnosis. It occurs as a complication of long-standing rheumatoid arthritis, usually present as nephrotic syndrome, sometimes chronic renal failure. The protein comprising amyloid is protein AA, which occurs in rheumatoid arthritis and other inflammatory conditions like inflammatory bowel disease, bronchiectasis, familial mediterranean fever, etc. This type of amyloid has a predilection for kidney, causing nephrotic syndrome, hematuria and renal failure. Usually normotensive, kidney may be enlarged and palpable. Splenomegaly, hypersplenism may occur. Rectal biopsy or involved organ biopsy is necessary for diagnosis. Amyloid stains red with Congo red and shows apple green birefringence under polarized light. Immunohistochemical staining can identify the type of amyloid fibril.

CASE NO. 060

a. Paroxysmal nocturnal hemoglobinuria (PNH).
b. Ham's acid serum test, flow cytometry to demonstrate CD 59 or RBC.
c. Deep venous thrombosis.
d. Due to reticulocyte.

Note: Blood picture with pancytopenia, hemolysis and dark urine (due to hemoglobinuria) is likely to be due to paroxysmal nocturnal hemoglobinuria (PNH). It is an acquired clonal abnormality of red cells, which are destroyed by activated complement resulting in intravascular hemolysis. Also, platelet and granulocyte are involved, resulting in thrombocytopenia and leukopenia. Commonly, the urine voided at night and in the morning on waking is dark-colored. Hemolysis may be precipitated by infection, surgery or iron therapy. Ham's acid serum test may be positive. There is tendency to thrombosis involving the mesenteric, portal (Budd-Chiari syndrome) or cerebral veins, also calf muscles. Cause of thrombosis is unknown, probably complement mediated activation of platelet deficient in CD_{55} and CD_{59}, resulting in hypercoagulability. Aplastic anemia may precede PNH in 25% cases and acute myeloid leukemia may occur. Other complications in PNH are increased susceptibility to infection, iron deficiency, pigment gallstone, etc.

Investigation: Flow cytometric analysis of red cells with CD_{55} and CD_{59} has replaced Ham's test. Bone marrow may be hypoplastic or aplastic.

Treatment: Supportive (blood transfusion, iron), prednisolone (in some cases). In marrow failure, antithymocyte globulin, cyclosporine or bone marrow transplantation. Recently, a recombinant humanized monoclonal antibody (eculizumab) may be helpful. Gene therapy. Survival—10 to 15 years.

CASE NO. 061

a. Microscopic polyangiitis, Wegener's granulomatosis, SLE (other Churg-Strauss syndrome).
b. P-ANCA, C-ANCA, ANA, anti-ds DNA, renal biopsy.

Note: In any disorder involving multiple systems of the body, always think of the above diagnosis. In Wegener's granulomatosis, the patient may consult with ENT or eye specialist. In chest, there may be migrating shadows, which appear or disappear that is seen in serial chest X-ray film, which may be confused with TB.

Renal involvement may occur specially in microscopic polyarteritis for which renal biopsy may be required.

CASE NO. 062

(See also case no. 45)
a. Addison's disease, salt loosing nephropathy.
b. Morning and midnight cortisol, serum ACTH, 24 hours urine for sodium, synacthen test.
c. Postural hypotension.

Note: Hyponatremia and hyperkalemia are typical of Addison's disease. Only hyponatremia is more important. Glucose may be in lower limit of normal. Low cortisol and high ACTH is highly suggestive. For investigation, first of all, test should be done to confirm Addison's disease, then other test to find out the causes. In some cases, high TSH and low T_4 may occur without hypothyroidism. With steroid, both TSH and T_4 revert to normal. Addisonian crisis may occur following surgery, trauma, infection, any major illness. Acute abdomen may occur. Other autoimmune diseases may be associated such as pernicious anemia, IDDM, vitiligo, primary ovarian failure, PBC, etc.

CASE NO. 063

a. Cushing's syndrome, primary aldosteronism, ectopic ACTH syndrome.
b. Cushing's syndrome.
c. Obesity, striae, plethoric face, skin is thin with bruise, proximal myopathy.
d. Serum morning and midnight cortisol, dexamethasone suppression test, ultrasonography of abdomen, CT scan or MRI of suprarenal glands.

Note: Hypertension with hypokalemia and diabetes mellitus is highly suggestive of Cushing's syndrome. In primary aldosteronism, diabetes mellitus is not common and hypokalemia is more severe.

To diagnose Cushing's syndrome, serum morning and midnight cortisol, 24 hours urinary-free cortisol, short overnight dexamethasone suppression test should be done, first to see whether Cushing's syndrome is present or not. Then further test should be done to find out causes (e.g. ACTH, X-ray chest, USG of suprarenal gland, CT or MRI of suprarenal glands and pituitary gland).

Pseudo-Cushing's may occur in depression, obesity and alcoholism. In these cases, there is increased urinary excretion of steroid, absent diurnal variation of cortisol and failure of suppression by dexamethasone. To differentiate from Cushing's syndrome, insulin-induced hypoglycemia is helpful. In Cushing's syndrome, almost no response, but in pseudo-Cushing's syndrome, there is excess cortisol secretion.

CASE NO. 064

a. Aplastic anemia, aleukemic leukemia.
b. Bone marrow study.
c. Blood transfusion.

Note: Blood picture indicates pancytopenia. Causes are aplastic anemia, aleukemic leukemia, megaloblastic anemia, hypersplenism, PNH. Cause may be found by bone marrow study.

Other investigation should be done according to the findings in bone marrow and clinical findings.

CASE NO. 065

a. Primary biliary cirrhosis.
b. Pruritus.
c. Antimitochondrial antibody.
d. Liver biopsy.
e. Orthotopic liver transplantation.

Note: Middle aged female patient presenting with pigmentation, cholestatic jaundice and hepatosplenomegaly, primary biliary cirrhosis is the likely diagnosis. Pruritus may precede the onset of jaundice by many years. PBC is an autoimmune disease, characterized by granulomatous destruction of interlobular bile ducts, inflammatory damage with fibrosis, cholestasis and eventual cirrhosis. Common in females, 40 to 60 years. Cause unknown, immunological mechanism plays a part. Environmental factor acts in genetically predisposed person. *E. coli* and other enterobacteria, retrovirus are probable triggering factors. Hypercholesterolemia is due to reduced biliary excretion, because of biliary obstruction. Xanthelasma and palmar xanthoma may be present, Osteomalacia is due to vitamin D deficiency resulting from fat malabsorption.

Antimitochondrial antibody is positive in 95% cases, antismooth muscle antibody is positive in 50%, antinuclear antibody is positive in 20%. There are 4 types of antimitochondrial antibody—M_2 (specific for PBC), M_4, M_8 and M_9.

Liver biopsy—infiltration of plasma cells and lymphocytes in portal tracts, granuloma (40%), and small bile duct destruction with ductal proliferation, piecemeal necrosis and cirrhosis.

Hepatic granulomas are found in PBC, sarcoidosis, TB, schistosomiasis, drug reaction, brucellosis, parasitic (strongyloidosis).

CASE NO. 066

a. Pheochromocytoma, drugs, food, clonidine withdrawal.
b. Urine for metanephrine, USG or CT scan of adrenal glands.

Note: Vanillymandelic acid (VMA) is a breakdown product of catecholamine. It is usually high in pheochromocytoma. Other causes are drugs (methyldopa, MAO inhibitor, phenothiazine, tetracycline), foods (tea, coffee, chocolate, banana, ice-cream, vanilla), clonidine withdrawal. Before performing VMA measurement, above drugs and food must be stopped. Also, antihypertensive drug should be stopped. 24 hours urine is collected for VMA measurement.

CASE NO. 067

a. Guillain Barre syndrome, Froin's syndrome, carcinomatous neuropathy, bacterial meningitis.
b. EMG, X-ray of vertebra, MRI of vertebral column.

Note: In this case, CSF shows high protein, but normal cells and also glucose. Very high protein in CSF occurs in Guillain Barre syndrome, Froin's syndrome, carcinomatous neuropathy, acoustic neuroma, meningitis (tuberculous, acute pyogenic, fungal).

CASE NO. 068

a. Infectious mononucleosis with hepatitis.
b. Paul-Bunnel test, antibody to EB virus, monospot test.

Note: Features of infections, hepatosplenomegaly, jaundice, high reticulocyte, low platelet are consistent with the diagnosis of infectious mononucleosis. This disease is caused by Epstein Barr virus. This virus infects and replicates in B lymphocytes. Transmission through oral contact. There is lymphadenopathy, splenomegaly, petechial rash in palate. Skin rash specially after ampicillin or amoxicillin occurs in 90% cases. In the peripheral blood, atypical lymphocyte is commonly found. False positive Paul-Bunnel test may be found in viral hepatitis, hydatid cyst and acute leukemia.

Causes of atypical lymphocyte are cytomegalovirus infection, toxoplasmosis, acute HIV or any viral infection can cause.

Complications: Commonly chronic fatigue syndrome. Rarely, mild hepatitis, thrombocytopenia, meningoencephalitis, myocarditis, hemolytic anemia, rupture of the spleen, etc.

Treatment: Symptomatic. Steroid may be indicated in encephalitis, meningitis, GBS, thrombocytopenia, hemolysis.

CASE NO. 069

a. Macrocytic anemia.
b. Bone marrow study.
c. Hypothyroidism, chronic liver disease, chronic alcoholism, (others are hemorrhage, hemolysis, azathioprine therapy).
d. Thyroid functions and liver function tests.

Note: High MCV with macrocytosis in peripheral blood film indicates macrocytic anemia. Commonly, it is due to B_{12} or folic acid deficiency. MCV >110 is usually associated with megaloblastic bone marrow. Macrocyte is found in the peripheral blood and megaloblast in the bone marrow. Macrocytic anemia may be found with either megaloblastic or normoblastic bone marrow.

Causes of macrocytosis with megaloblastic marrow—vitamin B_{12} or folic acid deficiency.

Causes of macrocytosis with normoblastic marrow—chronic liver disease, hypothyroidism, chronic alcoholism, hemolysis, azathioprine therapy, etc. In such cases, liver function tests and thyroid function tests should be done.

Hypothyroidism itself is associated with high MCV. But in 10% cases, autoimmune hypothyroidism may be associated with pernicious anemia. Drugs causing high MCV or macrocytosis are methotrexate, azathioprine, hydroxyurea, zidovudine.

CASE NO. 070

a. Hemolytic anemia.
b. Coomb's test, lymph node biopsy, bone marrow study.
c. Hodgkin's disease.

Note: High reticulocyte with high bilirubin, but normal liver enzymes indicates hemolytic anemia. In Hodgkin's disease, anemia may be due to autoimmune hemolytic anemia or bone marrow infiltration, which is associated with leukoerythroblastic blood picture. Hallmark in lymph node biopsy is presence of Reed Sternberg giant cell. Common age is adolescence and also after 50 years (bimodal). Pruritus may occur in 10% cases and Pel-Ebstein fever occurs in 10% cases. Before starting treatment, staging should be done, which will guide to therapy and prognosis.

CASE NO. 071

a. Septic arthritis. Gonococcal arthritis (or reactive arthritis).
b. Aspirated fluid for Gram stain and special culture for *Gonococcus*, urine C/S, blood C/S, high vaginal swab for C/S.

Note: In septic arthritis, there is high fever, leukocytosis, aspirated fluid shows high leukocyte, may be >50,000/cmm, glucose low and protein high. It is treated by—complete rest, NSAIDs, IV flucloxacillin (2 g 6 hourly). Joint aspiration may be necessary, occasionally surgical drainage.

Gonococcal arthritis usually involves large joints. Effusion may be present, associated with high fever and tenosynovitis involving the wrist, hand, feet and Achilles tendon. Skin rash is maculopapular at first, then pustular, then hemorrhagic and finally necrotic. History of urethritis, high fever, skin rash, arthritis of 1 or 2 joints, or tenosynovitis in a young person is highly suggestive of gonococcal arthritis. Routine C/S is negative.

Gonococcus is gram-negative intracellular *Diplococcus*. Organism is isolated by culture from urethral swab in man, and endocervical swab in woman, also from synovial fluid, blood, throat or skin lesion. In female, there is less symptoms and may act as a carrier. Gonococcal organism is difficult to isolate by culture. In disseminated gonococcal infection, organism is isolated from blood culture in <20%, joint aspirate 50% and from skin lesion 5 to 10%.

Treatment: IV ceftriaxone 1g daily for 1 week. Ciprofloxacin 500 mg 12 hourly may be given.

Causes of monoarthritis in young patient are trauma, septic, tuberculous, reactive arthritis, hemophilia, other seronegative arthritis.

CASE NO. 072

a. Restless leg syndrome (RLS) due to chronic renal failure (CRF).
b. Correction of iron deficiency, erythropoietin, dialysis must be proper, clonazepam.

Note: Restless leg syndrome (also called Ekbom's syndrome) is a common complication in chronic renal failure. It may occur in iron deficiency anemia. The patient has irresistible movement of limb.

RLS is a neuromuscular abnormality, characterized by discomfort or abnormal sensation in the calf or feet requiring irresistible and frequent movement of the affected limb. It is worse in the evening or at the onset of sleep at night, interfering with sleep. Commonly involves the lower limbs, may also involve upper limbs. Exaggerated by pregnancy, inactivity, caffeine, sleep disturbance, etc. It is common in normal population, 1 to 5% (average 2%) cases, in middle age. But frequency increases up to 20 to 30%, if occurs after 60 years. May be familial, in 1/3rd cases, multiple members in the family may be affected, occasionally inherited as autosomal dominant. When RLS is associated with iron deficiency anemia and CRF, it is called secondary RLS.

Treatment: Clonazepam (0.5 to 2.0 mg), levodopa (100 to 200 mg), dopamine agonist (pramipexole or ropinirole). Narcotics, benzodiazepine and anticonvulsant may be helpful. Treatment of primary cause should be done.

In CRF, correction of iron deficiency, proper dialysis, erythropoietin for correction of anemia. Kidney transplantation may cure the condition. Clonazepam and codeine phosphate may be helpful.

CASE NO. 073

a. Renal cell carcinoma with metastasis in liver and cervical lymph nodes.
b. Renal tuberculosis (or disseminated tuberculosis).
c. Hematuria and pain in the flank.
d. Renal mass.
e. Urine for malignant cells, urine for AFB, MRI of renal system.

Note: Hematuria with polycythemia with other features are the clue for the diagnosis of renal cell carcinoma or hypernephroma. It commonly presents with triad of painless hematuria, loin pain or heaviness and palpable mass in loin. Hematuria is present in 50% cases. In 20% cases, PUO may be the only manifestation, due to secretion of pyrogen by tumor. Usually, there is normocytic and normochromic anemia. Neoplastic cells may produce peptide hormones such as erythropoietin, renin, ADH, PTH-related peptide. There may be polycythemia due to excess erythropoietin, hypercalcemia due to bony metastasis or secretion of parathormone-like substance. Hypertension, hypokalemia may occur. The tumor is adenocarcinoma arising from proximal tubular epithelial cells, common in elderly, males affected twice more than females. In 10% cases, hypernephroma may be bilateral. Diagnosis is done by ultrasonography, IVP, CT scan or MRI.

Treatment: Radical nephrectomy that includes perirenal fascial envelope and ipsilateral para-aortic lymph nodes is done, if possible. Chemotherapy or radiotherapy is not helpful. Some benefit may be found with immunotherapy using interferon and interleukin-2.

CASE NO. 074

a. Thrombotic thrombocytopenic purpura, hemolytic uremic syndrome.
b. Renal biopsy.
c. Plasma exchange with transfusion of fresh-frozen plasma.

Note: Any patient presenting with fever, thrombocytopenia, microangiopathic hemolytic anemia and renal failure, differential diagnoses are thrombotic thrombocytopenic purpura and hemolytic uremic syndrome. The two conditions are probably the part of the same disorder. TTP is a disorder of unknown etiology characterized by fever, microangiopathic hemolytic anemia, thrombocytopenia, neurological signs and renal failure. Common in young females. Neurological features are common in TTP, which includes headache, seizure and coma. Neurological feature is absent in HUS.

Diagnostic pentad in TTP—(i) fever, (ii) thrombocytopenia, (iii) microangiopathic hemolytic anemia, (iv) renal failure, (v) neurological features.

Pathophysiology of TTP—initially endothelial damage, cell swelling, platelet adherence and thrombosis. There is severe microangiopathic hemolytic anemia with thrombocytopenia.

Renal disease is due to hyaline occlusion of capillaries and arterioles and proliferative change in glomeruli. Microscopically, there is microvascular hyaline thrombi. Thrombocytopenia is invariable. Also, there is increased reticulocytes, presence of fragmented RBC (schistocyte), prolonged bleeding time, raised bilirubin and LDH, reduced haptoglobin. Usually no DIC.

Treatment: Plasma exchange plus fresh-frozen plasma infusion. Steroid may be used in some cases. Platelet transfusion is avoided, as it may aggravate the disease. Mortality 90% in untreated, 10 to 30% in treated cases.

CASE NO. 075

a. Acute interstitial nephritis with ARF due to cefixime.
b. USG of kidney, renal biopsy.
c. Dialysis, prednisolone.
d. Renal biopsy.
e. Offending drug should be stopped.

Note: This patient presents with fever, skin rash, eosinophilia and renal impairment shortly after antibiotic therapy. These findings are consistent with acute interstitial nephritis. It is an acute inflammation of tubular interstitium, probably due to hypersensitivity reaction. It is characterized by fever, arthralgia, skin rash, bodyache and renal failure. There is also oliguria, salt and potassium loss, proteinuria, high eosinophil in the blood.

In urine, leukocyturia is common and eosinophils are high in 70%. Oliguria may be absent, despite moderately severe ARF.

Renal biopsy shows infiltration of eosinophil, polymorph and lymphocyte surrounding the tubules and blood vessels. Tubular necrosis may be seen. In some patients, linear deposition of IgG and C_3 along the tubular basement membrane may be seen.

Causes are (i) drugs (70%)—penicillin and NSAID commonest. Also, sulfonamide, allopurinol, cephalosporin, rifampicin, phenytoin, phenindione, diuretic (furosemide, thiazide), (ii) others—autoimmune, infection 15% (acute bacterial pyelonephritis, tuberculosis, CMV and hantavirus, leptospirosis), multiple myeloma, idiopathic 8%, tubulointerstitial nephritis with uveitis (TINU) 5%.

Treatment: (i) Prednisolone 60 mg/day, (ii) Offending drug should be stopped, (iii) Correction of electrolytes, (iv) Dialysis may be required.

CASE NO. 076

a. Bone marrow study, serum protein electrophoresis.
b. Waldenstrom's macroglobulinemia.
c. Plasmapheresis for hyperviscocity, chlorambucil or fludarabine.

Note: Waldenstrom's macroglobulinemia is a low grade lympho-plasmocytoid lymphoma, producing large quantities of IgM paraprotein. This leads to hyperviscosity syndrome (70%) as well as suppression of normal bone marrow activity. Plasma viscosity is high and protein electrophoresis shows IgM band.

Bone marrow shows lymphoid cells and prominent mast cells.

No lytic lesion in bone or no renal involvement (which are common in myeloma). Bence-Jones protein in urine occurs in 70% cases. Common in elderly, male slightly more than female. Median survival—5 years.

Causes of Bence-Jones proteinuria—multiple myeloma, Waldenstrom's macroglobuline-mia, benign monoclonal gammopathy, heavy chain disease, non-Hodgkin's lymphoma, CLL, amyloidosis.

CASE NO. 077

a. Hemosiderosis with CCF.
b. Anemia and cardiomyopathy due to hemosiderosis.
c. Serum ferritin.
d. Desferrioxamine.

Note: Features of CCF in hereditary hemolytic anemia, hemosiderosis is the likely cause. It may occur following repeated blood transfusion. Also, hemolysis may be a contributing factor. Iron is deposited in different parts of the body, especially in the heart causing cardiomyopathy, arrhythmia, heart failure, etc. Chelating agent such as desferrioxamine should be used to prevent this complication.

CASE NO. 078

a. Relapsing polychondritis.
b. ANA, biopsy of nasal or ear cartilage.
c. Prednisolone 40 to 60 mg/day.

Note: Recurrent ear, nose and eye involvement with progressive deafness is highly suggestive of relapsing polychondritis. It is an inflammatory disorder of unknown cause involving the cartilage, characterized by recurrent chondritis involving the cartilage of ear, nose, larynx and trachea. There is pain and redness of ear with progressive deafness, recurrent nasal involvement leads to saddle nose. Eye involvement causing conjunctivitis, episcleritis, scleritis, iritis. In heart, may be aortic regurgitation due to dilatation of aortic ring or destruction of valve cusp. Oral or genital ulcer may occur. Trachea and larynx involvement leads to hoarseness of voice, even stenosis may occur with difficulty in breathing. Acute focal glomerulonephritis may be found. This disease involves equally both male and female, common in elderly.

Investigations: Mild leukocytosis, very high ESR, RA factor and ANF may be positive. X-ray may show calcification of cartilage of nose, ear and trachea.

Diagnosis: Mainly by the history. Cartilage biopsy will show reduction of chondrocyte and infiltration of inflammatory cells.

Treatment: Nonsteroidal anti-inflammatory drug, prednisolone 40 to 60 mg/day, is the drug of choise. Dose is reduced with improvement. If no response, cyclophosphamide or azathioprine or cyclosporine, dapsone, MTX may be helpful. Reconstructive surgery for deformity of ear, nose or trachea.

CASE NO. 079

a. Leukoerythroblastic anemia.
b. Myelofibrosis.
c. Tear drop poikilocyte.
d. Bone marrow study and LAP score.

Note: In any elderly patient with huge splenomegaly and high WBC, differential diagnoses are myelofibrosis and CML. Myelofibrosis is a disorder of unknown cause, characterized by bone marrow fibrosis, extramedullary hemopoiesis and leukoerythroblastic blood picture, due to neoplastic proliferation of primitive stem cells. It is common above 50 years. There may be peptic ulcer, pruritus after hot bath, gout, etc. May transform to AML in 10 to 20% cases.

LAP score and uric acid are high.

Bone marrow study may be dry tap. Trephine biopsy is needed which shows increased megakaryocyte, increased reticulin and fibrous tissue. Initially, bone marrow is hypercellular, later fibrosis. Fibrosis is due to excess release of fibroblast stimulating factors from abnormal megakaryocyte, such as platelet-derived growth factor.

Treatment: Blood transfusion, folic acid. If leukocytosis, hydroxycarbamide (hydroxyurea) may be given. In young patient, bone marrow transplantation.

Radiotherapy for huge spleen. If evidence of hypersplenism and huge spleen with pressure symptoms, splenectomy may be necessary.

Median survival—4 years (1 to 20 years).

Causes of death: Cardiovascular disease, infection or GIT bleeding.

Huge splenomegaly and very high WBC may be found in both myelofibrosis and CGL, may be difficult to differentiate clinically. Differentiating points are:

Points	CML	Myelofibrosis
1. Blood film	High granulocytes of different stages	Leukoerythroblastic, tear drop poikilocytes
2. LAP score	Low	High
3. Philadelphia chromosome	Present in 90%	Absent
4. Bone marrow	Hypercellular with myeloid precursors	Fibrosis, stains black with reticulin

CASE NO. 080

a. Amiodarone therapy.
b. FT_3, FT_4.

Note: The patient has biochemical abnormality of thyroid function and he was on anti-arrhythmic drug, likely to be amiodarone toxicity. Long-term use of amiodarone may cause hyperthyroidism, hypothyroidism, goiter, etc. It inhibits the conversion of T_4 to T_3 in the periphery by blocking deiodinase activity. This results in low T_3, but high T_4.

Half-life of amiodarone is 28 days (may be 25 to 110 days). It does not impair ventricular function, so can be given in heart failure. This drug has delayed onset of action of 3 to 7 days, may take 50 days for maximum effects. Toxicity of amiodarone are corneal microdeposit, skin (slaty-gray pigmentation, hypersensitivity), thyroid (hypo- and hyperthyroidism), lung (allergic alveolitis, pulmonary fibrosis), GIT (nausea, vomiting, metallic taste), hepatitis, heart (prolonged QT, prominent U wave, torsades de pointes tachycardia). Others are neuropathy, myopathy, tremor. It potentiates the action of digoxin and warfarin. May promote digoxin toxicity by competing for digoxin binding sites, so increases plasma digoxin level, dose of digoxin should be half when amiodarone is given.

Amiodarone may cause prolongation of QT, which may be associated with ventricular tachycardia (or Torsades de pointes). In such cases, amiodarone should be stopped and IV magnesium should be given.

Patient on long-term amiodarone therapy should have an annual thyroid test, LFT and K co-estimation.

CASE NO. 081

a. Dimorphic anemia.
b. Combined iron and B$_{12}$ or folic acid deficiency, sideroblastic anemia, partial correction of anemia.
c. Serum iron and TIBC, serum B$_{12}$, folic acid, bone marrow to see ring sideroblast.

Note: Combination of macrocytic and microcytic anemia is called dimorphic anemia. Commonly, it is due to deficiency of iron, B$_{12}$ or folic acid. When anemia is treated, dimorphic picture may be found in the early stage. Sideroblastic anemia may also show dimorphic picture.

CASE NO. 082

a. Fundoscopy to see papilledema.
b. Benign (idiopathic) intracranial hypertension.
c. Iatrogenic Cushing's syndrome.

Note: Benign intracranial hypertension (BIH), also called idiopathic intracranial hypertension (IIH), is defined as symptoms of raised intracranial pressure without space occupying lesion or ventricular dilatation or focal neurological sign. It is common in young females, 18 to 40 years, obese, rarely familial. BIH may be associated with pregnancy, obesity, oral contraceptive pill, hypo- or hyperthyroidism, adrenal insufficiency, steroid use or withdrawal, drugs (sulfur, nitrofurantoin, nalidixic acid, tetracycline), hypervitaminosis A. The patient usually, presents with frequent headache and visual disturbance. 6th nerve palsy may be seen (false localizing sign). Usually no epileptic attack. Visual loss may occur due to optic atrophy. Lumbar puncture shows high CSF pressure, no other abnormality.

CT scan of brain is normal with no ventricular dilatation. MR angiography or cerebral venography may be done to exclude cerebral venous sinus thrombosis.

Actual cause of BIH is unknown, likely mechanism is reduction in the reabsorption of CSF by the arachnoid villi.

Treatment: (i) Weight reduction, (ii) Avoid offending drugs, (iii) Loop diuretics or acetazolamide may be given, (iv) Repeated lumbar puncture, (v) Occasionally, steroid may be used (it reduces intracranial pressure).

Surgical treatment: Ventriculoperitoneal shunt, especially if there is progressive visual loss. Optic nerve fenestration may be done.

CASE NO. 083

a. Acute cold hemagglutinin disease.
b. Hemoglobinuria.
c. Coomb's test and measurement of cold antibody (IgM).

Note: Features of hemolysis with hemoglobinuria after viral infection is likely to be due to cold hemagglutinin disease (CHAD). It is characterized by hemolytic anemia due to IgM antibodies (rarely IgA or IgG) directed against polysaccharide antigens on the red blood cell surface.

Hemolysis is due to cold autoantibody that reacts with red cells at temperature below 37°C (optimum 0 to 4°).

CHAD may be primary or secondary. Primary type occurs in adults, especially above 50 years and is rare in children. It occurs equally in both sexes. Secondary type occurs transiently in infectious mononucleosis, cytomegalovirus infection, *Mycoplasma pneumoniae*. Also, rarely in lymphoma, chronic lymphatic leukemia, SLE, Waldenstrom's macroglobulinemia.

Postinfectious CHAD is usually self-limiting, resolves in 2 to 3 weeks.

The diagnosis of cold agglutinin disease is made when the following are present:
❖ Presence of a high titer of cold agglutinins.
❖ Positive direct antiglobulin (Coombs) test .
❖ Other test to exclude *Mycoplasma* infection, infectious mononucleosis, or lymphoma.

Treatment: Avoidance of cold. Cytotoxic agents, cyclophosphamide and chlorambucil to reduce the production of antibody. Corticosteroid may be added. Rituximab alone or in combination with fludarabine, may be used in severe hemolysis not responding to treatment with conventional therapy. Plasmapheresis can be used as adjunctive treatment.

CASE NO. 084

a. Plummer-Vinson syndrome.
b. Koilonychia.
c. PBF to see microcytic hypochromic blood picture.
d. Serum iron, TIBC, ferritin.

Note: Combination of iron deficiency anemia, dysphagia and glossitis is called Plummer-Vinson syndrome (also called Paterson-Brown-Kelly syndrome). It is common in women, 4th to 6th decade, cause is unknown. There is constriction in upper esophageal sphincter in the postcricoid region and appears radiologically as a web. This web may be asymptomatic or may produce dysphagia. It may be difficult to see endoscopically. It is a premalignant condition, can predispose to carcinoma of esophagus, which needs to be excluded by endoscopy and biopsy. Blood picture will show features of iron deficiency anemia.

Treatment: Iron therapy. Rarely, dilatation may be required. If severe anemia, blood transfusion. Rarely, there may be squamous cell carcinoma.

CASE NO. 085

a. Dissociative (conversion) disorder.
b. Familial periodic paralysis.
c. Serum electrolytes, mainly to see potassium.

Note: In young female patient with no neurological abnormality, functional disorder is the likely diagnosis. In periodic paralysis, muscles are extremely weak with hypotonia and loss of reflexes. Sometimes, in dissociative disorder, there is rigidity, which increases more and more during more maneuver.

The term dissociative (conversion) disorder has replaced 'hysteria'. It is a disorder characterized by profound loss of awareness or cognitive ability without organic disease. Conversion means unresolved conflict is converted into symbolic physical symptoms as a defense against it, e.g. paralysis, sensory loss, abnormal movements, aphonia, gait disturbance. Dissociate means disintegration of different mental activity, e.g. amnesia, fugue, pseudoseizure.

CASE NO. 086

a. Hereditary fructose intolerance.
b. Measurement of glucose, after oral or IV fructose (will show hypoglycemia) and urine for fructose (fructosuria).
c. To avoid fructose-containing diet.

Note: GIT upset after drinking fruit juice is highly suggestive of hereditary fructose intolerance. It is an autosomal recessive disease. Symptoms develop after ingestion of fructose-containing diet. In infant, there is vomiting, retardation of growth, hypoglycemia, jaundice, hepatosplenomegaly, ascites, aminoaciduria, hyperuricemia, acidosis, etc.

Treatment: Avoid fructose-containing diets (e.g. fruits).

CASE NO. 087

a. Euthyroid Graves' disease.
b. TSH receptor antibody, orbital ultrasonography, CT scan of orbit.
c. Graves' ophthalmopathy.

Note: This patient has been suffering from Graves' disease, who is clinically and biochemically euthyroid. One should remember that the natural history of Graves' disease is hyperthyroidism, followed by euthyroid and later, hypothyroidism. Commonest cause of bilateral exophthalmos is Graves' disease, which may or may not be associated with other features such as diffuse goiter, dermopathy. Antimicrosomal (antiperoxidase) and antithyroglobulin antibody may be present in low titer. TSH receptor antibody (TR Ab) is high.

　　Causes of bilateral exophthalmos are Graves' disease, cavernous sinus thrombosis, caroticocavernous fistula, craniostenosis, hypertelorism, severe myopia, Hand-Schuller-Christian disease.

CASE NO. 088

a. Acute calculus cholecystitis, acute pancreatitis, splenic infarction.
b. Ultrasonography of abdomen, serum amylase.

Note: In hereditary hemolytic anemia, there may be pigment gallstone formation. There is splenomegaly and splenic infarction may occur, especially in sickle cell anemia in which repeated infarction may cause autosplenectomy by the age of 16 years. Gallstone may be associated with acute pancreatitis.

CASE NO. 089

a. Hyperchloremic hypokalemic metabolic acidosis with normal anion gap.
b. Distal renal tubular acidosis, ureterosigmoidostomy, acetazolamide therapy.
c. Distal renal tubular acidosis.
d. Hypokalemia.

Note: Usually, hypokalemia is associated with alkalosis. In some cases, hypokalemic acidosis may occur. Hyperchloremic hypokalemic metabolic acidosis with normal anion gap is common in distal RTA.

Anion gap is measured by $(Na + K) - (Cl + HCO_3)$. Here it is $(136 + 3.1) - (110 + 14) = 15.1$. Normal anion gap is 8 to 15.9. Other cause is bicarbonate loss in severe persistent diarrhea.

CASE NO. 090

a. Goodpasture's syndrome, microscopic polyarteritis, Wegener's granulomatosis, SLE.
b. P-ANCA and C-ANCA, anti-GBM antibody, kidney biopsy.
c. Goodpasture's syndrome.

Note: In young patient with renal and lung involvement, the commonest cause is Goodpasture's syndrome. Other causes are microscopic polyarteritis, Wegener's granulomatosis, SLE. In elderly, bronchial carcinoma with metastasis in the kidney or membranous glomerulonephritis may occur.

Goodpasture's syndrome is a clinical syndrome of glomerulonephritis and pulmonary hemorrhage mediated by anti-GBM antibody. It starts with upper respiratory tract infection, followed by cough, hemoptysis and glomerulonephritis or renal failure. The patient usually presents with recurrent hemoptysis and progressive, proliferative glomerulonephritis. In one-third cases, no lung injury, only glomerulonephritis is present. Lung hemorrhage is more in smokers.

Goodpasture's syndrome is more in males, age 20 to 40 years. Females are affected more, if it occurs after the age of 60. Systemic features like fever, malaise, arthritis, headache, weight loss are not common, but may occur. Hypertension is usually not a feature. Chest pain and pleurisy are also rare.

P-ANCA is positive in 30%, ANA is negative and complements are normal. Associated influenza A_2 virus may be found. Lung function test—Increased CO transfer due to pulmonary hemorrhage and restrictive lung disease may occur in advanced stage. In sputum, hemosiderin-laden macrophage may be present.

Anti-GBM antibody is positive (usually IgG. Occasionally, may be IgA or IgM).
Kidney biopsy shows proliferative or crescentic glomerulonephritis.

Treatment: Plasmapheresis and methylprednisolone (1 to 2 g/day for 3 days). Cyclophosphamide 2 to 3 mg/kg/day may be given. Occasionally, kidney transplantation may be considered. Recurrence may occur in transplantted kidney.

CASE NO. 091

a. Laboratory error.
b. The test should be repeated.

Note: When discrepancy between the clinical and laboratory findings is present, laboratory error should be suspected. If any doubt, the test must be repeated immediately before any therapy.

CASE NO. 092

a. Wilson's disease.

b. Serum ceruloplasmin, serum and urinary copper.
c. Kayser-Fleischer ring.

Note: In a young patient, if presents with prolonged jaundice or recurrent hepatitis or CLD or neurological features like involuntary movement or abnormal speech, etc. or psychiatric manifestations, Wilson's disease should be excluded. Wilson's disease is an inborn error of copper metabolism, inherited as autosomal recessive, characterized by failure of biliary excretion of copper and its deposition in and damage of different organs, such as liver, basal ganglia of brain, cornea, kidney and skeleton. There is less ceruloplasmin production of unknown mechanism.

Presentation—age of 5 to 30 years. In child, commonly hepatitis and in adult, commonly neurological features.

Liver diseases are acute hepatitis which may be recurrent, fulminating hepatic failure, chronic persistent hepatitis, chronic active hepatitis and eventually cirrhosis.

Neurological abnormalities are extrapyramidal (Parkinsonism, batwing tremor, dysarthria, chorea, athetosis, dystonia), cerebellar syndrome, dementia. Usually never sensory abnormality. Unusual clumsiness for age may be an early symptom.

In the eye, KF ring, commonly in 10 to 12 o'clock position (upper periphery), due to deposition of copper in the Descemet's membrane of cornea. It is greenish brown pigmentation at the sclerocorneal junction. Occasionally, seen by slit lamp examination, may be absent or less in young children, but always present in neurological Wilson's disease. Rarely, sunflower cataract due to deposition of copper in lens (does not impair vision).

Occasionally, the patient may present with psychiatric problem such as personality change, suicidal tendency, MDP, etc.

Investigations: (i) Low ceruloplasmin, (ii) High serum-free copper, (iii) High 24-hour urinary copper (Normal <40 mg, in Wilson's disease—100 to 1000 mg or 0.6 mmol/24 hrs). 24-hour urinary copper following penicillamine therapy >25 mmol is a confirmatory test. Hemolytic anemia, aminoaciduria or Fanconi syndrome, osteoporosis may occur. Liver biopsy with quantitative measurement of copper (high hepatic copper, usually not done).

Treatment: Penicillamine (drug of choice) or trientine. Zinc may be helpful. Liver transplantation in fulminating hepatic failure or in advanced cirrhosis.

Prognosis is excellent, provided the treatment is started before irreversible damage. Sibling and children must be investigated and treatment should be given, even they are asymptomatic.

CASE NO. 093

a. Polycythemia rubra vera with iron deficiency anemia.
b. Red cell mass, LAP score, serum iron and TIBC, bone marrow study.
c. Venesection.

Note: Clue for the diagnosis of polycythemia is high RBC, WBC and platelet. In this case, low hemoglobin, low MCV, MCH, MCHC and hypochromic blood pictures indicate associated iron deficiency.

Polycythemia rubra vera is the stem cell disorder in which there is excess proliferation of erythroid, myeloid and megakaryocyte progenitor cells.

The hematological findings in PRV are high hemoglobin, hematocrit and RBC. Also neutrophilic leukocytosis in 70%, high basophil and platelet in 50%. Others are high LAP score, high vitamin B_{12} and B_{12} binding protein transcobalamin 1. Iron deficiency may occur following venesection. Erythropoietin is low or absent (high in secondary polycythemia). Bone marrow shows erythroid hyperplasia and increased megakaryocyte.

PRV is common in males, after 40 years. Common features are hyperviscosity syndrome (headache, dizziness, blackout), pruritus after hot bath or with warm body. Plethoric deep dusky cyanosis, splenomegaly (70%), hepatomegaly (50%). Thrombosis (CVD, peripheral vascular disease) is common. There may be hypertension, angina, intermittent claudication and tendency to bleed. Peptic ulcer is common, bleeding may occur.

Red cell mass measured with radioactive ^{51}Cr labeled red cells—increased (>36 mL/kg in male, >32 mL/kg in female).

Diagnosis: Plethoric appearance, splenomegaly, increased WBC and increased platelets are highly suggestive of PRV.

PRV may transform to myelofibrosis (15%), acute myeloid leukemia and refractory state with anemia.

Treatment: (i) Venesection (400 to 500 mL of blood, every 5 to 7 days) until hematocrit is <45% and platelet <400 × 10^9/L, (ii) Radioactive phosphorus is reserved for elderly patient (5 mCi of ^{32}P IV, may cause acute leukemia 6 to 10-fold), (iii) Other drugs are hydroxycarbamide (hydroxyurea) or interferon may be used, (iv) Aspirin reduces risk of thrombosis.

Median survival—10 years, some 20 years.

Criteria for diagnosis of PRV—High red cell mass and normal PO_2 with either splenomegaly or two of the following:
  i. WBC >12,000/cmm.
 ii. Platelet >400,000/cmm.
iii. High B_{12} binding protein.
 iv. High LAP score.

CASE NO. 094

a. Von Willebrand's disease (D/D—mild hemophilia).
b. Serum vWF factor, platelet aggregation by ristocetin, factor VIII level.
c. Aspirin.

Note: Von Willebrand's disease is an inherited disorder of hemostasis. It is inherited as autosomal dominant, rarely recessive, equally affects both sexes. There is defective platelet function and factor VIII: C deficiency, which are due to deficiency or abnormality of vWF. Coagulation defect is due to the deficiency of factor VIII activity in plasma.

Bleeding tendency is usually mild, such as easy bruising, epistaxis, which follow upper respiratory infection. Sometimes, severe bleeding may occur, prolonged bleeding up to 36 hours following minor laceration, tooth extraction may occur.

Investigations: (i) Platelet is normal and prothrombin time is also normal, (ii) Prolonged both bleeding time and APTT, (iii) Failure of aggregation of platelet by ristocetin, (iv) Factor VIII:C activity may be reduced, (v) von Willebrand's antigen is reduced or absent, (vi) Tourniquet test is positive.

VWD is confused with mild hemophilia.

Differentiating points are:

Features	Mild hemophilia	vWD
1. Sex	Male	Male and female
2. Ecchymoses and epistaxis	Rare	Common
3. Traumatic bleeding	Delay onset, persist for days to weeks	Immediate onset, persist for 1 to 2 days
4. Bleeding time	Normal	Prolonged
5. APTT	Abnormal	Abnormal
6. Prothrombin time	Normal	Normal
7. Factor VIII:C	Reduced	Normal or reduced
8. vWD antigen	Normal	Reduced

Remember: vWF is a protein synthesized by endothelial cells and megakaryocyte. Its functions, (i) Acts as a carrier protein for factor VIII. So, its deficiency results in low factor VIII, (ii) Forms bridge between platelet and endothelial component (collagen), allowing platelet adhesion to damaged vessel wall.

CASE NO. 095

a. de Quervain's thyroiditis (subacute thyroiditis).
b. FNAC of thyroid gland.
c. Postpartum thyroiditis, factitious hyperthyroidism, iodine-induced hyperthyroidism.

Note: After any viral infection, fever with pain in the thyroid associated with features of thyrotoxicosis is likely to be due to de Quervain's thyroiditis. It is a virus-induced transient inflammation of thyroid gland, usually self-limiting thyroiditis. Commonly by Coxsackie B$_4$, also may be associated with influenza, infectious mononucleosis, measles, mumps, common cold. Common in females, 20 to 40 years. Presents with pain over thyroid, radiate to jaw, ear, worse by coughing, swallowing or movement of neck. Systemic features are common. Thyroid gland is enlarged and tender. FNAC shows presence of giant cells. ESR is typically high.

Inflammation of thyroid releases thyroid hormones, which are high in the blood, responsible for the features of thyrotoxicosis. This may persist for 4 to 6 weeks.

Iodine uptake is low, because damaged follicular cells are unable to trap iodine. Low titer of thyroid autoantibody appears transiently. Hyperthyroidism followed by transient hypothyroidism may occur. Complete recovery occurs in 4 to 6 months.

Treatment: Symptomatic (NSAID). Propranolol may be used. Prednisolone 40 mg/day for 3 to 4 weeks may be needed. Antithyroid drug should not be given.

CASE NO. 096

a. Acute lymphoblastic leukemia (ALL).
b. Bone marrow study, cytochemical test on blast cell.

Note: ALL is common in children, peak age is 1 to 5, whereas AML is 4 times more common in adult, lowest incidence in young adult life and there is striking rise over the age of 50 years. Clinical features are due to anemia, bleeding or infection. The patient may present with flu-like illness, bleeding manifestations such as purpura, ecchymoses, gum bleeding, epistaxis. There may be sore throat, mouth ulcer, herpes labialis.

For the diagnosis, blood film shows blast cells. Sometimes, blast cell count may be very low in the peripheral blood and bone marrow is the most valuable test for the diagnosis and the material is used for cytology, cytogenetics and immunological phenotyping. The marrow is usually hypercellular with replacement of normal elements by the blast cells.

ALL are of 2 types: (i) Precursor B ALL, (ii) Precursor T ALL.

CASE NO. 097

a. Hypogonadotropic hypogonadism.
b. Anterior pituitary, hypothalamus.
c. Pituitary tumor.
d. MRI of brain.

Note: Hypogonadism may be primary (in testis) or secondary (anterior pituitary or hypothalamus). Causes are:
  i. Primary—congenital (anorchia, Leydig cell agenesis, 5 α-reductase deficiency), acquired (mumps orchitis, tuberculosis, leprosy, castration, hemochromatosis, radiation or chemotherapy, cirrhosis of liver or alcoholism).
  ii. Secondary—hypopituitarism, Kallmann's syndrome (isolated GnRH deficiency), hyperprolactinemia. Causes of primary hypogonadism in females are (i) Turner's syndrome, (ii) Ovarian dysgenesis, (iii) Autoimmune oophoritis, (iv) Oophorectomy, (v) Chemotherapy, (vi) Swyer's syndrome.

CASE NO. 098

a. Leukoerythroblastic anemia.
b. X-ray chest, bone marrow study, CT scan (or ultrasonography of abdomen), MT.
c. Secondary deposit, lymphoma, tuberculosis.

Note: Leukoerythroblastic anemia is characterized by presence of immature myeloid and nucleated red cells in the peripheral blood, usually secondary to disturbance in the bone marrow. Key feature of the disease is presence of nucleated red cells.

Causes are myelofibrosis, secondary deposit in the marrow, active hemolytic anemia, thalassemia major (especially after splenectomy). Rarely, it may occur in multiple myeloma, lymphoma, Gaucher's disease, Niemann-Pick's disease, marble bone disease.

CASE NO. 099

a. Chronic lymphatic leukemia and autoimmune hemolytic anemia.
b. Increased reticulocyte count.
c. Coomb's test, bone marrow study.

Note: High WBC with predominant lymphocytes is mostly due to CLL. It is common in middle age and elderly. Clinical features are insidious, diagnosis sometimes may be incidentally done in routine blood examination. In CLL, anemia may be due to autoimmune hemolytic and bone marrow suppression by increased lymphocyte. Because of high lymphocyte, during preparation of smears, lymphocytes are deranged producing smudge cells or basket cells. Most of the lymphocytes are B type. Not all cases or even high WBC is not an indication for therapy. Patient who presents with low platelets has advanced disease and a poor prognosis rarely, CLL may transform to high grade lymphoma called Richter's transformation.

Treatment: Depends on stage. It is necessary when evidence of marrow failure, massive or progressive lymphadenopathy or splenomegaly, symptoms (weight loss, night sweat), rapidly increasing lymphocyte, etc. Usually, oral chlorambucil is given. Fludarabine is also helpful. If there is bone marrow failure or autoimmune hemolytic anemia, steroid may be given. Other treatment is radiotherapy for huge lymphadenopathy causing obstruction or discomfort, also for symptomatic splenomegaly. Sometimes, splenectomy may be necessary for autoimmune hemolytic anemia or hypersplenism.

Median survival—5 to 6 years, depending on stage.

CASE NO. 100

a. Serum morning and midnight cortisol serum ACTH, dexamethasone suppression test, CT scan of adrenal glands.
b. Cushing's syndrome.
c. BP, hirsutism, striae.
d. History of steroid intake.

Note: Combination of diabetes mellitus, hypokalemic alkalosis, hypertension, obesity, polycythemia is highly suggestive of Cushing's syndrome. If there is weight loss, severe muscular weakness, more pigmentation and severe hypokalemic alkalosis, it is suggestive of ectopic ACTH syndrome. High ACTH >200 ng/L and high cortisol >1000 nmol/L is highly suggestive of ectopic ACTH syndrome.

In Cushing's syndrome, first of all, investigation should be done to confirm the diagnosis, then other investigations should be done to find out the causes.

CASE NO. 101

a. DIC with microangiopathic hemolytic anemia with iron deficiency anemia with septicemia.
b. Septicemia, retained product of conception or amniotic fluid embolism.

Note: Thrombocytopenia with prolonged prothrombin time and APTT, low fibrinogen is likely to be due to DIC. It is a hemorrhagic disorder in which diffuse intravascular clotting causes a hemostatic defect resulting from utilization of coagulation factor and platelet in the clotting process. For this reason, this is also called consumption coagulopathy. There is secondary activation of fibrinolysis, leading to production of fibrin degradation products (FDP). The consequence of these changes is a mixture of initial thrombosis, followed by bleeding tendency due to consumption of coagulation factors and fibrinolytic activity.

Causes of DIC are (i) obstetrical (abruptio placenta, amniotic fluid embolism, abortion), (ii) surgery (especially heart and lung), (iii) hemolytic transfusion reaction, (iv) septicemia (which is due to gram-negative and meningococcal), (v) pulmonary embolism, (vi) others are falciparum malaria, malignant disease, liver disease, trauma, burn, snake bite, heat stroke, etc. Chronic DIC may occur in (i) acute leukemia (usually promyelocytic), (ii) IUD, (iii) septicemia, (iv) disseminated malignancy.

CASE NO. 102

a. SLE.
b. Echocardiography, ANA, anti-ds DNA.
c. Antiphospholipid syndrome.

Note: Clue for the diagnosis of SLE in this case are high ESR, low platelet and X-ray features of pericardial effusion. In a patient with SLE, if associated with antiphospholipid syndrome, there may be persistent bleeding following delivery. Other systemic features including pericardial effusion are highly suggestive of SLE. Other causes to be excluded are tuberculosis, myxedema (though in these cases, there will be no thrombocytopenia).

CASE NO. 103

a. Senile purpura, scurvy, drug-induced purpura, paraproteinemia, amyloidosis.
b. Arterial biopsy.

Note: Non-thrombocytopenic purpura or bleeding or bruise or ecchymoses may occur following vascular defect.

Causes are senile purpura, drugs (NSAID, steroid), Henoch-Schonlein purpura, Cushing's syndrome, Ehlers-Danlos syndrome, pseudoxanthoma elasticum.

CASE NO. 104
(See also case no. 85)
a. Dissociative (conversion) disorder.
b. Reassurance, sedation, followed by psychotherapy.

Note: In any young patient, there may be HCR or panic attack presenting as difficulty in breathing. Because of hyperventilation, there is respiratory alkalosis and tetany.

Reassurance, sedation followed by psychotherapy is important.

CASE NO. 105

a. Myasthenia gravis, opium poisoning.
b. For myasthenia gravis, IV edrophonium bromide 10 mg.
   For opium poisoning, IV naloxone.

Note: Edrophonium IV relieves the symptoms of myasthenia gravis in 30 seconds. This is also used as a test called Tensilon test for the diagnosis of myasthenia gravis. Naloxone is an antidote to opium, which counteracts the action of opium.

Tensilon test—2 mg edrophonium bromide IV. If no side effect, 8 mg IV after half minute is given. Symptoms improve in 30 seconds, last for 2 to 3 minutes. This test should be done where there is resuscitation facility. It can cause bronchoconstriction and syncope.

CASE NO. 106
a. SLE.
b. ANA, anti-ds DNA.

Note: Blood picture is suggestive of ITP. However, splenomegaly is not common in ITP. Sometimes, SLE may present initially as ITP. Later on, other manifestations of SLE may occur. In any patient presenting as ITP, SLE must be excluded.

CASE NO. 107
a. Syndrome of inappropriate ADH secretion (SIADH) with tuberculous meningitis (or bronchial carcinoma).

b. X-ray chest, plasma and urine osmolality, CT scan or MRI of brain.
c. Restriction of water.

Other investigations: Serum ADH, water load test (oral water 20 mL/kg given. Urine collected for next 5 hours. In SIADH, there is impaired excretion of water. Normally, 80% water is excreted).

Note: In SIADH, clue for the diagnosis is everything in serum may be low (such as low sodium, chloride, bicarbonate, urea, creatinine, total protein, uric acid, etc.). Plasma renin and aldosterone are also low. Usually no hypokalemia, no edema, no hypertension or no postural hypotension. Plasma osmolality is low, urine osmolality is high, urine sodium is high (>30 mmol/L).

Treatment: (i) Restriction of water (500 to 1000 mL daily), (ii) Demeclocycline 900 to 1200 mg daily may be used to make iatrogenic nephrogenic diabetes insipidus. (iii) Occasionally, hypertonic saline 5% 200 cc may be given plus furosemide IV (hypertonic saline may be dangerous, may cause central pontine myelinolysis). (iv) Treatment of the primary cause should be done.

The commonest cause of SIADH—oat cell carcinoma of lung.

CASE NO. 108

a. Hemolytic uremic syndrome.
b. PBF to see schistocyte or fragmented RBC, serum FDP, serum electrolytes.

Note: Hemolytic uremic syndrome (HUS) is characterized by rapid onset of microangiopathic hemolytic anemia, thrombocytopenia and acute renal failure (triad) due to thrombosis in small arteries and arteriole. HUS is caused by verotoxin-producing organism, such as enterotoxigenic *E. coli* 0157 and H7. It occurs in up to 6% patients infected with this organism, by infected food (undercooked beef) or unpasteurized milk. The organisms excrete a toxin, responsible for the gastrointestinal effect, such as colicky abdominal pain diarrhea, may be bloody.

Pathogenesis: Infection triggers damage to the endothelial cells of microcirculation and derangement of hemostatic coagulation system. This is followed by cell swelling, platelet clumping, fibrinogen deposition, thrombosis and occlusion. Common in glomerular capillaries and renal arterioles. Other features are intravascular hemolysis, high bilirubin, high LDH, reduced haptoglobin and increased reticulocyte count. Confused with DIC, but coagulation tests are normal in HUS.

The HUS is common in children, <3 years. It usually follows upper respiratory tract or gastrointestinal infection. There is fever, vomiting and diarrhea, often bloody called diarrhea associated HUS (D-HUS). Intravascular hemolysis is followed by oliguria or anuria. Purpura, anemia, bleeding, drowsiness and hypertension may occur.

Peripheral blood film shows schistocyte, spherocyte and thrombocytopenia.

Treatment: Supportive (transfusion, hydration, control of hypertension), FFP, plasmapheresis, dialysis. Heparin or antiplatelet drug may be helpful. No role of antibiotic. 5% die in acute episode, 5% develop CRF and 30% develop persistent proteinuria.

CASE NO. 109

a. Porphyria cutanea tarda (PCT).
b. Serum ferritin, liver biopsy.
c. Use sunscreen, alcohol must be stopped.

Note: Blistering skin lesion associated with biochemical evidence of liver disease is suggestive of PCT. It is the commonest porphyria, may be hereditary (autosomal dominant) or sporadic, due to abnormality of hepatic uroporphyrinogen decarboxylase, which catalyzes the conversion of uroporphyrin to coproporphyrin.

PCT may be acquired in cirrhosis of liver, benign or malignant hepatic tumor, chronic alcoholism. May be precipitated by hepatitis C, HIV, iron overload, estrogen therapy.

The patient presents with painless bullous eruption or blister on dorsal surface of hands. This may be followed by scarring. Also, there is hypertrichosis and hyperpigmentation. Abnormal liver functions, high iron and high transferrin saturation may occur. Liver biopsy will show evidence of CLD and iron stain will show iron overload.

Features of porphyria cutanea tarda are (i) Urine shows coral pink fluorescence under Wood's light, (ii) Urine total uroporphyrin is increased, (iii) Stool for coproporphyrin is increased, (iv) Urine α ALA is increased, (v) Biopsy of local skin lesion shows subepidermal blister, (vi) Liver function test—abnormal, (vii) Serum ferritin—high. Blisters on the skin lesion contain PAS-positive material.

Treatment: Treatment of primary cause. Sunscreen, venesection—one unit every 2 to 4 weeks, until hemoglobin is <12 g/dL, low dose chloroquine or hydroxychloroquine—200 mg twice weekly (it increases urinary excretion of porphyrin). Desferrioxamine is given, if ferritin is high. Alcohol must be stopped.

CASE NO. 110

a. Pseudopolycythemia.
b. Red cell mass and plasma volume.
c. Venesection.

Note: In pseudopolycythemia, both Hb and PCV are high due to hemoconcentration resulting from any cause of reduced extracellular volume (dehydration or diuretic therapy). A type of pseudopolycythemia, also called Gaisbock's syndrome, is a disorder of unknown etiology. It is also called polycythemia of stress, as half of the patients are in anxiety state or neurotic. Common in middle-aged males and have a smoking history, associated with obesity, hypertension, peripheral vascular disease. It may cause myocardial infarction, cerebral ischemia. In this type of polycythemia, only red cells are high and WBC and platelet are normal, plasma volume is low and red cell mass is normal (in contrast to PRV, red cell mass and plasma volume are high, other cells such as WBC and platelet are also high).

Treatment: Venesection. Smoking must be stopped.

CASE NO. 111

a. Hypokalemic alkalosis.
b. Hypomagnesemia.

Note: Tetany may occur secondary to metabolic alkalosis, hypocalcemia, hypomagnesemia or hypokalemic alkalosis. Never forget hypomagnesemia as a cause of tetany other than hypocalcemia.

Features of hypomagnesemia are mostly neurological such as tremor, chorea, confusion, agitation, fit, hallucination, etc.

Causes of hypomagnesemia are prolonged diarrhea, less intake as in protein calorie malnutrition, prolonged parenteral nutrition without magnesium, vomiting, aspiration, fistula, laxative abuse, renal loss in diabetic ketoacidosis, renal tubular acidosis, diuretic phase of acute tubular necrosis. Others are chronic alcoholism, hyperparathyroidism, primary aldosteronism, Bartter's syndrome, acute pancreatitis, drugs (loop diuretic, cisplatin, gentamicin).

Treatment: It should be corrected by giving IV infusion of magnesium.

CASE NO. 112

a. Left renal vein thrombosis.
b. Left renal artery embolism.
c. Ultrasonogram of kidney, isotope renogram, IVP (also Doppler ultrasound study of renal veins).

Note: In nephrotic syndrome, if there is loin pain, hematuria and deterioration of renal function, it is highly suggestive of renal vein thrombosis.

In nephrotic syndrome, there is hyperlipidemia, commonly high LDL and cholesterol, high VLDL and triglyceride. So, more atherosclerosis. There is hypercoagulable state due to increased fibrinogen and factor VIII, also reduction of antithrombin III. Thrombosis may occur, especially in renal vein. Other complications in nephrotic syndrome are loss of TBG resulting in low T_3 and T_4, loss of transferrin and iron, loss of vitamin D binding protein, infection such as pneumococcal peritonitis and septicemia.

Renal vein thrombosis is more common membranous nephropathy, mesangiocapillary glomerulonephritis and amyloidosis.

Factors for thrombosis in nephrotic syndrome are (i) Loss of fibrinolytic factors in urine commonly antithrombin III, also protein C and S, plasminogen, (ii) Increased synthesis of clotting factors—factor V, VIII and fibrinogen, (iii) Thrombocytosis, (iv) Over diuresis causes dehydration, reducing renal blood flow and increasing viscosity.

CASE NO. 113

a. Catheterization to evacuate the urinary bladder.
b. Hyponatremia.
c. Water intoxication secondary to psychogenic water drinking.
d. Restriction of water intake.

Note: Catheterization to evacuate the urinary bladder is the first therapeutic measure to be done. Then correction of electrolyte imbalance. Excess intake of water is due to polydipsia, resulting in dilutional hyponatremia. It may be confused with SIADH, but polydipsia and polyuria are not common in SIADH.

CASE NO. 114

a. Tertiary hyperparathyroidism.
b. Serum parathormone, X-ray of bone (skull, hands), isotope bone scan.
c. Parathyroidectomy.
d. Renal osteodystrophy.

Note: Tertiary hyperparathyroidism means development of apparently autonomous parathyroid hyperplasia after long-standing secondary hyperparathyroidism. In this case, CRF is the cause. In tertiary hyperparathyroidism, serum calcium and phosphate are very high, latter is more.

USG, CT scan, MRI of the parathyroid gland may be done. Renal osteodystrophy is a group of metabolic bone disease in chronic renal failure, which consists of osteoporosis, osteomalacia, osteosclerosis and osteitis fibrosa cystica.

Treatment: Parathyroidectomy is usually done.

CASE NO. 115

a. Hereditary angioedema.
b. Serum C_2 and C_4, C_1 esterase inhibitor (C_1-INH) measurement.

Note: Hereditary angioedema, inherited as autosomal dominant, is due to deficiency of C_1 esterase inhibitor (C_1-INH), a component of complement system. As a result, there is uncontrolled activation of C_1. It is characterized by angioedema in skin, larynx but no urticaria, no itching. There may be recurrent acute abdomen (due to intestinal edema).

Rarely, this condition may be acquired, associated with lymphoma or SLE. However, in such cases, there are low C_1-INH and also low C_1, C_2. Acquired form usually occurs in older age.

Diagnosis: Common in late childhood or early adolescence. Attack may follow trauma, infection, dental procedures or emotional stress. Also, there is increasing frequency and severity during puberty, menstruation and ovulation. Usually family history is present. Patient can present with any combination of cutaneous angioedema, abdominal pain or acute airway obstruction. Serum C_4 and C_2 are low, but C_1 and C_3 are normal. Barium meal and follow-through show intestinal sacked coin appearance during attack. Confirmed by measurement of serum C_1-INH.

Treatment: Purified C_1-INH infusion during acute attack. Fresh-frozen plasma may be used. Steroid and adrenaline are ineffective.

For prevention, danazol or stanozolol may be given, which increase C_1-INH, C_2 and C_4 by hepatic synthesis.

CASE NO. 116

a. History of taking steroid.
b. Secondary adrenocortical failure.
c. MRI of pituitary fossa, USG or CT scan of adrenal gland.

Note: Progressive increase of cortisol after high dose dexamethasone is typical of secondary adrenocortical failure. This may be due to prolonged use of steroid. However, disease secondary to pituitary may also cause this type of response.

CASE NO. 117

a. Microcytic hypochromic with leukoerythroblastic blood picture.
b. Venesection and transformation to myelofibrosis.
c. Venesection.

Note: In PRV, depletion of iron store or iron deficiency is usual. After venesection, iron deficiency occurs. Peptic ulcer is also common, hematemesis may occur. Venesection should be done carefully if platelet count is very high, because of risk of thrombosis. PRV may transform to refractory anemia, myelofibrosis or acute leukemia.

CASE NO. 118

a. Nephrogenic diabetes insipidus (NDI).
b. History of intake of lithium.

Note: During water deprivation test, normally urine osmolality should rise. In nephrogenic diabetes insipidus, there is impairment of active chloride transport in the ascending loop of Henle. Following desmopressin, failure to concentrate urine indicates renal insensitivity to ADH. In NDI, there is insensitivity of the renal tubule to ADH. In cranial diabetes insipidus, there is also failure to rise the urine osmolality during water deprivation test, but following desmopressin, there is rise of urine osmolality.

Causes of NDI: (i) Familial or hereditary, (ii) Drugs—lithium, demeclocycline, glibenclamide, (iii) Hypokalemia and hypercalcemia (act in part by antagonizing the effects of desmopressin on the collecting duct), (iv) Sickle cell disease, (v) Idiopathic.

CASE NO. 119

a. Giant cell arteritis (GCA).
b. Temporal artery biopsy.
c. Infective endocarditis, disseminated tuberculosis, SLE, para-neoplastic syndrome.

Note: Giant cell arteritis or temporal arteritis is an important cause of PUO in elderly. Giant cell arteritis and polymyalgia rheumatica may present either separately or in combination, involves large artery with an internal elastic component causing arterial occlusion. Unilocular blindness may occur due to retinal artery occlusion, binocular blindness may also occur. Visual loss in 25% cases. Posterior ciliary artery occlusion causes acute anterior ischemic optic neuropathy, the disk is pale and swollen. GCA can cause sudden blindness, brainstem ischemia, cortical blindness, TIA and stroke (see also Case No. 27).

CASE NO. 120

a. Primary hyperparathyroidism.
b. Serum PTH, hydrocortisone suppression test, X-ray of hand, CT scan of neck, thallium and technetium subtraction scan of parathyroid and thyroid.

Note: High calcium, low phosphate and high alkaline phosphatase are typical of primary hyperparathyroidism. In secondary hyperparathyroidism, which is secondary to chronic renal failure, there is high phosphate and calcium is low or near normal, also high urea and creatinine. In tertiary hyperparathyroidism, autonomous parathyroid hyperplasia occurs, which develops after secondary hyperparathyroidism.

CASE NO. 121

a. Chronic subdural hematoma.
b. CT scan of brain.

Note: Previous history of trauma followed by increasing headache is the clue for the diagnosis of chronic subdural hematoma. Accumulation of blood in subdural space is due to rupture of the vein, commonly during head injury, even mild. Interval between the injury and symptoms may be days or weeks or months. Symptoms may be delayed in elderly or alcohol abuse.

Common features are headache, drowsiness, confusion. There may be hemiparesis, sensory loss, epilepsy, stupor, even coma.

Treatment: Spontaneous resolution may occur. Otherwise, neurosurgical intervention (burr hole drainage).

CASE NO. 122

a. Multiple myeloma, polymyalgia rheumatica, secondary deposit in lumbosacral region.
b. For each case, likely investigations are:
     i. Multiple myeloma—bone marrow study.
    ii. Polymyalgia rheumatica—therapeutic trial with prednisolone.
   iii. Secondary deposit in the lumbosacral region—X-ray of lumbosacral spine or MRI.
         High ESR and pancytopenia are suggestive of bone marrow infiltration.

Note: Other causes are osteoarthrosis, osteomalacia, osteoporosis, Paget's disease. However, these are not associated with pancytopenia.

CASE NO. 123

a. Multiple myeloma.
b. Bone marrow study.
c. Serum protein electrophoresis, X-ray of skull.

Note: Elderly patient with high ESR, hypercalcemia, renal failure, high protein, etc. is highly suggestive of multiple myeloma, which is characterized by neoplastic proliferation of plasma cells in bone marrow with production of monoclonal paraprotein.

In PBF, marked rouleaux formation is common. There may be leukoerythroblastic blood picture. Bone marrow shows atypical plasma cells >30%. Serum electrophoresis may show M band. Bence-Jones proteinuria is present in 20% cases.

X-ray shows lytic lesion (due to production of cytokines, which stimulate osteoclast responsible for bone resorption).

Treatment: (i) Supportive (correction of anemia, control of infection, etc.). (ii) Thalidomide, or more recently bortezomib is highly effective. In older patient, thalidomide plus melphalan plus prednisolone. (iv) Autologous stem cell transplantation in < 65 years. Allogenic bone marrow transplantation in < 55 years.

Bad prognostic factors are high urea, low hemoglobin, high α_2 microglobulin, low albumin and high calcium at presentation.

CASE NO. 124

a. Sinus bradycardia, complete heart block.
b. Repeat ECG.
c. Injection atropine IV or temporary pacemaker.

Note: Sinus bradycardia or complete heart block are quite common complications in acute inferior myocardial infarction. There is usually complete recovery from complete heart block after 10 to 14 days.

CASE NO. 125

a. Water intoxication due to psychogenic excess drinking, SIADH.
b. Plasma and urinary osmolality, serum ADH (low).

Note: In psychogenic polydipsia, both plasma and urinary osmolality will be low. In SIADH, plasma osmolality is low, but urinary osmolality is high. In nephrogenic diabetes insipidus, plasma osmolality is high or normal, but urinary osmolality is low. Chronic intake of a large amount of water impairs renal concentrating mechanism making the difference between primary polydipsia and true diabetes insipidus more difficult. Water deprivation test is helpful to differentiate between these two. A psychiatric history is also helpful.

CASE NO. 126

a. Lag storage curve.
b. Partial gastrectomy.
c. Hypoglycemia.
d. Combined iron deficiency anemia and deficiency of vitamin B_{12} or folic acid (less intake of food).

Note: Following gastric ulcer surgery, there may be dumping syndrome. Initially, increased glucose is due to rapid absorption. Later, there is increased insulin secretion, responsible for hypoglycemia, causing fainting attack.

In lag storage GTT, after 30 minutes, glucose level is high which exceeds renal threshold. This stimulates insulin secretion, which results in subsequent hypoglycemia.

Causes of lag storage GTT are (i) reactive hypoglycemia (normal variant), (ii) thyrotoxicosis, (iii) severe liver disease, (iv) gastrectomy or gastrojejunostomy.

Causes of flat glucose tolerance curve (failure to rise glucose in OGTT) are (i) normal (ii) malabsorption state, (iii) Addison's disease, (iv) hypopituitarism (with growth hormone deficiency).

CASE NO. 127

a. Paracetamol.
b. Hepatic failure due to toxic metabolite of paracetamol.
c. Hepatic coma, sedative, hypoglycemia.
d. Serum paracetamol level, blood glucose, prothrombin time.

Note: Intake of 15 g of paracetamol is considered potentially serious in most cases. Toxic metabolite of paracetamol is NAPQI, which is normally conjugated with glutathione and is excreted. In paracetamol poisoning, there is production of excess toxic metabolite and deplete cellular glutathione. The liver is unable to excrete NAPQI, which is harmful to the liver, causes massive hepatic necrosis and hepatic failure (not by the drug itself). No liver damage until 18 hours. If blood level of paracetamol is >200 mg/mL, it indicates severe poisoning. Maximum liver damage occurs after 72 to 96 hours of ingestion. There is increased prothrombin time and aminotransferase activity (AST or ALT). There may be hypo- and hyperglycemia, metabolic acidosis, arrhythmia, GIT bleeding, cerebral edema, lactic acidosis and coma. Brainstem coning may occur after 96 hours.

Three important risk or prognostic markers for severe hepatic injury are (i) prothrombin time is >20 sec in 24 hours, (ii) pH <7.3, (iii) serum creatinine >300 mmol/L. If a peak prothrombin time is >180 sec, mortality is 90%. If creatinine is >300 mmol/L, mortality is 70%. If pH <7.3, mortality is 85%. Without treatment, a few patients may develop fulminant hepatic failure. Renal failure may develop, due to acute tubular necrosis in 25% cases.

Treatment: (i) Gastric lavage within 4 hours, (ii) N-acetylcysteine IV or methionine orally. More effective, if given within 10 hours. Protective effects decline rapidly and ineffective after 15 to 16 hours, (iii) If PT prolonged, fresh-frozen plasma, (iv) Glucose may be needed. Forced diuresis and dialysis have no role. Dialysis only if renal failure.

Monitor: LFT (ALT and PT), electrolytes, glucose and creatinine.

CASE NO. 128

a. Severe insulin resistance.
b. Due to antibody against insulin receptor.

Note: This type of insulin resistant diabetes mellitus is rarely found in young female, associated with acanthosis nigricans and androgenic features (hirsutism, acne, oligomenorrhea). Also in older women, circulating immunoglobulin binds to insulin receptor and reduces their affinity to insulin.

Insulin resistance is defined as defective glucose disposal associated with raised glucose and insulin concentration.

Causes are (i) Physiological (puberty, pregnancy, old age, bed rest), (ii) Metabolic (type 2 DM, obesity, PCOS, syndrome X or insulin resistance syndrome), (iii) Endocrine (acromegaly, Cushing's syndrome, thyrotoxicosis, glucagonoma, pheochromocytoma), (iv) Others are acanthosis nigricans, myotonic dystrophy, cirrhosis of liver, hemochromatosis.

Insulin resistance syndrome: It is a metabolic derangement characterized by (i) Insulin resistance, (ii) Hypertension, (iii) Dyslipidemia (high TG, low HDL), (iv) Obesity, (v) Type 2 DM, (vi) Accelerated cardiovascular disease. This syndrome is also called metabolic syndrome or syndrome X or CHAOS (coronary artery disease, hypertension, atherosclerosis, obesity, stroke).

CASE NO. 129

a. Salicylate poisoning.
b. Serum salicylate, serum electrolytes, CT scan of brain.

Note: There is severe metabolic acidosis with respiratory alkalosis, likely cause in this early age is salicylate poisoning. Low $PaCO_2$ indicates respiratory alkalosis, which is due to hyperventilation and wash out of carbon dioxide by direct stimulation of respiratory center by salicylate.

Later on, a combined respiratory and metabolic acidosis may occur due to (i) Depression of respiratory center by the increased level of salicylate (respiratory acidosis), (ii) Retention of organic metabolic acids by the kidney because of hypotension and dehydration, (iii) Salicylate impairs carbohydrate metabolism with accumulation of acetoacetate, lactic acid and pyruvic acid.

In salicylate poisoning, urine for ferric chloride test is positive (shows presence of reducing substance). Salicylate interferes with metabolism of carbohydrate, lipid, protein and amino acid. Ketone bodies are increased due to excess of fat metabolism. Lactic acid and pyruvic acid are also increased, because of inhibition of Krebs cycle by salicylate.

Other causes of severe metabolic acidosis are (i) diabetic ketoacidosis, (ii) renal failure, (iii) lactic acidosis.

CASE NO. 130

a. Cervical cord compression at C_6 level.
b. Cervical myelopathy, motor neuron disease, multiple sclerosis.
c. Sensory sign and its level.
d. X-ray of cervical spine, MRI of cervical spine.

Note: Progressive increase of neurological sign is highly suggestive of cord compression. Loss of biceps and exaggerated triceps indicates lesion at C_6. At the level of lesion, there is lower motor neuron (LMN) sign and below the level, upper motor neuron (UMN) sign. This type of reflex is called inversion of reflex.

CASE NO. 131
(See also case no. 99)
a. Chronic lymphatic leukemia.
b. Autoimmune hemolytic anemia and bone marrow infiltration.
c. Coomb's test, bone marrow study.

Note: High leukocyte with high lymphocyte is likely to be due to CLL. It may be asymptomatic in 25% cases, diagnosed incidentally in routine investigation. There may be generalized lymphadenopathy, hepatosplenomegaly. Huge splenomegaly may occur if there is auto-immune hemolytic anemia. Coomb's test is positive in 20% cases.

CLL is common in males (M:F = 2:1), usually after 45 years, involving B lymphocyte. Hemolysis is usually by warm autoantibody and Coomb's test is positive.

CASE NO. 132

a. Diabetic ketoacidosis (DKA).
b. Blood sugar and urine for ketone bodies.

Note: Dry tongue, weight loss, severe metabolic acidosis are the clue for the diagnosis of DKA. It is common in IDDM (type 1). The patient may present first time with DKA in younger age.

Three main problems in DKA are (i) hyperglycemia, (ii) hyperketonemia and (iii) metabolic acidosis. Marked dehydration is common. 5% cases develop coma in DKA. Average loss of fluid and electrolytes are (i) Water—6 liters, (ii) Sodium—500 mmol, (iii) Chloride—400 mmol, (iv) Potassium—350 mmol. Half of the lost fluid is intracellular. If bicarbonate is <12 mmol/L, it indicates severe acidosis.

Treatment: IV normal saline rapidly, IV soluble insulin preferably with pump, potassium therapy, control of infection, correction of acidosis by sodium bicarbonate, if arterial pH is <7 (complete correction of acidosis is avoided, because there is correction of extracellular acidosis with isotonic, 1.26%, but acidosis in brain is persistent, which aggravates cellular dysfunction in brain).

Complications of DKA: Cerebral edema, ARDS, DIC, thromboembolism, acute circulatory failure. Mortality is 5 to 10%, more in elderly.

CASE NO. 133

a. Primary hemochromatosis.
b. Serum ferritin, liver biopsy for iron studies.
c. Chondrocalcinosis.
d. Cardiomyopathy.

Note: Combination of diabetes mellitus, cardiac abnormality, hepatic problem with arthritis, and pigmentation are highly suggestive of hemochromatosis. It may be primary or secondary. Primary hemochromatosis is a hereditary disorder, inherited as autosomal recessive, characterized by increased iron absorption by the intestine, increased total body iron and deposition of iron in different organs of body with its dysfunction. Commonly, iron is deposited in liver, heart, pancreas, endocrine organs, joints, testis, skin, etc. Common in males, >40 years, females are protected by menstruation and pregnancy, but hemchromatosis occurs after menopause. Chondrocalcinosis may occur. Deposition of iron in liver leads to cirrhosis and may cause hepatoma in 33% cases. Leaden gray skin pigmentation is called bronze diabetes. Cardiac involvement leads to dilated or restrictive cardiomyopathy, abnormal ECG. Hypogonadism occurs due to deposition of iron in gonads, also hypopituitarism may occur.

Investigations: High iron, ferritin, high saturation of TIBC. CT scan or MRI of hepatobiliary system may be done. Liver biopsy for iron staining and quantitative measurement of iron (>180 mmol/g liver tissue).

Treatment: Weekly venesection of 500 mL of blood (it reduces 250 mg of iron) should be done until ferritin comes to <50 ng/mL. May take 2 to 3 years. Alcohol and vitamin C must be avoided (cause more absorption of iron).
　　Causes of secondary hemochromatosis are (i) repeated blood transfusion (>50 liters), (ii) chronic hemolytic disease, (iii) sideroblastic anemia, (iv) porphyria cutanea tarda, (v) alcoholism, (vi) Bantu siderosis (in Africa).

CASE NO. 134

a. SLE.
b. TPHA, ANA, anti-ds DNA.

Note: In this female patient, splenomegaly, thrombocytopenia, high ESR are the good clue for the diagnosis of SLE. False positive VDRL may be present in SLE, especially when there is high antiphospholipid. False positive VDRL may also be found in leprosy, narcotic abuse, old age. High ASO titer is not significant, it indicates previous streptococcal infection.

CASE NO. 135

a. Adrenal carcinoma and ectopic ACTH syndrome (oat cell carcinoma of bronchus in smokers is the likely cause).

b. X-ray chest, ultrasonography to see suprarenal gland, serum ACTH, CT scan of adrenal glands.
c. Hypokalemia, proximal myopathy, carcinomatous myopathy.
d. Secondary deposit from bronchial carcinoma, osteoporosis.

Note: Cushing's syndrome may present in any carcinoma, commonly oat cell carcinoma of bronchus, ovarian carcinoma, etc. In ectopic ACTH syndrome, the patient is emaciated, pigmented with severe hypokalemic alkalosis. ACTH is very high and also cortisol is very high.

CASE NO. 136

a. Subacute combined degeneration of spinal cord with pernicious anemia.
b. Serum B_{12} assay, bone marrow study.
c. Vibration and position sense, fundoscopy to see optic atrophy.

Note: Anemia, peripheral neuropathy, loss of knee and ankle jerk but extensor plantar are all suggestive of SCD. It is characterized by combination of peripheral neuropathy, signs of posterior column lesion (loss of vibration and position sense) and signs of pyramidal lesion (due to involvement of lateral column). Romberg sign may be positive. SCD occurs as a sequela to Addisonian pernicious anemia and rarely due to other causes of vitamin B_{12} deficiency. Other evidences of B_{12} deficiency such as anemia, glossitis, optic atrophy, dementia may be present.

Pathological change in spinal cord are (i) demyelination of peripheral nerve, (ii) degeneration of ascending tract in posterior column, (iii) degeneration of descending pyramidal tract in lateral column of spinal cord.

Treatment: Injection vitamin B_{12}, 1000 µg IM daily for one week, then weekly for one month, then every 3 months. Treatment of primary cause.

CASE NO. 137

a. Metabolic acidosis and metabolic alkalosis.
b. Chronic renal failure (CRF).
c. CRF with severe vomiting, CRF with bicarbonate therapy.

Note: Low bicarbonate indicates acidosis and high pH indicates alkalosis. In CRF, metabolic acidosis is common. Because of repeated vomiting, there may be metabolic alkalosis. If sodium bicarbonate is given, there is also correction of acidosis.

CASE NO. 138

a. Spontaneous pneumothorax.
b. X-ray of chest (PA view).

Note: In any young patient, common cause of sudden severe chest pain is spontaneous pneumothorax. Other causes of chest pain may be pleurisy, reflux esophagitis, costochondritis, pneumonia and pulmonary embolism. Acute myocardial infarction and dissecting aneurysm are other rare possibilities.

CASE NO. 139

a. Bleeding in the iliopsoas muscle and retroperitoneal bleeding.

b. Iliopsoas hematoma causing compression of left femoral nerve.

c. Insufficient dose, poor quality antihemophilic factor, antibody against factor VIII.

d. Abdominal ultrasonography or CT scan.

Note: Iliopsoas bleeding may occur in hemophilia. The patient has difficulty in flexion of hip and paresthesia along the distribution of femoral nerve due to compression. Muscle bleeding may occur in any muscle causing ischemic damage to the nerve by entrapment, leading to muscle necrosis or Volkman's ischemic contracture. In hemophilia, clotting time and APTT are prolonged, but bleeding time, prothrombin time, platelet, fibrinogen are all normal.

CASE NO. 140

a. Mixed respiratory alkalosis and metabolic acidosis.

b. Portosystemic encephalopathy.

c. Respiratory alkalosis is due to hypoxia and elevated diaphragm due to ascites. Metabolic acidosis is due to diarrhea.

Note: Diarrhea in cirrhosis is a cause of hyperchloremic acidosis. Hypoxia and elevated diaphragm are responsible for hyperventilation, resulting in respiratory alkalosis.

CASE NO. 141

a. Partially treated bacterial meningitis, tuberculous meningitis, brain abscess, fungal infection.

b. AFB staining, culture and sensitivity, immunoelectrophoresis for bacterial antigen, PCR.

c. CT scan or MRI of brain, blood for C/S, serum electrolytes, urine for ketone bodies, X-ray chest.

Note: Causes of increased lymphocyte in CSF are (i) infection (tuberculous, viral, fungal, meningovascular syphilis), (ii) neoplastic (lymphoma, leukemia, secondary deposit), (iii) sarcoidosis, (iv) sometimes, chronic brain abscess, (v) partially treated bacterial meningitis.

CASE NO. 142

a. Familial periodic paralysis, thyrotoxic periodic paralysis.

b. Thyrotoxic periodic paralysis.

c. Whether patient feels weakness with activity.

Note: History is suggestive of periodic paralysis. Systolic hypertension, tachycardia are in favor of thyrotoxicosis. In familial periodic paralysis, inherited as autosomal dominant, there is membrane abnormality. Three types are (i) hypokalemic—lasts for days. (ii) hyperkalemic—lasts for hours (in hyperkalemic type, myotonia of tongue and eye may occur, common in <10 years of age), (iii) normokalemic.

Hypokalemic periodic paralysis is rare, characterized by episodic extreme weakness, progress from proximal to distal. Cranial and respiratory muscles are spared. It usually occurs during rest after prolonged exercise, also while the patient is asleep. Precipitating factors are increased carbohydrate meal, cold, rest after exercise, alcohol, anxiety or tension and cause of hypokalemia is unknown, but shift of potassium from extracellular fluid to the intracellular fluid is responsible. Symptoms can be precipitated by intravenous glucose and insulin into this patient which would support the diagnosis of potassium shift theory. Long-term treatment with potassium supplement or potassium sparing diuretic are given.

Thyrotoxic periodic paralysis (TPP): If a thyrotoxic patient develops sudden or periodic weakness, it is called thyrotoxic periodic paralysis. It is due to hypokalemia (caused by entry of potassium into the cell), common in Asians. May occur following excess carbohydrate or glucose or heavy exercise. Persists up to 7 to 72 hours. Treatment of thyrotoxicosis improves the condition.

CASE NO. 143

a. Acute myocardial infarction, spontaneous pneumothorax, pulmonary embolism.
b. Repeat ECG, X-ray of chest (PA view), serum troponin 1 (and ventilation/perfusion scan).

Note: Following any chest surgery, if the patient develops sudden respiratory distress or chest pain, always exclude the above disorders. In pulmonary edema, PO_2 is usually much lower. ECG may appear normal in early case of myocardial infarction. Enzymes such as troponin I, CPK, SGOT test should be done.

CASE NO. 144

a. Pulmonary hypertension.
b. Atrial fibrillation with pulmonary embolism.
c. Pulmonary infarction.
d. Eisenmenger's syndrome.
e. Heart lung transplantation.

Note: This patient is suffering from VSD, now develops CCF, secondary to pulmonary hypertension. Pulmonary hypertension with reversal of shunt is called Eisenmenger's syndrome. When it is due to VSD, then it is called Eisenmenger's complex. If there is Eisenmenger's syndrome, surgical closure should not be done. Only supportive treatment is given. Heart and lung transplantation may be considered.

CASE NO. 145

a. Prerenal acute renal failure.
b. Vomiting.
c. Correction of electrolytes by intravenous normal saline with potassium, also bicarbonate.

Note: Prerenal acute renal failure may occur in severe vomiting, diarrhea, bleeding, burn, excess aspiration, etc. If properly treated, it is reversible.

Remember the urea/creatinine ratio in relation to renal failure. In some cases, urea is very high, but creatinine is normal which does not indicate renal failure. Conversely, in some cases, urea is normal or low, but creatinine is high indicating renal failure. Causes of high urea (but normal creatinine), *high urea/creatinine ratio*—(i) High protein diet, (ii) Dehydration, (iii) Gastrointestinal hemorrhage, (iv) Steroid therapy. Causes of high creatinine (but normal urea), *low urea/creatinine ratio*—(i) Vomiting (more urea loss), (ii) Liver disease (less urea production), (iii) Peritoneal or hemodialysis (urea reduces quickly), (iv) Rhabdomyolysis, (v) Drug (trimethoprim), (vi) Protein restricted diet.

CASE NO. 146

a. Cirrhosis of liver with erythropoietin secreting hepatoma with secondary polycythemia.
b. Cirrhosis of liver with secondary polycythemia due to pulmonary A-V shunting.
c. USG of hepatobiliary system, serum α-fetoprotein, CT scan of hepatobiliary system, liver biopsy.

Note: This patient developed hepatoma secondary to CLD, also there is high hemoglobin and RBC, which indicates secondary polycythemia. 80% hepatoma is secondary to cirrhosis of liver. Metabolic abnormalities in hepatoma are polycythemia, hypercalcemia, hypoglycemia, porphyria cutanea tarda. α-fetoprotein is commonly high in hepatoma, >500 ng/mL is highly suggestive. Hepatorenal syndrome may occur.

CASE NO. 147

a. Myelodysplastic syndrome (refractory anemia).
b. Ring sideroblast.

Note: This patient has been suffering from transfusion dependent anemia, which is likely to be myelodysplastic syndrome. This is a group of acquired bone marrow disorders due to defect in stem cells, characterized by increasing marrow failure with quantitative and qualitative abnormality of all three cell lines. There are anemia, neutropenia and thrombocytopenia, usually with hypercellular or normocellular marrow. Common in elderly, transform to AML in 30% cases.

In MDS, blood picture shows—cytopenia (thrombocytopenia and leukopenia), hypogranular neutrophil, hyposegmented neutrophil (Pelger cells) or hypersegmented neutrophil, MCV—high (macrocytic) or normal.

Bone marrow—hypercellular with dysplastic change despite pancytopenia. Megaloblastic changes, ring sideroblast in all types, dyserythropoiesis, granulocyte precursor and megakaryocyte show abnormal morphology.

Chromosome analysis reveals abnormality in chromosome 5 or 7.

The patient presents with anemia, infection or bleeding manifestations. Secondary MDS may be seen in any patient treated with radiotherapy, chemotherapy or combination (as in lymphoma).

Types of diseases in MDS:
(i) Refractory anemia (RA)—blast <5%, erythroid dysplasia only, (ii) Refractory anemia with sideroblast (blast <5%, ring sideroblast >15%), (iii) Refractory cytopenias with multilineage dysplasia—(blast <5%, 2 to 3 lineage dysplasia), (iv) Refractory anemia with excess blast (blast 5 to 20%, 2 to 3 lineage dysplasia), (v) Refractory anemia with excess blast in transformation (blast 20 to 30%), (vi) MDS with 5q-MDS with del (5q) cytogenetic abnormality blasts <5%, normal or increased blood platelet, (vii) MDS unclassified—none of the above or inadequate material.

Treatment:
A. If blast <5%—(i) Supportive therapy with platelet, red cell transfusion, (ii) Erythropoietin and G-CSF may be given.
B. If blast >5%—(i) Supportive therapy, (ii) Chemotherapy—low dose hydroxyurea or etoposide, (iii) Lenalidomide (a thalidomide analog) may be effective in early stage of MDS with

chromosome 5q deletion (iv) Allogenic stem cell transplantation in young <55 years, (v) A new hypomethylating agent Azacytidine may be given, use especially not eligible for transplantation.

Prognosis: Slowest in refractory anemia, rapidly progresses in refractory anemia with ring sideroblast.

CASE NO. 148

a. Ovarian androgen secreting tumor.
b. Ultrasonography of abdomen, CT scan of abdomen to see ovarian mass, laparoscopy.

Note: Failure of testosterone to fall after low dose dexamethasone suppression test indicates that this is not a polycystic ovary or congenital adrenal hyperplasia. In ovarian androgen secreting tumor, there is failure of suppression by dexamethasone.

CASE NO. 149

a. Distal renal tubular acidosis.
b. Osteomalacia with myopathy and hypokalemia.
c. Osteomalacia.
d. Ammonium chloride test (other test—pH of overnight urine).
e. Sodium bicarbonate therapy.

Note: Hypokalemia is usually associated with alkalosis. In distal RTA, hypokalemia is associated with acidosis. High chloride, low potassium with metabolic acidosis is highly suggestive of RTA. Muscular weakness is due to severe hypokalemia and hypocalcemia.

CASE NO. 150

a. Restrictive lung disease.
b. Interstitial lung disease with chronic cor pulmonale.
c. Chest X-ray, CT scan of chest, ABG (arterial blood gas analysis), bronchoscopy and bronchoalveolar lavage, transbronchial or open lung biopsy.

Note: FEV_1 and FVC are proportionately low and the ratio between these is normal. CO transfer is also low. There may be hyperventilation with hypocapnea, hypoxemia. X-ray chest will show reticulonodular shadow and honeycomb lung. Bronchoalveolar lavage may show high neutrophil and high eosinophil.

CASE NO. 151

a. Cushing's disease (due to pituitary dependent bilateral adrenal hyperplasia).
b. Serum ACTH, MRI of pituitary fossa.

Note: Features are suggestive of Cushing's syndrome. The commonest cause of Cushing's syndrome is iatrogenic. Otherwise in 80% cases, it is due to Cushing's disease. It is characterized by increased production of ACTH from pituitary gland, commonly microadenoma, < 10 mm. Dexamethasone suppression indicates Cushing's disease. Failure of dexamethasone suppression occurs in ectopic ACTH syndrome and adrenal carcinoma.

Treatment: Transphenoidal removal of adenoma, if possible. Pituitary irradiation may be helpful. Occasionally, bilateral adrenalectomy may be necessary (later on, there may be Nelson's syndrome, which can be prevented by pituitary irradiation).

CASE NO. 152

a. Idiopathic thrombocytopenic purpura.
b. Bone marrow study, antiplatelet antibody.
c. SLE.

Note: Bleeding or bruise with low platelet after viral fever is suggestive of Idiopathic thrombocytopenic purpura. In ITP, low platelet, increased megakaryocyte in bone marrow, prolonged bleeding time, normal clotting time are common. There may be antiplatelet antibody and anticardiolipin antibody. Initially, SLE and antiphospholipid syndrome may present like ITP. In 10% cases, ITP may be associated with autoimmune hemolytic anemia, called Evan's syndrome.

ITP is due to autoantibody directed against platelet membrane glycoprotein IIb-IIIa, responsible for removal of platelet by monocyte-macrophage system.

Treatment: In child-usually self-limiting. If no improvement, (1) Prednisolone (2 mg/kg), (2) if persistent bleeding, IV immunoglobulin. (3) platelet transfusion, if persistent bleeding (epistaxis, GIT bleeding, retinal hemorrhage, intracranial bleeding) (4) If thrombocytopenia persists more than 6 months, it is chronic. In that case, splenectomy should be considered. In adult, persistent thrombocytopenia is common. (1) Prednisolone—1 mg/kg for 4 to 6 weeks, then taper the dose. Relapse is common after withdrawal of steroid. Then, steroid dose should be increased. (2) If persistent bleeding, IV immunoglobulin may be given (1 g/kg for 3 to 5 days). Its effect is temporary, persists for 1 to 2 weeks. (3) In frequent relapse (usually more than 2 times), splenectomy may be considered (effective in 70% cases). But, if bleeding or purpura after splenectomy, low dose prednisolone (5 mg daily) should be continued. (4) In 30% cases, no response to splenectomy. Then, if the patient is asymptomatic and platelet count >40,000 to 50,000, follow-up the case. But if bleeding or purpura, low dose prednisolone (5 mg daily) should be continued. (5) If still no response, other therapy—danazol 600 mg daily. Or repeated IV immunoglobulin, azathioprine, cyclophosphamide, vincristine, vinblastine, cyclosporine, anti-D infusion, interferon-α.

If no response after splenectomy, may be accessory spleen (confirm by radionuclide scan). After splenectomy, infection by *Pneumococcus, Meningococcus* and *H. influenzae* (vaccination against these is essential).

CASE NO. 153

a. Failure to rise urinary osmolality after 8 hours water deprivation test. After desmopressin, there is rise of urinary osmolality.
b. Cranial diabetes insipidus.
c. Diabetes mellitus, primary polydipsia.
d. Head injury, sarcoidosis, hemochromatosis, histiocytosis X, idiopathic.

Note: Cranial diabetes insipidus is responsive to desmopressin, but nephrogenic diabetes insipidus does not respond to desmopressin. In CDI, plasma osmolality is usually

> 300 mOsm/kg and urine osmolality is <600 mOsm/kg. If urine osmolality rises by at least 50% after DDAVP, it is diagnostic of CDI.

Other causes of cranial diabetes insipidus—craniopharyngioma, pituitary tumor with suprasellar extension, basal meningitis, surgery, encephalitis, DIDMOAD syndrome (diabetes insipidus, diabetes mellitus, optic atrophy, deafness).

In cranial diabetes insipidus, if associated cortisol deficiency is present, there may not be any features until steroid replacement is given.

CASE NO. 154

a. Chronic pancreatitis with malabsorption.
b. Chronic alcoholism.
c. Plain X-ray abdomen to see pancreatic calcification, pancreatic CT scan, ERCP.

Note: High MCV and γ-GT, both occur in chronic alcoholism, which is the likely cause of chronic pancreatitis. Diabetes mellitus secondary to chronic pancreatitis is common. Vitamin B_{12} deficiency may occur in chronic pancreatitis.

CASE NO. 155

a. Tuberculous meningitis with SIADH.
b. Chest X-ray, CT scan or MRI of brain.
c. SIADH, Addison's disease.

Note: In tuberculous meningitis, low sodium may occur as a part of SIADH. Low sodium may also occur, if there is involvement of adrenal glands by tuberculosis, causing Addison's disease. Fundoscopy may show choroid tubercle.

CASE NO. 156

a. Acetazolamide therapy.
b. Hyperchloremic hypokalemic metabolic acidosis.
c. Urine for ketone bodies, serum lactate level.

Note: Long-term use of carbonic anhydrase inhibitor such as acetazolamide is an important cause of hyperchloremic metabolic acidosis associated with hypokalemia. Sugar is not so high to cause DKA. Lactic acidosis should be excluded also.

CASE NO. 157

a. Antiphospholipid syndrome.
b. ANA, anti-ds DNA, serum antiphospholipid or anticardiolipin.

Note: In any young patient, if presents with features like CVA or TIA, antiphospholipid syndrome should be excluded. In this case, clue for the diagnosis is prolonged APTT, which is not corrected by addition of normal plasma. Antiphospholipid syndrome is characterized by the presence antiphospholipid antibody, causing thrombosis by an effect on platelet membrane, endothelial cell and clotting components such as prothrombin, protein C and S.

Antiphospholipid antibody collectively included lupus anticoagulant and anticardiolipin antibody. In some patients, only one of these is positive and in others, both are positive.

Presence of this antibody may be associated with thrombosis (venous or arterial), recurrent abortion, thrombocytopenia, neurological (stroke, TIA, epilepsy, migraine, chorea), sterile endocarditis (Liebmann Sach's), livedo reticularis, pulmonary hypertension, avascular necrosis of head of femur. Renal involvement with proteinuria in 50%, in some cases, lupus nephritis (membranous) like lesion may be seen. Recurrent abortions are thought to be due to placental infarction.

Indirect evidence of antiphospholipid antibody—false positive VDRL, thrombocytopenia, prolonged prothrombin time, prolonged APTT (not corrected by normal plasma).

It may be primary or secondary to other disease. Secondary causes are SLE, rheumatoid arthritis, systemic sclerosis, Behcet's syndrome, temporal arteritis, Sjogren's syndrome, psoriatic arthropathy.

Treatment: Low dose aspirin (in mild to moderate case), warfarin in severe case. In pregnancy, heparin and low dose aspirin may be used.

CASE NO. 158

a. Obstructive airway disease.
b. Emphysema.
c. α_1 antitrypsin deficiency, cigarette smoking.

Note: Antitrypsin (antiproteinase) has a protective action for lung tissue. In smoking, damage of lung tissue occur due to an imbalance between proteinase and antiproteinase, release of oxidants and proteinase from inflammatory cells, which are responsible for damage to the supporting connective tissue of alveolar septa. Also, there is increased proteinase synthesis and inactivation of antiproteinase.

CASE NO. 159

a. Serum electrolytes, Tensilon test.
b. Alveolar hypoventilation.
c. Myasthenia gravis, Guillain-Barre syndrome (GBS), hypokalemia.

Note: In myasthenia gravis, weakness of muscles usually occur after exercise, not associated with muscular pain. Respiratory muscle involvement may cause dyspnea, respiratory failure, etc. Hypokalemia may be associated with severe muscular weakness or even paralysis. Respiratory muscle paralysis may occur in GBS. Repeated measurement of vital capacity and peak expiratory flow rate (PEFR) should be done, may require intermittent positive-pressure respiration (IPPR).

CASE NO. 160

a. Acute myocardial infarction, pulmonary edema, pulmonary embolism, severe bronchial asthma.
b. Chest X-ray, ECG, troponin 1.

Note: Hypocapnia is due to hyperventilation. Hypoxemia is due to ventilation/perfusion defect.

■ CASE NO. 161

a. Leukemoid reaction.
b. Neoplastic infiltration in bone marrow.
c. Bone marrow study, isotope bone scan.

Note: High WBC count with few premature series are suggestive of leukemoid reaction. It means the peripheral blood picture resembles leukemia, but there is no leukemia. It may be myeloid or lymphatic.

Causes of myeloid leukemoid reaction are leukoerythroblastic anemia, infection, malignancy, acute hemolysis (LIMA).

Causes of lymphatic leukemoid reaction are viral (infectious mononucleosis, cytomegalovirus infection, measles, chicken pox), whooping cough. Rarely, tuberculosis and carcinoma.

■ CASE NO. 162

a. Addisonian crisis.
b. Serum cortisol and ACTH.

Note: This patient used to take steroid for long time. Sudden stopping of steroid or following infection or stress, there may be Addisonian crisis. It is an acute severe adrenocortical insufficiency, characterized by features of collapse, with nausea, vomiting, diarrhea, acute abdomen, even unconsciousness. There is profound hypotension and hypoglycemia, electrolyte imbalance.

Causes are sudden withdrawal of steroid, if the patient was on steroid for long time. Others are stress (infection, operation).

Treatment: Three problems in Addisonian crisis—(i) Hyponatremia, (ii) Hypoglycemia, (iii) Cortisol deficiency.

So, IV normal saline, glucose, hydrocortisone 200 mg 6 hourly should be given. Control of infection, if any.

■ CASE NO. 163
(See also case no. 68)

a. Infectious mononucleosis, cytomegalovirus infection, dengue, typhus fever.
b. Antidengue antibody, monospot test, antibody to EBV, antibody to CMV (others—urinary isolation of CMV, Weil Felix reaction).

Note: Infectious mononucleosis is caused by EB virus. Cervical lymphadenopathy (commonly posterior), splenomegaly and skin rash especially after ampicillin or amoxicillin are typical features.

Other diseases caused by EB virus are—Burkitt's lymphoma, nasopharyngeal carcinoma, hairy leukoplakia in AIDS, immunoblastic lymphoma in AIDS, post-transplant lymphoma and Hodgkin's lymphoma.

Causes of fever with skin rash—chicken pox, scarlet fever, measles, rubella, typhus, enteric fever, dengue fever, drugs.

CASE NO. 164

a. Black water fever.
b. Chloroquine or quinine, blood transfusion, steroid.
c. Hemolytic uremic syndrome.

Note: In a patient with high fever, signs of hemolysis with black urine in endemic area, suggest black water fever. It is a severe manifestation of falciparum malaria that occurs in previously infected person. It is characterized by sudden intravascular hemolysis and hemoglobinuria. Urine looks black. Occurs in those who took anti-malarial drug irregularly or in non-immune person, who took irregular anti-malarial drug prophylaxis. It is due to antibody production formed against red cells that have been altered by drug, parasite or both.

Treatment: Quinine IV, 20 mg/kg (maximum 1.4 g), with 5% D/A, for 4 hours, then 10 mg/kg 8 hourly (maximum 700 mg) for 7 days, until patient can take orally. Injection artemether is a suitable alternative. Dose—80 mg IM twice daily for one day, followed by 80 mg daily for 4 days or 80 mg IM twice daily for 3 days (it is a synthetic anti-malarial, derived from artemisinin. It should be avoided in pregnancy, unless strongly indicated). Blood transfusion may be necessary. Prednisolone may be helpful.

CASE NO. 165

a. Clubbing, signs of polycythemia (plethoric face, blood shot eyes).
b. Cyanotic congenital heart disease, cystic fibrosis.
c. Chest X-ray, echocardiogram.

Note: Fallot's tetralogy is the commonest congenital heart disease, which presents with short stature, cyanosis and clubbing. Other diseases are transposition of great vessels, tricuspid atresia, aortic and mitral atresia.
   Cystic fibrosis may be associated with bronchiectasis, cyanosis and clubbing.

CASE NO. 166

a. Sarcoidosis, hypervitaminosis D, hypercalcemia associated with malignancy.
b. Primary hyperparathyroidism.

Note: Failure of suppression of calcium after hydrocortisone is suggestive of primary hyperparathyroidism. In tumor associated hypercalcemia, calcium may not fall in 50% cases. In other cases, there is suppression of calcium.

CASE NO. 167

a. Myxedema coma.
b. Serum TSH and cortisol.

Note: In this patient, typical history, low voltage ECG and cardiomegaly is likely to be due to myxedema, associated with pericardial effusion. Myxedema coma is rare, common in elderly, characterized by depressed level of consciousness, low body temperature, even convulsion. Coma may be due to SIADH, hypoxemia, hypercapnia, hypothermia, hypoglycemia, infection. Cardiac failure may occur. 50% mortality. CSF shows high pressure with high protein.

Treatment: IV T$_3$ (20 µg) eight hourly. After 48 to 72 hours, oral thyroxine may be given. If T$_3$ is not available, oral thyroxine, hydrocortisone IV 100 mg 8 hourly.

Other treatment: Oxygen, slow rewarming, antibiotic, glucose infusion, assisted ventilation.

■ CASE NO. 168

a. DIC.
b. Serum FDP, D-dimer, serum fibrinogen.

Note: Bleeding associated with low platelet, prolonged prothrombin time, APTT, thrombin time indicates DIC. After myocardial infarction, there may be release of thromboplastic substance into the circulation, which activates extrinsic clotting system. In DIC, prothrombin time, APTT, thrombin time are prolonged. Platelet count and fibrinogen are all low. FDP and D-dimer are high. Other clotting factors are also low.

■ CASE NO. 169

a. Juvenile hypothyroidism.
b. Thyroxine.

Note: Prolactin is high in hypothyroidism. Pituitary fossa may be enlarged in hypothyroidism due to increased thyrotroph. Hyperprolactinemia may occur secondary to multiple causes. The commonest cause is prolactinoma of the pituitary gland. Other causes—(i) Physiological-pregnancy, lactation, sleep, stress, (ii) Pathological—disease of pituitary gland (prolactinoma, acromegaly), hypothalamic disorder (tumor, trauma, radiation), hypothyroidism, renal failure, chest wall injury, ectopic production by non-endocrine tumor (bronchial carcinoma, renal cell carcinoma), drug (metoclopramide, domperidone, phenothiazine, butyrophenones, antidepressant, pimozide, methyldopa, estrogen), idiopathic. Hyperprolactinemia may present with—(i) In female—amenorrhea, galactorrhea, infertility, dyspareunia (ii) In male—decreased libido, reduced frequency of shaving, lethargy. Prolactin stimulates milk secretion, not breast development. So, galactorrhea never occurs in male. Gynecomastia is present, if hypogonadism.

Causes of enlarged sella turcica (i) Pituitary macroadenoma, (ii) Hypothalamic mass or cyst, (iii) Aneurysm, (iv) Primary hypothyroidism, (v) Hypogonadism, (vi) Increased intracranial pressure, (vii) Empty sella syndrome.

Empty sella syndrome—it is characterized by enlargement of pituitary fossa due to herniation of suprasellar sub-arachnoid space through incomplete diaphragma sella, so the sella is filled with CSF with arachnoid sac. The pituitary gland is pushed to one side, but function normally. The patient is usually obese, multipara having headache, hypertension (30%), hyperprolactinemia, CSF rhinorrhea, pseudotumor cerebri, visual field defect, etc. Endocrine function is normal. *Diagnosis*—MRI. *Treatment*—reassurance.

■ CASE NO. 170

a. Restrictive lung disease.
b. Fibrosing alveolitis, sarcoidosis, lymphangitis carcinomatosa.

Note: In restrictive lung disease, the ratio of FEV_1/FVC is normal, but low PEF and low TLC, low transfer factor for carbon monoxide.

CASE NO. 171

a. Hyperkalemia.
b. It is more likely to be spurious or pseudohyperkalemia. Probable cause is blood sample having been left for long time before biochemical analysis. As a result, red cell potassium leaks into the plasma, leading to falsely high level of potassium.
c. Repeat serum potassium.

Note: Pseudohyperkalemia commonly occurs, if the blood sample is kept for long time. This may also be found in chronic lymphatic leukemia, myeloproliferative disorders, etc. in which leakage of potassium from high leukemic cells leads to high potassium. Rarely, high potassium may occur in familial pseudohyperkalemia and hypoaldosteronism.

CASE NO. 172

a. Essential thrombocythemia with pulmonary embolism.
b. Chest X-ray PA view, bone marrow study.
c. Pleurisy.
d. Pleural rub.

Note: Thrombocytosis may occur in—acute blood loss, hemolysis, postsplenectomy, CGL.

Essential thrombocythemia is a myeloproliferative disease with very high production of platelet. Platelet aggregation is impaired, blood film shows large or atypical platelet and megakaryocyte fragments. Bone marrow shows increased megakaryocyte. There is splenomegaly, hemorrhage and thromboembolic episodes.

CASE NO. 173

a. MEN type 2a.
b. Thyroid function test (radioiodine uptake test, FT3, FT4 and TSH, FNAC), USG of abdomen to see suprarenal gland, 24 hours urine for VMA, subtraction scan of thyroid and parathyroid (with thallium and technetium).

Note: In this patient, there is goiter, more likely to be medullary carcinoma of thyroid (MTC), high calcium (hyperparathyroidism) and periodic hypertension (pheochromocytoma), which suggest MEN type 2a. It consists of primary hyperparathyroidism, medullary carcinoma of thyroid and pheochromocytoma, also called Sipple's syndrome.

In MTC, serum calcitonin is high.

In hyperparathyroidism, high calcium, low phosphate and high alkaline phosphatase.

In pheochromocytoma, high serum catecholamines, high 24 hours urine VMA, etc.

Treatment: Individual tumor should be treated surgically.

MEN type 2b: When there is associated Marfanoid body habitus, skeletal abnormality, multiple mucosal neuroma, abnormal dental enamel.

MEN type I (Werner's syndrome): Pituitary tumor, primary hyperparathyroidism and pancreatic neuroendocrine tumor (glucagonoma, insulinoma).

CASE NO. 174

a. Turner's syndrome.
b. Karyotyping.

Note: Turner's syndrome is associated with primary amenorrhea and short stature. It is characterized by a single X chromosome (45, X0). The main abnormality is gonadal dysgenesis, there is aplasia of ovaries (streak gonad), responsible for primary amenorrhea and infertility.

It is diagnosed by karyotyping from buccal smear, which shows 45 (X0), occasionally 46 (XX) mosaic. There is low estrogen, high LH and FSH. USG shows small uterus, small fallopian tube and streak gonad.

Features of Turner's syndrome are:

1. Skeletal: Short stature, short and webbing of neck, small lower jaw (micrognathia), mouth is small and fish like, high arched palate. Chest—broad, widely apart nipples (shield-like chest). Hand—short 4th metacarpal (other metacarpals may be short), lymphedema of hands (also feet), nails- hypoplastic. Elbow—increased carrying angles (cubitus valgus).
2. Cardiac abnormality: Coarctation of aorta (10 to 20% cases), ASD, VSD, AS, hypertension.
3. Renal abnormality: Horseshoe shaped kidney, hydronephrosis.
4. Miscellaneous: Low hairline and redundant skin fold on the back of neck, low set and deformed ears. Others (incidence is more)—diabetes mellitus, Hashimoto's thyroiditis (may be frank hypothyroidism in 20% cases), lymphedema in infancy, red-green color blindness, strabismus and ptosis, premature osteoporosis, pigmented nevi, mental retardation (rare).

CASE NO. 175

a. Budd-Chiari syndrome.
b. Chronic constrictive pericarditis, congestive cardiac failure, inferior vena caval obstruction.
c. LFT (bilirubin, SGPT, alkaline phosphatase, prothrombin time), USG of HBS, CT scan or MRI of liver, technetium scan of liver.

Note: SLE with recurrent abortion is associated with antiphospholipid syndrome, which may cause venous thrombosis. Sudden and rapid enlargement of liver with ascites is highly suggestive of hepatic venous obstruction, called Budd-Chiari syndrome.

Other causes of thrombosis causing this syndrome are polycythemia rubra vera, PNH, oral contraceptive pill, deficiency of antithrombin III, protein C and S, malignancy (such as hepatic, renal or adrenal carcinoma, posterior wall abdominal sarcoma), congenital venous web, hydatid cyst, radiotherapy, trauma to liver. It is idiopathic in 30% cases. There may be cirrhosis of liver.

Investigations: Color Doppler USG or CT scan or MRI will show hepatic venous occlusion with diffuse abnormal parenchyma on contrast enhancement, sparing caudate lobe because of its independent blood supply and venous drainage. Technetium scan of liver shows low uptake, but there may be excess uptake in caudate lobe, because it has separate venous drainage from the rest of the liver. Other investigations should be done to find out causes.

Treatment: (i) Treat primary cause, (ii) For ascites—diuretic, sodium and water restriction, paracentesis, (iii) Thrombolytic, such as streptokinase may be given in acute case, (iv) TIPSS—transjugular intrahepatic portosystemic shunt, (v) Liver transplantation may be necessary in chronic case and for fulminant failure.

CASE NO. 176

a. SLE.
b. ANA, anti-ds DNA.

Note: Flitting arthritis associated with high ESR, thrombocytopenia, positive VDRL in young female is highly suggestive of SLE. Flitting arthritis may occur in rheumatic fever, SLE, viral fever, lyme disease, chronic active hepatitis, secondary syphilis, etc. False positive VDRL may occur in atypical pneumonia, malaria, bacterial or viral infection, SLE, leprosy, rheumatoid arthritis, primary biliary cirrhosis.

CASE NO. 177

a. Von Hippel-Lindau syndrome.
b. MRI of brain.

Note: Von Hippel-Lindau syndrome is characterized by combination of cerebellar signs and polycythemia. It is inherited as autosomal dominant, due to defective gene on chromosome 3p25-26. There is retinal and intracranial (cerebellar) hemangioma and hemangioblastoma associated with increased erythropoietin production causing polycythemia. Extracranial hamartoma lesion may occur, which may undergo malignant change. 10% posterior cranial fossa tumors are hemangioblastoma.

CASE NO. 178

a. DIC.
b. Serum FDP, D-dimer, serum fibrinogen, prothrombin time, APTT.
c. Antibody to CMV, antibody to EB virus, isolation of CMV from urine.
d. Post-transfusion cytomegalovirus infection, infectious mononucleosis.

Note: Massive blood transfusion with development of low platelet indicates DIC. Blood transfusion may be associated with any infection, such as CMV, infectious mononucleosis, hepatitis B and C, HIV, etc. DIC may occur after massive blood transfusion.

CASE NO. 179

a. Primary hyperaldosteronism.
b. Serum aldosterone and renin, 24 hour urine potassium, CT scan (or MRI of adrenal glands).

Note: Hypertension with hypokalemic alkalosis is highly suggestive of primary hyper-aldosteronism, also called Conn's syndrome. It is an aldosterone secreting tumor, responsible for <1% cause of hypertension. Excess aldosterone secretion leads to sodium retention, hypokalemia and combination of hypertension with hypokalemia. It is due to adrenal adenoma in 60% (Conn's syndrome) and 30% bilateral adrenal hyperplasia. Adrenal adenoma is usually small, common in young female. Adrenal hyperplasia is common in male, after 40 years. Serum renin is low in primary aldosteronism, whereas renin is high in secondary aldosteronism.

Investigations: (i) High sodium, low potassium and high bicarbonate (metabolic alkalosis), (ii) Urine potassium >30 mmol in 24 hours, (iii) High aldosterone and low renin, (iv) Failure of suppression of aldosterone by giving 0.9% sodium chloride 300 cc for four hours, (v) CT or MRI to localize tumor, (vi) [131]Iodine cholesterol scanning of adrenal may be done, (vii) Selective venous catheter of adrenal for aldosterone measurement, (viii) Urine for 18-OH cortisol is increased.

Simultaneous measurement of renin and aldosterone measurement should be done in lying and standing position. Renin is low and aldosterone is high in supine position. On standing suddenly, there is paradoxical drop of aldosterone in patient with adenoma and exaggerated rise in aldosterone in patient with hyperplasia.

Treatment: If adenoma, surgery. If hyperplasia—spironolactone 100 to 400 mg daily. For hypertension, amiloride and calcium channel blocker may be used.

Rare tumor with hypokalemia and hypertension occur in 11-β-hydroxylase deficiency in CAH, which respond to prednisolone and dexamethasone. Still rare, 17-hydroxylase deficiency (CAH plus hypokalemia plus hypogonadism), also respond to steroid.

Causes of hypokalemic alkalosis and hypertension—primary hyperaldosteronism (Conn's syndrome), Cushing's syndrome, Liddle's syndrome, accelerated hypertension, hypertension treated with diuretics, renal artery stenosis, carbenoxolone therapy, liquorice abuse, congenital adrenal hyperplasia (11-β-hydroxylase deficiency).

CASE NO. 180
(See also case no. 276)

a. Microangiopathic hemolytic anemia.
b. Sulfasalazine induced.

Note: Anemia, jaundice, high reticulocyte count indicates hemolytic anemia. When associated with fragmented RBC (schistocyte, helmet cell) indicate microangiopathic hemolytic anemia. Sulfasalazine may cause blood dyscrasia such as agranulocytosis, megaloblastic anemia, hemolytic anemia, occasionally Heinz body hemolytic anemia. It can also cause GIT upset, skin rash, Stevens Johnson syndrome, reversible sterility in male. Causes of microangiopathic hemolytic anemia are—DIC, TTP, HUS, disseminated malignancy, vasculitis, metallic valve prosthesis, malignant hypertension.

CASE NO. 181

a. Polycystic ovarian syndrome, late onset congenital adrenal hyperplasia, Cushing's syndrome, virilizing tumor of ovary or adrenal.
b. Ultrasonography of ovary and suprarenal glands.
c. Serum testosterone, LH, FSH, androgen (androstenedione, dihydroepiandrosterone), sex hormone-binding globulin (SHBG), 17-hydroxyprogesterone.

Note: Any patient with hirsutism, first the above hormones should be measured. Combination of obesity, hirsutism and amenorrhea or oligomenorrhea, infertility is highly suggestive of polycystic ovarian syndrome. There may be insulin resistance.

In PCOS, there is high testosterone, low SHBG, high LH, normal or low FSH and LH:FSH >2. Free androgen are also high. Mild rise of prolactin.

PCOS may be confused with late onset congenital adrenal hyperplasia, in which serum 17-hydroxyprogesterone and ACTH are high, urine pregnanetriol is also high.

It is also confused with virilizing tumor of adrenal or ovary.

CASE NO. 182

a. Malabsorption syndrome.
b. Barium meal and follow-through X-ray, jejunal biopsy, fecal fat estimation.
c. Osteomalacia.

Note: Frequent diarrhea, weight loss with combination of nutritional deficiency should always raise the possibility of malabsorption syndrome. In this case, both macrocytic and microcytic anemia, low calcium, low albumin indicate malabsorption. Proximal myopathy is due to osteomalacia.

CASE NO. 183

a. Acute promyelocytic leukemia with DIC.
b. Serum fibrinogen, FDP.
c. Relatively good.

Note: Initial blood picture shows pancytopenia. Bone marrow is hypercellular with predominant promyelocyte, which indicates acute promyelocytic leukemia (AML type 3). DIC occurs only in this type of leukemia. Bone marrow may show hypergranular blast cells. The granules contain a procoagulant, which triggers DIC. Reciprocal translocation of the long arms of chromosome 15 and 17 is the basic genetic defect in the type of leukemia.

Treatment: **All-transretinoic acid (ATRA)** plus anthracycline-base (idarubicin) chemotherapy. Combination of arsenic trioxide plus ATRA, when anthracycline therapy cannot be given. Allogenic transplantation may be necessary. Complete remission in 80% cases in young, 60% may be cured. Lysis of blast cells during chemotherapy may worsen DIC, which needs appropriate support with platelet and fresh frozen plasma. Once in remission, acute promyelocytic leukemia has good prognosis.

CASE NO. 184

a. Acromegaly.
b. Wilson's disease, renal failure, heroin abuse.

Note: Normally, during GTT, with the rise of glucose, there is fall of growth hormone. Paradoxical rise of growth hormone during GTT occurs in acromegaly in 50% cases. However, it may occur in other cases such as—Wilson's disease, renal failure, heroin abuse, etc.

CASE NO. 185

a. Hypopituitarism due to Sheehan's syndrome.
b. Serum LH, FSH, ACTH, TSH and FT_3, FT_4, MRI of pituitary.

Note: Postpartum pituitary necrosis is called Sheehan's syndrome, which develops following severe postpartum hemorrhage and features of hypopituitarism. There is failure of lactation, persistent amenorrhea, atrophy of breast, reduced pubic, axillary and body hair, skin is pale, soft, fine and wrinkled. With progressive hypopituitarism, at first there is loss of growth hormone, then LH, FSH, ACTH, TSH. Fatigue and loss libido are early features of gonadotropin deficiency. Gradual loss of secondary sexual characters and reduced muscle bulk occur later. Secondary hypothyroidism occur without myxedema. Diabetes insipidus develops due to lack of ADH, though impaired glomerular filtration caused by cortisol deficiency may mask the symptoms. Coma in hypopituitarism may be due to—(i) Hypoglycemia, (ii) Hyponatremia, (iii) Water intoxication, (iv) Hypothyroidism, (v) Hypothermia.

Low sodium in hypopituitarism is due to SIADH, caused by cortisol deficiency. Potassium is usually normal, as aldosterone is normal or high.

Treatment: (i) Hydrocortisone 15 mg in morning and 5 mg in afternoon, (ii) Thyroxine (it is dangerous to start thyroxine without giving hydrocortisone, Addisonian crisis may occur), (iii) Hormone therapy in premenopause—estrogen (1 to 21 days) plus progesterone (day 14 to 21), (iv) For fertility—gonadotropin may be used.

CASE NO. 186

a. Aspirin therapy.
b. Stop the aspirin.

Note: Prolonged use of low dose aspirin may be associated with bleeding tendency, prolonged prothrombin time, prolonged bleeding time, prolong APTT, etc.

CASE NO. 187

a. Lateral medullary syndrome (also called Wallenberg syndrome).
b. MRI of brain.
c. Horner's syndrome in left eye, cerebellar sign in left side, pain and temperature on opposite side.

Note: Lateral medullary syndrome is characterized by ipsilateral—(i) Horner's syndrome (lesion in descending spinothalamic tract lesion), (ii) Cerebellar signs (lesion in cerebellum and its connection), (iii) Palatal palsy and diminished gag reflex (dysphagia and hoarseness due to IXth, Xth nerve involvement, (iv) Decreased pain and temperature (Vth nerve nucleus and its descending tract lesion).

Contralateral decrease of pain and temperature (spinothalamic tract lesion).

This syndrome is produced by infarction of small wedge of lateral medulla posterior to inferior olivary nucleus, due to occlusion of posterior inferior cerebellar artery (PICA). Occlusion of any of the vessels may be responsible—(i) vertebral, (ii) posterior inferior cerebellar, (iii) superior, middle or inferior lateral medullary arteries.

In the majority of cases of lateral medullary syndrome, there is also occlusion of vertebral artery and pyramidal signs are present.

Vomiting is due to the involvement of nucleus ambiguous, hiccough is due to the lesion in reticular formation and vertigo is due to the involvement of vestibular nuclei.

Rarely, occlusion of lower basilar artery, vertebral artery or one of its medial branches produce medial medullary syndrome, characterized by contralateral hemiplegia, which spares the face, contralateral loss of vibration and joint position sense and ipsilateral paralysis and wasting of tongue.

CASE NO. 188

a. Hypothyroidism.
b. Serum TSH estimation.

Note: Gradual weight gain, ascites, pericardial effusion, high MCV low sodium and hyperlipidemia with high CPK, all suggest hypothyroidism. Polyserositis may occur in myxedema. Muscular pain, arthralgia, effusion in any serous cavity may occur. SIADH, high CPK, SGPT, SGOT, LDH may occur in myxedema.

Other causes of polyserositis—disseminated TB, SLE, polyarteritis nodosa, disseminated malignancy and viral fever (dengue).

CASE NO. 189

a. Mixed connective-tissue disease (MCTD) (or overlap syndrome).
b. ANA, anti-ds DNA, anti-scl 70.
c. Anti-RNP antibody.

Note: MCTD is a group or combination of features of systemic sclerosis, SLE and polymyositis (or other collagen disease, e.g. rheumatoid arthritis). It is better to be called overlap syndrome. Commonly occurs in female, third to fourth decade, rare in children and elderly. Usual features are synovitis, edema of hands, Raynaud's phenomenon and muscular pain or weakness.

Lung involvement occurs in 85% cases, but frequently asymptomatic. CO transfer is diminished only. Pleurisy is common. Pulmonary hypertension is the common cause of death. In 25% cases, renal disease usually membranous glomerulonephritis may occur. Gastrointestinal involvement occurs in 70% cases. In heart, pericarditis (30%), myocarditis, arrhythmia, mitral valve prolapse may occur.

The serum shows high anti-RNP antibody. ANA may be positive with a speckled nucleolar pattern. There may be positive anti-scl 70, CPK may be high. Other investigations are—CBC (ESR is high), X-ray chest (may show reticulonodular shadow), barium swallow, skin biopsy etc.

Treatment: Prednisolone, which responds quickly. 10 years survival in 80% cases.

CASE NO. 190

a. Endoscopy and biopsy, serum CPK, EMG, muscle biopsy.
b. Dermatomyositis with carcinoma of esophagus.

Note: This patient is likely to be suffering from carcinoma of esophagus. His skin manifestations is due to dermatomyositis. It is associated with malignancy that occurs in 5 to 8% cases, as non-metastatic manifestation of malignancy. More in male. It occurs commonly in oat cell carcinoma of bronchus. There is also association with malignancy of ovary, breast, stomach, which may predate the onset of myositis. Associated cancer may not become apparent for 2 to 3 years. Recurrent or refractory dermatomyositis should prompt a search for occult malignancy.

Muscular pain and tenderness are found in 50% cases. Proximal myopathy, wasting are common. Ocular muscle involvement is rare.

Treatment of the primary cause may improve dermatomyositis.

CASE NO. 191

a. Pheochromocytoma.

b. 24 hour urinary VMA, urinary metanephrine, abdominal CT scan or MRI.

Note: Recurrent or paroxysmal attack of hypertension in young is highly suggestive of pheochromocytoma. It is characterized by recurrent, paroxysmal attack of hypertension due to increased release of catecholamines. It is the rare tumor of chromaffin tissue, that secretes catecholamines responsible for 0.1% cases of hypertension. Commonly in adrenal medulla (90%), but may occur in any part of sympathetic chain.

Rule of '10'—10% malignant, 10% extra-adrenal (in sympathetic chain), 10% familial. May be associated with MEN Type II. (primary hyperparathyroidism, medullary carcinoma of thyroid and pheochromocytoma, also called Sipple's syndrome) or MEN Type II b (above plus Marfanoid habitus, skeletal deformity, neuroma of lip, tongue, conjunctiva, eyelid). 25% may be multiple. Hypotension may occur with dopamine secreting tumor.

It may present with pallor, fear of death or anxiety or panic attack or acute medical crisis (myocardial infarction, CVA, acute renal failure, paralytic ileus). Postural hypotension occurs in 70%, glycosuria in 30%.

Most tumors release adrenaline and noradrenaline, but extra-adrenal and large tumor release mainly noradrenaline. Pheochromocytoma may occur in urinary bladder and micturition can precipitate an attack. Commonest extra-adrenal tumor is at bifurcation of aorta (organ of Zuckerkandl).

Other investigations: Serum and urine catecholamines, meta-iodobenzyl-guanidine scan (MIBG) helpful for extra-adrenal tumor (it is selectively taken by adrenergic cells).

Treatment: Surgical resection. For hypertension, α-blocker (phenoxy-benzamine 10 to 20 mg 6 to 8 hourly). If tachycardia, β-blocker may be added (only β-blocker should not be given, as it may cause crisis). Malignant pheochromocytoma is a slowly growing tumor and the patient may survive for long time.

CASE NO. 192

a. Anorexia nervosa.

b. Psychotherapy, controlled supervised diet (to increase the weight 1 kg weekly).

Note: It is common in young girl, onset between 16 to 17 years, rare after 30 years. Less in male (M:F = 1:10). More in higher social class, the girl is hard working, perfectionist and ambitious. Endocrine abnormality is present, which reverts to normal after improvement of the disease.

Diagnostic criteria are (i) Weight loss of at least 15% of the expected body weight, (ii) Avoidance of high calorie diet, (iii) Distortion of body image, so the patient regards herself fatty even when she is thin or grossly underweight, (iv) Amenorrhea for at least 3 months (in male, loss of sexual interest replaces amenorrhea).

There is profound body image disturbance so that despite emaciation, patient still feels overweight and terrified of weight gain. The patient may hide her emaciation by using loosely fitting clothes. Physically overactive, performs excessive exercise, may use laxative or diuretic and sometimes vomit after meal. There may be downy, lanugo hair on trunk and limb. Hypotension, bradycardia, increased sensitivity to cold, constipation, peripheral cyanosis may be found. Anxiety, depression are common. Psychosexual immaturity present. Osteoporosis may occur due to less estrogen. Bilateral parotid enlargement may be present.

Low LH, low FSH, low estradiol, low T_3, but normal T_4 and TSH, high cortisol and high GH are present. In male, low LH and testosterone. Dexamethasone suppression test may be abnormal. All revert to normal after therapy. Glucose intolerance may occur due to starvation.

Treatment: (i) In mild case—treated in outdoor basis, (ii) Moderate to severe case—hospitalization, (iii) Controlled diet to increase the weight 1 kg weekly, (iv) Psychotherapy.

Prognosis: 50% full recovery, 30% partial recovery and 20% none. 2 to 5% death from suicide or physical complication.

CASE NO. 193

a. Carcinoid syndrome.
b. USG of abdomen (to see hepatic metastasis), color Doppler echocardiography, 24 hours urine for 5-HIAA (hydroxy-indolo acetic acid).

Note: In this patient, recurrent attack of diarrhea associated with flushing of face and respiratory distress is consistent with the diagnosis of carcinoid syndrome. Presence of firm, irregular liver is suggestive of metastasis in the liver. Carcinoid tumor is derived from enterochromaffin cells, 90% found in GIT (common in ileum, also appendix, rectum) and 10% in the lung. In appendix, it is usually benign, presents as appendicitis (10%).

Carcinoid tumors are asymptomatic, until metastasis. Only 5% develop carcinoid syndrome, when there is metastasis to the liver. Episodic release of 5-HT and other neuroendocrine mediators (such as bradykinin, histamine, tachykinin, prostaglandin) released from the tumor produce the symptoms, when enter into the systemic circulation.

The features are—recurrent attack of flushing, wheezing, abdominal pain, recurrent diarrhea, vomiting, pellagra and photosensitive dermatitis may occur. Flushing is hallmark. There may be hypotension, bradycardia, facial edema. Cardiac abnormalities are found in 50%, such as tricuspid regurgitation, pulmonary stenosis and endocardial plaques, which may lead to heart failure. Left sided cardiac valves are not affected, but bronchial carcinoid causes left sided valvular lesion. Cardiac involvement is a very poor prognostic marker.

Unexplained right sided heart failure with periodic flushing, wheezing and hypotension is highly suggestive of carcinoid syndrome.

Diagnosis: 24 hours urine for 5-HIAA (5-hydroxy-indole-acetic acid).

Treatment: Surgery or embolization for solitary liver metastasis or bronchial carcinoid. Octreotide or lanreotide improves the syndrome in 90%. Long acting octreotide sometimes inhibits tumor growth. Interferon and chemotherapy may be used which reduces tumor growth, but does not prolong survival. Cyproheptadine and methysergide may help in diarrhea.

Nicotinamide is helpful for pellagra. Survival is 5 to 10 years.

CASE NO. 194

a. Turner's syndrome.
b. Karyotyping from buccal smear.
c. Coarctation of aorta.

Note: This patient presents with persistent amenorrhea with short stature. Estrogen is low, but LH and FSH are high, which suggests primary hypogonadism. The most probable diagnosis is Turner's syndrome, which is a sex chromosomal abnormality, characterized by the absence of one X chromosome (45, X0). Diagnosis is confirmed by a buccal smear, which reveals an absent Barr body. The patient presents with amenorrhea and short stature. Other features are—(i) Neck—short, webbing, low hair line, (ii) Face—small lower jaw, small fish like mouth, low set ears, (iii) Chest—shield like, (iv) Hand- short 4th metacarpal, lymphedema, (v) Elbow—increased carrying angle. Normal IQ.

Investigations: (i) Karyotyping from buccal smear (45, X0 is classical, 46 XX in mosaic), (ii) Ultrasonogram (small uterus, fallopian tube, streak gonad), (iii) Low estrogen, but high LH and FSH.

Association with Turner's syndrome—coarctation of aorta (10 to 20%), horseshoe shaped kidney, diabetes mellitus, Hashimoto's thyroiditis and hypothyroidism.

CASE NO. 195

a. Multiple sclerosis.
b. MRI of brain.
c. Retrobulbar neuritis.

Note: This patient has optic neuritis, nystagmus (cerebellar), scanning speech, monoplegia (UMN type), also history of previous attack is highly suggestive of multiple sclerosis. History of recurrent attack is common (relapsing and remitting in 80 to 90%).

Multiple sclerosis is a demyelinating disorder characterized by the involvement of optic tract, pyramidal tract, cerebellar peduncle and posterior column of spinal cord. Usual presentations are—(i) Weakness of one or more limbs, (ii) Spastic paraplegia (confused with spinal cord compression), (iii) Cerebellar signs, (iv) Brainstem dysfunction—vertigo, diplopia, nystagmus, dysphagia, pyramidal signs in limbs, (v) Bladder dysfunction—incontinence, dribbling, hesitency, (vi) Others (rarely)—epilepsy, trigeminal neuralgia, facial palsy (may be recurrent), 6th nerve palsy, tonic spasm or brief spasm of limbs, dementia, organic psychosis, depression, (vii) Euphoria despite of disability.

Diagnosis of multiple sclerosis is usually clinical. It should be considered in any patient who presents with neurological features that are scattered in time (2 or more separate episodes) and space (2 or more separate locations). There is no single test for diagnosis, but MRI with clinical findings are highly suggestive. CSF study shows oligoclonal bands.

Treatment: Acute attack—intravenous methylprednisolone 1 g/day for 3 to 5 days or oral high dose steroid.

Treatment of aggressive disease—immunomodulating agent and biological agent—Natalizumab, Alemtuzumab and oral fingolimod. Interferon beta SC or IM injection. Glatiramer acetate is similar to interferon beta. Mitoxantrone (5 mg/m^2) in the early aggressive disease.

CASE NO. 196

a. Alzheimer's disease (AD).
b. Multi-infarct dementia, Creutzfeldt-Jakob disease.

Note: AD is a primary degenerative brain disease of unknown cause characterized by gradual deterioration of memory and progressive dementia.

Key features: Inability to remember information acquired in the past. Both short and long-term memory are involved, commonly short-term. In early stage, patient may complain of problem, but in later stage, usually deny of any problem (anosognosia).

Pathology: Macroscopically, there is diffuse atrophy of brain, particularly cerebral cortex and hippocampus with secondary enlargement of ventricular system. Microscopically— (i) Neuritic senile plaque containing Ab amyloid, (ii) Silver staining neurofibrillary tangles in neuronal cytoplasm of cerebral cortex, (iii) Accumulation of Ab amyloid in arterial wall of cerebral blood vessels.

Biochemical abnormality: Impairment of acetylcholinesterase transmission. Other neuro-transmitters, such as noradrenaline, 5HT, glutamate and substance P are also involved.

Treatment: Usually acetylcholinesterase inhibitor drugs are used (donepezil, galantamine, rivastigmine). Another drug—memantine (affects glutamine transmission) may be used. Anti-depressant may be needed.

CASE NO. 197

a. MRI of brain, EEG, lumbar puncture and CSF study (also TPHA).
b. Multiple sclerosis, Alzheimer's disease and Creutzfeldt-Jakob disease.
c. Creutzfeldt-Jakob disease.

Note: Creutzfeldt-Jakob disease is a slow viral encephalopathy, which leads to rapidly progressive dementia with myoclonus, multifocal neurological signs including aphasia, cerebellar ataxia, cortical blindness, spasticity and extrapyramidal signs. Common in middle aged and elderly.

It is characterized by profound neuronal loss, astrocytosis, and a typical spongiform degeneration of the brain. EEG is typical, which shows repetitive slow wave complex.

Iatrogenic transmission to human may occur by surgical specimen, autopsy, corneal graft, depth EEG electrode, neurosurgery (cadaveric dura mater graft), pooled cadaveric growth hormone.

No treatment is available. Quinacrine is in trial. The disease usually rapidly progresses, leading to death within 4 to 6 months.

One variant of CJD called vCJD, rare variety common in young age, slowly progressive, prolonged course. Early symptoms are neuropsychiatric, followed by ataxia, dementia, myoclonus or chorea.

CASE NO. 198

a. Pseudomembranous colitis (secondary to antibiotic).
b. Stool for RME and C/S, isolation of *Clostridium difficile* toxin (A or B) from stool by ELISA, colonoscopy.

c. Antibiotic is stopped, correction of dehydration. Add metronidazole 400 mg TDS or vancomycin 125 mg QDS.

Note: If a patient following antibiotic therapy develops bloody diarrhea, pseudomembranous colitis should be considered. It is an inflammatory condition due to *Clostridium difficile*. 5% healthy adults and 20% elderly are healthy carrier of this organism. Occurs by using any antibiotic, commonly cephalosporin, ampicillin, amoxicillin and clindamycin. Common in the first few days of using antibiotic or even up to 6 weeks after stopping drug. Two types of toxins—A (enterotoxin) and B (cytotoxic) are responsible. It is common (80%) in elderly, above 65 years. Colonic mucosa may be ulcerated, occasionally covered by creamy white membrane like material, so it is called pseudomembranous colitis. May be confused with ulcerative colitis. Complications such as toxic dilatation, perforation, ileus may occur.

Diagnosis: (i) Detecting A or B toxin in stool by ELISA, (ii) Stool culture is positive in 90% cases, (iii) Colonoscopy—erythema, wide plaque, adherent pseudomembrane. Biopsy should be taken.

Treatment: (i) Offending drug should be stopped, (ii) Metronidazole 400 mg 8 hourly or vancomycin 125 mg qds for 7 to 10 days, (iii) In severe case, IV immunoglobulin may be given.

CASE NO. 199

a. Ulcerative colitis, Crohn's disease, angiodysplasia of the colon.
b. Barium enema, colonoscopy and biopsy, color Doppler echocardiogram (others—prothrombin time, APTT).
c. Angiodysplasia of colon.

Note: Angiodysplasia is characterized by vascular malformation, which consists of ectatic areas of mucosal microvessels, especially of capillaries and venules associated with dilatation of submucosal veins. It is common in cecum and ascending colon, but may occur in upper and lower intestine.

Common in elderly, >70 years. The patient usually presents with fresh blood per rectum, which is acute and profuse, usually stops spontaneously but commonly recurs. Angiodysplasia may be associated with aortic stenosis, chronic renal failure, von Willebrand's disease.

Cause—unknown. Dysplasia are degenerative lesions arise from chronic colonic muscular contraction that obstructs the venous mucosal drainage. Later, mucosal capillaries dilate and incompetent with formation of arteriovenous communication.

Best way of diagnosis is by colonoscopy, which shows vascular spots like spider nevi. Selective mesenteric angiography may be helpful.

Treatment: Vessels are obliterated by electrocautery or laser therapy during colonoscopy. In some severe cases, hemicolectomy may be required, if bleeding continues.

CASE NO. 200

a. Antibody against factor VIII, insufficient dose, poor quality factor VIII.
b. Porcine factor VIII, or activated clotting factors—VIIa or Feiba (Factor eight inhibitor bypassing activity—an activate concentrate of II, IX and X).

Note: Following repeated transfusion of factor VIII, there may be production of antifactor VIII antibody, occurs in 20 to 30% cases of severe hemophiliac. This antibody neutralizes the factor VIII, reducing its efficacy. This case is difficult to treat. Factor VIII from other species such as porcine factor VIII may be helpful. Activated clotting factors may be necessary. Other options are—immunosuppressive therapy (steroid, cytotoxic drugs) may be helpful.

CASE NO. 201

a. Infective endocarditis with left sided septic cerebral embolism or left atrial myxoma with left sided cerebral embolism.
b. Full blood count, blood for C/S, echocardiography and CT scan of brain.

Note: Any patient with low grade continuous fever and cardiac murmur should suggest the possibility of infective endocarditis. However, with other systemic features, myxoma should also be excluded. Myxoma is a gelatinous, benign, polypoid, pedunculated, friable tumor arising from the heart. 75% from the left atrium, arises from fossa ovalis or its rim of atrial septum. May arise from mitral valve leaflet, posterior wall of left atrium, right atrium and rarely from ventricle. Involves any sex, any age, may be familial.

Clinical features: Three groups of features (i) Systemic features—fever, malaise, weight loss, arthralgia, Raynaud's phenomenon, skin rash, clubbing, (ii) Obstructive features—like mitral stenosis as it obstructs the valve. In addition to loud 1st heart sound and MDM, tumor plop (3rd sound). Patient may have breathlessness, PND, arrhythmia, syncope or sudden death, (iii) Embolic—cerebral, splenic, kidney or any part of the body.

ESR is high, there may be anemia, may be hemolytic, polycythemia, leukocytosis, thrombocytopenia or thrombocytosis, abnormal serum protein, hypergammaglobulinemia may occur.

Confused with mitral stenosis, but there is no opening snap and the murmur is variable with postural change.

It is confirmed by transthoracic echocardiography, but a transesophageal echocardiogram is more accurate.

Treatment: Surgical excision as early as possible. In 5%, chance of recurrence.

CASE NO. 202

a. Lumbar puncture and CSF study, CT scan or MRI of brain, EEG, antibody to HSV.
b. Herpes simplex encephalitis.
c. Brain abscess, viral encephalitis, meningitis.

Note: Herpes simplex type 1 may cause encephalitis, type 2 may cause benign recurrent lymphocytic meningitis. The virus usually affects the inferior aspect of frontal lobes and medial aspect of temporal lobe.

Herpes simplex encephalitis is characterized by flu-like illness, followed by fever, severe headache, altered consciousness, behavior abnormality and speech disturbance. There may be focal neurological deficit, such as dysphasia, hemiparesis, focal or generalized seizure, commonly temporal lobe seizure. Olfactory and gustatory hallucinations and impairment of memory are recognized. There may be multiple cranial nerve palsy and ataxia. Untreated patient develop convulsion and laps into comatose state. Mortality is high.

Diagnosis: Serum anti-HSV antibody. CSF study, which shows lymphocytic leukocytosis, normal protein and sugar. In CSF, HSV-DNA polymerase chain reaction (PCR) is highly sensitive for rapid diagnosis. EEG shows distinctive periodic pattern in some cases. CT scan shows low density lesion in temporal lobes, that enhance with contrast. MRI shows orbitofrontal and medial temporal lobe involvement (not found in other virus).

Treatment: Acyclovir 10 mg/kg 8 hourly IV for 10 days. Anticonvulsant may be necessary. Dexamethasone for raised intracranial pressure.

CASE NO. 203

a. SLE.
b. Liebmann-Sach's endocarditis.
c. ANA, anti-ds DNA, echocardiography.

Note: In young female with unexplained fever, polyarthralgia, mouth ulcer, persistently high ESR, SLE should be excluded.

In heart, it can cause non-infective, atypical verrucous endocarditis, called Liebmann-Sach's endocarditis, which itself remains asymptomatic, but may cause valvular insufficiency. Commonly involves mitral valve, causing mitral regurgitation, which may be a source of systemic embolism. Anti-phospholipid antibody may be associated with this.

Treatment: High dose steroid is given.

CASE NO. 204

a. Bronchial carcinoma with non-metastatic extrapulmonary manifestations (or paraneoplastic syndrome).
b. Sputum for malignant cells, CT guided FNAC.

Note: Low sodium, chloride, urea are due to SIADH and high calcium is due to PTH like secretion of substance from bronchial carcinoma. Non-metastatic extrapulmonary manifestations of bronchial carcinoma, occurs in 15 to 20% cases. These are (i) Endocrine—SIADH, ectopic ACTH secretion, carcinoid syndrome, hypercalcemia, gynecomastia, (ii) Neurological—peripheral neuropathy, subacute cerebellar degeneration, cortical degeneration, MND, (iii) Musculoskeletal—polymyositis or dermatomyositis, myasthenic myopathic syndrome (Eaton Lambert syndrome), clubbing and hypertrophic osteoarthropathy, (iv) Hematological—anemia, migrating thrombophlebitis, DIC, thrombotic thrombocytopenic purpura, (v) Marantic endocarditis (non-bacterial thrombotic endocarditis), (vi) Skin—acanthosis nigricans, dermatomyositis, (vii) Kidney—nephrotic syndrome (membranous glomerulonephritis).

CASE NO. 205

a. JIA (Still's disease).
b. SLE.
c. RA test, ANA, FNAC of lymph nodes.

Note: Fever, arthritis, neck stiffness, lymphadenopathy, hepatosplenomegaly and leukocytosis in early age should suggest the possibility of JIA, Still's variety. However, other possibilities such as-lymphoma, SLE, disseminated tuberculosis, acute aleukemic leukemia, infection should be excluded.

Still's disease is characterized by systemic features, such as high swinging fever, evanescent pink maculopapular skin rash with fever called Salmon rash, arthralgia or arthritis, myalgia, pleurisy, pericarditis, hepatosplenomegaly, lymphadenopathy. Equally affects both the boys and girls up to 5 years, after that more in female. Leukocytosis, lymphocytosis, thrombocytosis, high ESR and CRP may be present. Autoantibody—negative.

Treatment: (i) To relieve pain—NSAID, (ii) Disease modifying drugs in all cases (such as methotrexate sulfasalazine is used, if enthesitis), (iii) Steroid may be required, if systemic features are present (pulse methylprednisolone), (iv) Anti-TNF agents may be used if methotraexate fails (e.g. etanercept, infliximab, adalimumab), (v) Others—physiotherapy, passive movement to prevent contracture, orthopedic measures, if needed.

CASE NO. 206

a. Visceral leishmaniasis.
b. ICT for leishmaniasis, urine for latex agglutination test (Katex), bone marrow for LD body, FNAC of lymph node.
c. Lymphoma, malaria.

Note: Prolonged fever, hepatosplenomegaly, increased monocyte and low albumin are all in favor of visceral leishmaniasis.

CBC, if repeated, will show progressive leukopenia. There may be pancytopenia, granulocytopenia and increased monocyte. For definitive diagnosis, isolation of LD body from splenic puncture (98%), bone marrow or aspiration from lymph node. Among the non-invasive tests, ICT and urine for latex agglutination test are highly sensitive and specific for early diagnosis. Other tests—DAT, CFT, hemagglutination, ELISA, PCR may be done.

IgG is markedly increased, IgM less so. Total protein is also very high, with low albumin. Cell mediated immunity to visceral leishmaniasis is undetectable.

Treatment: Sodium stibogluconate 20 mg/kg, IV for 30 days. Miltefosine is the only oral drug for leishmaniasis, 50 mg if <25 kg weight, 100 mg in > 25 kg, or 2.5 mg/kg in children.

CASE NO. 207

a. Pyogenic liver abscess.
b. USG of hepatobiliary system.
c. Blood for C/S, fluorescent antibody test, indirect hemagglutination test, ELISA.

Note: High fever, hepatomegaly, high alkaline phosphatase, low albumin, leukocytosis indicates pyogenic liver abscess. PUO may be the only presentation.

Common organisms in pyogenic liver abscess are *E. coli, Streptococcus* (*S. milleri*). Others are *S. faecalis, Staph. aureus,* anaerobic organism, Bacteroides. It may single,more common in right love of liver or multiple, which are due infection in biliary obstruction. Treatment-broad spectrum antibiotic with metronidazole for 3–4 weeks. If large abscess, ultrasonography guided aspiration may be done.

Amebic liver abscess also occurs commonly. In 50% cases, no history of intestinal disease. Abscess are usually large, single in the right love, multiple in advance cases. 5 to 10% cases will have negative serology. USG or CT scan is diagnostic to see the abscess. Aspiration of the pus may demonstrate the organism. Rupture of the abscess into the lung and development of hepatobronchial fistulae is a recognized complication (with anchovy-sauce sputum production). Peritonitis, pericarditis and cutaneous sinus formation are recognized rare complications.

Local intercostal tenderness in right lower chest, local edema should be looked for. Abnormality in right lung base occurs in 25% cases.

Treatment of amebic liver abscess—metronidazole 500 to 750 thrice daily for 7 to 10 days. Other drug—tinidazole or ornidazole 2 g daily for 3 days or nitazoxanide 500 mg twice daily for 3 days. After treatment—diloxanide furoate or paromomycin 500 mg three times daily to 10 days (to eradicate luminal cyst). Sometimes aspiration of large abscess.

CASE NO. 208

a. Sarcoidosis.
b. Cardiomyopathy.
c. MT, serum calcium, serum ACE, gollium-67 scanning, lung biopsy.

Note: Polyarthritis, skin rash, reticulonodular shadow in the lung, lymphopenia are all in favor of sarcoidosis. Dilated cardiomyopathy may also occur. 5% cases of sarcoidosis affect the heart with arrhythmia, conduction disturbance, pericarditis, dilated cardiomyopathy, ventricular aneurysm in presence of normal angiogram. Lymphopenia is characteristic, high serum ACE (may be done to monitor the activity rather than the diagnosis). Anergy is common with negative MT. Lung functions show restrictive pattern and impaired gas exchange.

X-ray of hands may show cystic change in the bone.

CASE NO. 209

a. Proximal renal tubular acidosis (type 2).
b. Ammonium chloride test, serum and urinary pH, USG of renal system.

Note: Proteinuria, glycosuria with low potassium and hyperchloremic acidosis indicate proximal renal tubule dysfunction. In this condition, the amount of bicarbonate that can be reabsorbed is lower than the normal, resulting in bicarbonate loss and acidosis. Proximal RTA may present with myopathy, osteomalacia, etc.

Causes of proximal RTA—(i) Fanconi syndrome (ii) Wilson's disease, (iii) Cystinosis, (iv) Degraded tetracycline, (v) Hyperparathyroidism, (vi) Multiple myeloma, (vii) Amyloidosis, (viii) Drugs—carbonic anhydrase inhibitor, ifosfamide, (ix) Heavy metal poisoning—Pb, Hg, Cd.

CASE NO. 210

a. Chronic constrictive pericarditis.
b. ECG, echocardiography, CT scan or MRI of heart.
c. Cardiac catheterization.

Note: Chronic constrictive pericarditis is suggested by raised JVP, no cardiomegaly, enlarged, tender liver and ascites. Liver function tests may be slightly abnormal, because of passive venous congestion. Serum protein may be low, because of protein losing enteropathy.

Chronic constrictive pericarditis is due to progressive thickening, fibrosis and calcification of the pericardium.

Signs of chronic constrictive pericarditis are (i) Pulse—low volume, tachycardia, pulsus paradoxus may be present, (ii) JVP—raised, Kussmaul's sign may be positive, rapid Y descent, (iii) No cardiomegaly, (iv) Third sound (pericardial knock), (v) Hepatomegaly, (vi) Ascites— earlier than edema.

Differential diagnosis—restrictive cardiomyopathy and CCF.

Chest X-ray—pericardial calcification in 50% cases, no cardiomegaly.

Echocardiography shows thickening of pericardium. Cardiac MRI is more useful than echocardiography.

Cardiac catheter—pericardial constriction encompasses the whole heart, so right and left end diastolic pressures are equal, also the same atrial pressures (shows equal diastolic pressure in all the chambers of heart).

Treatment: Surgery plus treatment of causes.

CASE NO. 211

a. Phenytoin induced SLE.
b. ANA, anti-ds DNA, skin biopsy.
c. Anti-histone antibody.

Note: Drug induced SLE is suggested by history of taking drug, fever, mild systemic features, polyarthralgia, skin rash and pericarditis. There is positive ANA, but negative anti-ds DNA, normal complements. Sex ratio—equal. Lung involvement is common, but renal and neurological involvement are rare. Anti-histone antibody is positive in 95% cases.

Treatment: (i) Withdrawal of the drug, (ii) Occasionally, short course steroid.

Drugs causing SLE are hydralazine, procainamide, anticonvulsant (phenytoin, carbamazepine), phenothiazine, INH, oral contraceptive pills, penicillamine, methyldopa, ACE inhibitor, monoclonal antibody, minocycline.

CASE NO. 212

a. Pneumatosis cystoides intestinalis.
b. Plain X-ray abdomen in erect posture, stool for R/M/E and C/S, sigmoidoscopy.
c. Blind loop syndrome.
d. High flow oxygen.

Note: In any patient with systemic sclerosis, if there is severe abdominal pain, always exclude pneumatosis cystoides intestinalis. It is a rare disease, characterized by presence of air filled pseudocysts in the bowel wall, either submucosal or subserosal, commonly colon. May cause severe colicky abdominal pain, diarrhea, tenesmus, bleeding and intestinal obstruction. Causes unknown, in some cases, may be associated with other diseases, such as COPD, necrotizing enterocolitis, ischemic colitis, systemic sclerosis, etc. Rupture of cyst produces pneumoperitoneum. Characteristic presence of pneumoperitoneum without signs of peritoneal irritation is a clue that surgery is not required immediately. In idiopathic type, sigmoidoscopy may show blue sessile polyp with normal overlying mucosa. Plain X-ray will show gas pockets in bowel, which is highly characteristic.

Treatment: (i) High concentration of oxygen, in some cases, hyperbaric oxygen (ii) Broad spectrum antibiotic IV with metronidazole.

CASE NO. 213

a. Aspirin induced platelet dysfunction.
b. Aspirin should be stopped.

Note: Prolonged use of some drugs such as aspirin, other NSAID, antiplatelet drugs may cause bleeding due to functional abnormality of platelet. Following any bleeding, there may be high leukocyte, platelet, etc. without infection (as in this case).

Other causes of bleeding should be excluded such as DIC, collagen diseases, hemophilia, Christmas disease, von Willebrand's disease, chronic liver disease from the history and physical findings.

Causes of prolonged bleeding time—(i) Thrombocytopenia due to any cause, (ii) Abnormal platelet function (drug—Aspirin, NSAID, ticlopidine), (iii) von Willebrand's disease, Glanzmann's syndrome, dysproteinemia, etc. (iv) Factor V deficiency, (v) Liver failure.

Causes of prolonged prothrombin time: It measures extrinsic pathway (I, II, V, VII, X) and it is prolonged with deficiency of these factors.

Other causes are (i) Anticoagulant therapy (Warfarin), (ii) Hepatic failure, (iii) DIC, (iv) Malabsorption of vitamin K, (vi) Hemorrhagic disease of newborn. PT is most sensitive to deficiency of the factors V, VII and X.

Causes of prolonged APTT: Also called PTTK (partial thromboplastin time with kaolin). It measures intrinsic pathway (I, II, V, VIII, IX, X, XI) and it is prolonged with deficiency of these factors. Other causes are—(i) Hemophilia, (ii) Christmas disease, (iii) von Willebrand's disease (iv) Anticoagulant (heparin), (v) Hepatic failure, (vi) DIC, (vii) Lupus anticoagulant.

Causes of prolonged thrombin time: (i) Hypofibrinogenemia, (ii) Liver failure, (iii) Heparin therapy (but not warfarin), (iv) DIC.

APTT is not prolonged by low molecular weight heparin.
TT is used to monitor heparin therapy.

CASE NO. 214

a. Hemolysis caused by dapsone.
b. Heinz body.
c. Estimation of serum methemoglobin and sulfhemoglobin.
d. Hemolysis, vitamin B_{12} deficiency, folic acid deficiency.

Note: Macrocytic anemia with high reticulocyte count indicate hemolysis, more likely caused by dapsone. Other causes of macrocytosis may be due to vitamin B_{12} or folic acid deficiency, as the patient also looks malnourished. Dapsone may cause mild hemolysis. It can also cause methemoglobinemia and sulfhemoglobinemia, responsible for chemical cyanosis.

Treatment of leprosy: (i) Paucibacillary (2 to 5 skin lesions)—rifampicin 600 mg monthly (supervised) plus dapsone 100 mg daily (self-administered) for 6 months, (ii) Multibacillary (>5 skin lesions)—rifampicin 600 mg and clofazimine 300 mg monthly (supervised) plus dapsone 100 mg and clofazimine 50 mg daily (self-administered) for 12 months, (iii) Paucibacillary single lesion—ofloxacin 400 mg plus rifampicin 600 mg plus minocycline 100 mg- in single dose.

Note: First line drugs in leprosy—rifampicin, clofazimine and dapsone.
Second line drugs—pefloxacin, ofloxacin, minocycline and clarithromycin.

CASE NO. 215

a. Occupational asthma.
b. Pneumoconiosis.
c. Serial measurement of PEFR, serum IgE antibody, skin prick test.
d. Avoid exposure to the responsible agents, use of mask during working, step care treatment of bronchial asthma.

Note: Clue for the diagnosis of occupational asthma in this patient—(i) Textile mill worker, (ii) Relief of symptoms while at home, (iii) Normal X-ray. It is more in smoker.
Poor response of reversibility test indicates severe asthma, not necessarily COPD.
Occupational asthma may be defined as "asthma induced at work by exposure to occupation-related agents, which are mainly inhaled at the work place". The most characteristic features in the medical history is symptoms that worsens on workdays and improves on rest days or holidays. It comprises about 5% of all adult onset bronchial asthma.
This type of asthma may be found in chemical workers, pharmaceutical workers, farmers, grain handlers, cigarette manufacturers, fabric, dye, cosmetics workers, press and printing workers, laboratory workers, poultry breeders, textile workers, wood workers and bakery workers, etc. Atopic individuals and smokers are at risk of developing occupational asthma.
The diagnosis of occupational asthma is made by demonstrating improvement of peak expiratory flow rate or lung volumes when the patient is away from allergen. Measurement of 2 hourly peak flow at and away from work is helpful for diagnosis. In some cases, IgE antibody is increased, especially in atopic individuals.
Keystone of effective management is cessation of further exposure, appropriate work place measure like masks, barriers. If no response, step care asthma management plan should be done.

CASE NO. 216

a. Gitelman's syndrome.
b. 24 hours urine potassium, serum renin and aldosterone (others— 24 hours urinary calcium).
c. Bartter's syndrome, diuretic abuse.

Note: Gitelman's syndrome is characterized by hypokalemia, metabolic alkalosis, normal blood pressure, hypocalciuria, hypomagnesemia, high renin and high aldosterone.

Diagnosis: Low serum potassium (<3 mmol) and high 24 hours urine potassium (>20 mmol) plus high renin and high aldosterone, hypocalciuria, hypomagnesemia.

Treatment: Potassium plus potassium sparing diuretic (spironolactone).

Gitelman's syndrome—variant of Bartter's syndrome, but hypocalciuria, hypomagnesemia are present in Gitelman's syndrome, not in Bartter's syndrome.

CASE NO. 217

a. History of induced vomiting that relieves the symptom.
b. Hypochloremic hypokalemic metabolic alkalosis.
c. Gastric outlet obstruction due to chronic duodenal ulcer.
d. Endoscopy.

Note: Long history of indigestion or dyspepsia may be due to chronic duodenal ulcer. In young patient with vomiting, is highly suggestive of gastric outlet obstruction. In such a case, vomiting of acid stomach contents leads to loss of H^+ and Cl^-. HCO_3 generated in extracellular fluid leads to hypochloremic alkalosis. Hypokalemia is due to vomiting, secondary aldosteronism, alkalosis (enhance entry of potassium into cell), increased renal loss in exchange of sodium. Serum pH is high and urine pH is low (acidic).

CASE NO. 218

a. Acute pyelonephritis.
b. Perinephric abscess.
c. Loss of concavity in right flank or bulging in right flank with scoliosis.
d. Ultrasonography of abdomen, especially renal system.
e. Involvement of L_3 and L_4, deep venous thrombosis of right calf.

Note: Classic triad of pyelonephritis are—fever, loin pain and tenderness over kidney. Fever may be very high, associated with chill and rigor. Urinary complaints like dysuria, frequency, urgency are present.

Perinephric abscess is characterized by severe pain and tenderness in loin, may be bulging and very high fever. Urinary symptoms may be absent and urine examination may be entirely normal.

Other causes of dull or severe loin pain—renal stone, renal tumor, acute pyelonephritis, obstruction in renal pelvis, renal tuberculosis, congenital anomaly of pelviureteric junction (pain increased after drinking more fluid).

CASE NO. 219

a. Pemphigus vulgaris.
b. Erythema multiforme, bullous pemphigoid, bullous lichen planus.
c. Skin biopsy for histopathology and immunofluorescence test (an early intact bullae < 12 hours duration with perilesional area) should be taken.

Note: Pemphigus are a group of autoimmune blistering diseases of skin and mucous membranes, which include pemphigus vulgaris (PV), pemphigus foliaceus and paraneoplastic pemphigus.

PV is an autoimmune blistering disease affecting the skin and mucous membranes, mediated by circulating autoantibodies, directed against keratinocyte cell surfaces. It is characterized by thin walled, flaccid, easily ruptured, intra-epidermal bullae that appear in apparently normal skin and mucous membrane or on erythematous base (associated with mouth ulcer). Causes—unknown. Probable factors—autoimmunity, suggested by intercellular deposition of IgG and C3 complement in epidermis, genetic predisposition (associated with HLA DR4 and DR6), drugs (penicillin, penicillamine, captopril, rifampicin), ultraviolet light, PUVA, ionizing radiation, increased incidence in myasthenia gravis and thymoma. There is recognized association with human leukocyte antigen DR4 and DRw6.

PV presents with oral lesions in the majority of patients and most patients develop cutaneous lesions. Nikolsky sign—rubbing of uninvolved skin results in separation of epidermis.

Treatment: (1) High dose prednisolone—100 to 200 mg daily. When remission occurs with no new blister, taper the dose. Maintenance dose for long time (may require life long). If new blister during treatment, increase the dose of prednisolone. (2) Other therapy—Intravenous methylprednisolone—1 g/day for 5 days (pulse therapy). Mycophenolate mofetil 1 to 1.5 g twice a day (commonly used as steroid sparing drug). Other drugs—azathioprine, cyclophosphamide, methotrexate, cyclosporin, dapsone. In resistant case—intravenous immunoglobulin may be tried. Biologic agents (infliximab, rituximab, etanercept). Extracorporeal photochemotherapy. (3) General treatment—Topical—daily bath, 1% silver sulfadiazine, antiseptic mouth wash, care of eye. Antibiotic, fluid and electrolyte balance blood transfusion (if necessary). Prognosis— bad, recurrence is common with high mortality.

CASE NO. 220

a. Renal tuberculosis partially treated bacterial UTI.
b. MT, urine for AFB and mycobacterial culture and sensitivity, ANA and anti-ds DNA.

Note: Renal or genitourinary tuberculosis is quite common. This lady has a sterile pyuria, which could be due to partially treated bacterial infection. However, genitourinary tuberculosis should be excluded. Genitourinary TB develops in approximately 5% cases of pulmonary TB and is usually due to hematogenous spread to the renal cortex during the primary phase of infection. The cortical lesion may ulcerate, ultimately involving the pelvis, bladder, also in male seminal vesicles and prostate. Other clinical features include hematuria, urethral strictures, cold abscess and chronic epididymo-orchitis. Renal failure may occur due to extensive destruction of the kidneys or by obstruction secondary to fibrosis. The diagnosis can be made with ultrasound or CT scan, intravenous urography, in combination with several early morning urine samples for mycobacterial culture.

Treatment: Like pulmonary TB, to be continued for 9 months to 1 year.

CASE NO. 221

a. Central pontine myelinolysis (CPM).
b. MRI of brain.

Note: Rapid correction of hyponatremia by hypertonic saline results in central pontine myelinolysis (CPM), which is a dangerous complication. There may be various types of neurological deficits, from quadriparesis to coma and death. In CPM, there is demyelination of central basal pons or other areas of brain. Magnetic resonance imaging is the investigation of choice to demonstrate classical demyelination. Usually, rapid correction of hyponatremia by hypertonic saline should be avoided. Correction with IV normal saline and oral salt may be sufficient.

CASE NO. 222

a. Analgesic nephropathy.
b. CT scan of renal system, IVU, renal biopsy.
c. Withdrawal of offending drug, maintaining a fluid intake of 2 to 3 liter per day, control of hypertension and biochemical correction.

Note: The patient was suffering from long-standing arthritis for which she used to take multiple analgesic, which are responsible for chronic tubulointerstitial nephritis with papillary necrosis. It is twice as common in women, and is an important cause of chronic renal failure. 60% of patients are hypertensive at presentation. Sloughing of renal papillae can cause urinary tract obstruction, which may precipitate acute renal failure. Recurrent urinary tract infections are common. There may be sterile pyuria, also occasionally a salt-losing nephropathy. Diagnosis can be made by the history and characteristic appearances on intravenous urography, urine microscopy and biochemical evidence of tubular dysfunction. Renal biopsy is sometimes performed, which shows interstitial fibrosis and tubular atrophy. There is risk of tumors of uroepithelium. Total recovery of renal function occur in 25% patients.

CASE NO. 223

a. Churg-Strauss syndrome, Wegener's granulomatosis, microscopic polyangiitis (also polyarteritis nodosa).
b. Churg-Strauss syndrome.
c. P-ANCA, C-ANCA, kidney biopsy, ANA and anti-ds DNA.

Note: It is likely to be a case of Churg-Strauss syndrome, as suggested by asthma, hypertension, glomerulonephritis, and eosinophilia. It is associated with positive p-ANCA.

Churg-Strauss syndrome is a small-vessel granulomatous vasculitis characterized by cutaneous vasculitic lesions, respiratory involvement giving asthmatic symptoms, eosinophilia, mononeuritis or polyneuropathy and rarely glomerulonephritis. Gastrointestinal and cardiac involvements are recognized. Nasal polyp, allergic rhinitis and adult onset asthma usually occur before vasculitis by many years.

Diagnosis is usually clinical and supported by the presence of necrotizing granulomatous vasculitis with extravascular eosinophilic infiltration in lung, renal or sural (calf) muscle biopsy.

American College of Rheumatology (ACR) has defined criteria for the diagnosis of Churg-Strauss syndrome. Presence of 4 or more is highly indicative of Churg-Strauss syndrome:

1. Asthma. 2. Eosinophilia (10% on WBC differential). 3. Mononeuropathy or polyneuropathy. 4. Migratory or transient pulmonary infiltrates. 5. Systemic vasculitis (cardiac, renal, hepatic). 6. Extravascular eosinophils on a biopsy including artery, arteriole or venule.

Treatment: High dose steroid and cyclophosphamide, followed by maintenance therapy with low dose steroid and azathioprine, MTX, mycophenolate mofetil (MMF). Major life-threatening organ involvement may require treatment with pulse doses of IV methylprednisolone.

Other treatments include intravenous immune globulin; interferon-alpha, and plasma exchange, rituximab, hydroxyurea, Anti I L5 antibody (mepolizumab), omalizumab, plasma exchange has not improved the course of the disease.

CASE NO. 224

a. Heparin induced thrombocytopenia (HIT).
b. Heparin should be stopped, and alternative drug like lepirudin or a heparinoid such as danaparoid should be started.

Note: Thrombocytopenia may occur as a complication of heparin therapy. Two types of heparin induced thrombocytopenia. Type 1 usually occurs within 48 to 72 hours after therapy with unfractionated heparin, and platelet count rarely falls below 1,00,000. Platelet count usually normal over the next 4 days and there is no increased risk of thromboembolism. Type 2 is much rare and usually occurs 5 to 10 days after treatment with heparin and platelet count usually drops below 1,00,000. It is thought to be immune mediated, resulting in the formation of antibodies against heparin-platelet factor 4 complexes. There may be thromboembolism, venous more than arterial. Also, there may be skin necrosis. This condition is suspected in patient who develops thrombocytopenia or >50% drop from the original platelet count with thrombosis, few days after starting heparin. Type 2 HIT can be prevented by using low molecular weight heparin or limiting the use of heparin not >5 days.

All heparin products should be stopped and the patient should be commenced on alternative drug such as lepirudin or a heparinoid such as danaparoid.

CASE NO. 225

a. Pseudo-Cushing's syndrome.
b. Insulin induced hypoglycemia.

Note: Cortisol excess due to other illness is called pseudo-Cushing's syndrome. There is increased urinary excretion of steroid, absent diurnal variation of cortisol and failure of suppression by dexamethasone. This disorder may occur in chronic alcoholic, severe depression and in simple obesity. All revert to normal after removal of the cause.

To differentiate from Cushing's syndrome—insulin induced hypoglycemia is helpful. In Cushing's syndrome—almost no response, but in pseudo-Cushing's syndrome, there is excess cortisol secretion.

Overnight dexamethasone suppression test is usually used as a screening test for Cushing's syndrome. This test has a false-positive rate of up to 2 to 12%, Dexamethasone is primarily metabolized by the cytochrome P-450 system. Considerable increase in cytochrome P-450 enzyme can be seen in regular smokers and people who drink alcohol regularly. Several drugs such as phenobarbital, primidone, ethosuximide, carbamazepine and rifampicin induce the activity of the enzyme and can lead to false-positive dexamethasone suppression test.

CASE NO. 226

a. Diabetic nephropathy with retinopathy.
b. Losartan therapy.

Note: The patient is suffering from type 2 diabetes mellitus with moderate proteinuria and renal failure, highly suggestive of diabetic nephropathy. For the control of hypertension, ARB is thought to be more effective, especially in nephropathy. ACE inhibitor is helpful to reduce microalbuminuria in patient without overt nephropathy and retard progression of nephropathy in Type 1 diabetes mellitus.

Control of hypertension and good glycemic control are effective in retarding nephropathy in both Type 1 and Type 2 diabetes mellitus.

CASE NO. 227

a. Nonalcoholic fatty liver disease.
b. Supervised exercise program to reduce body weight, metformin, statin.
c. Liver biopsy.

Note: Nonalcoholic fatty liver disease (NAFLD) should be considered in obese individuals with abnormal liver function tests without evidence of alcohol excess. It is often asymptomatic, but hepatic enlargement due to lipid deposition within hepatocytes is common.

The NAFLD usually strongly associated with obesity, insulin resistance, dyslipidemia and type 2 DM. Patient with NAFLD are therefore at high risk of developing cardiovascular disease. Good control of diabetes and hyperlipidemia will reduce mortality and morbidity. Statins are not contraindicated in NAFLD despite the widespread misconception that these cause significant derangement of LFTs.

Nonalcoholic fatty liver disease (NAFLD) is subdivided into nonalcoholic fatty liver (NAFL) and nonalcoholic steatohepatitis (NASH). In NAFL, hepatic steatosis is present without evidence of inflammation, whereas in NASH, hepatic steatosis is associated with hepatic inflammation that histologically is indistinguishable from alcoholic steatohepatitis. NASH may lead progressive liver fibrosis, cirrhosis and liver cancer also cardiovascular risk.

Treatment: Rapid weight loss may increase fat deposition in liver and may precipitate NASH. Weight loss of 1 kg/week with an initial target loss of 10% body weight has been shown to be effective at restoring normal liver function. Exercise programs are an effective way to aid weight loss and reduce insulin resistance.

Various drugs have been used in the treatment of NAFLD, without proved benefit. Metformin is recommended for the treatment of insulin resistance associated with NAFLD and has been shown to reduce transaminases and lead to histological improvement. Insulin has little proven benefit over oral agents in the treatment of Type 2 diabetes. Orlistat for obesity and type 2 diabetes mellitus with NASH. Atorvastatin in dyslipidemia and NASH. Omega-3 fatty acids—may be used.

CASE NO. 228

a. Disseminated tuberculosis, lymphoma, neurosarcoidosis, SLE.
b. Neurosarcoidosis.
c. MT, ANA and anti-ds DNA, FNAC or biopsy from lymph node (Others—serum calcium, lung biopsy).

Note: This patient has neurological findings with dehydration, pyrexia, bilateral iritis and also lymphopenia, X-ray shows reticulonodular shadow. These findings are all consistent with neurosarcoidosis. Cerebral involvement in sarcoidosis is rare; features are cranial nerve lesions, aseptic meningitis, psychosis, multiple sclerosis type syndrome, etc. Mononeuritis multiplex is a recognized manifestation in peripheral nervous system.
(See also Case Nos 007 and 208).

CASE NO. 229

a. Myasthenic crisis.
b. Plasmapheresis.
c. Arterial blood gas analysis, serial measurement of FVC.

Note: The patient's history and physical findings support the diagnosis of myasthenia gravis. Severe generalized muscle weakness and respiratory failure, deterioration suddenly is due to myasthenic crisis. This may be precipitated by intercurrent illness or may occur spontaneously or with drugs.

Plasmapheresis directly removes anticholinergic receptor antibodies from the circulation. Treatment is given for up to 2 weeks and is effective for 1 to 2 months. Intravenous immunoglobulin is as effective as plasmapheresis in acute myasthenic crisis. Anticholinesterase drug therapy may cause cholinergic crisis that is also characterized by muscle weakness. Differentiation between cholinergic crisis and myasthenic crisis is based upon the presence of muscle fasciculation, pallor, abdominal cramps, excessive sweating, excessive salivation, small pupil and bradycardia in the former. Anticholinesterase drugs are withdrawn in myasthenia gravis, who present with severe generalized muscle weakness.

CASE NO. 230

a. Wegener's granulomatosis (WG).
b. Microscopic polyangiitis (or polyarteritis nodosa).
c. c-ANCA, biopsy from nasal crust.

Note: Wegener's granulomatosis is a necrotizing granulomatous vasculitis, involving the upper and lower respiratory tract and kidneys. It causes epistaxis, sinusitis, destruction of the nasal cartilage and glomerulonephritis and renal failure. c-ANCA is positive. It may involve any organ system.

Wegener's granudomatosis (WG), microscopic polyangiitis (MPA) and Churg-Strauss syndrome (CSS) are associated with primary systemic small-to-medium-sized vessel vasculitis associated with antineutrophil cytoplasmic antibodies (ANCA). However, WG can also affect medium and even large arteries, and may lack an association with ANCA. Usually, Wegener's granulomatosis is characterized by the presence of c-ANCA (antigen is proteinase 3), whereas microscopic polyangiitis is characterized by p-ANCA (antigen is myeloperoxidase).

Diagnosis of WG is based on combination of clinical, laboratory and, if necessary, pathological features. If typical clinical picture is associated with positive ANCA, with specificity for proteinase 3 (PR3), the diagnosis of WG can be presumed. Biopsy of the involved tissue will show necrotizing granulomatous lesion in small vessels (biopsy taken from nasal crust, lung or kidney, if these are involved).

Treatment: High dose steroid and cyclophosphamide, followed by maintenance therapy with low dose steroid and azathioprine, MTX, mycophenolate mofetil (MMF). Major life-threatening organ involvement may require treatment with pulse doses of IV methylprednisolone.

Other treatments—rituximab with high dose steroid, plasma exchange, intravenous immune globulin.

To monitor – CBC, ESR, CRP and c-ANCA should be measured periodically.

CASE NO. 231

a. Postural hypotension, hypoglycemic attack, pacemaker failure, pacemaker syndrome.
b. Pacemaker syndrome.
c. Dual chamber pacing should be done.

Note: Following single chamber pacing, there may be pacemaker syndrome. It is a disorder characterized by transient hypotension, fatigue, dizziness, syncope and distressing pulsation in the neck and chest. This occurs at the onset of ventricular contraction due to loss of atrio-ventricular synchrony. It occurs in single chamber pacing, which can be prevented by dual chamber pacing or by reducing the pacemaker rate so that, sinus rhythm predominates. However, as the patient is diabetic and hypertensive, other causes as mentioned above should be excluded.

CASE NO. 232

a. Occupational asthma, extrinsic allergic alveolitis (EAA).
b. Hypersensitivity pneumonitis (previously called extrinsic allergic alveolitis)
c. Lung function test, CT scan of the chest, bronchoscopy with bronchoalveolar lavage.

Note: This is likely to be a case of hypersensitivity pneumonitis evidenced by her work in the farm, with the symptoms. Recently, she has developed progressive breathlessness, suggesting parenchymal lung disease. Repeated episodes of pneumonitis progress to pulmonary fibrosis. In chronic cases, CXR is similar to cryptogenic fibrosing alveolitis except that in EAA, fibrosis is usually more pronounced in the upper zones. Also in such cases, usually there are clubbing with bilateral end inspiratory coarse crepitations.

Hypersensitivity pneumonitis results from inhalation of wide variety of organic antigen which give rise to widespread diffuse inflammatory reaction in the alveoli and bronchioles. Commonest causes are farmers lung and bird fancier's lung.

Investigations: (i.) CXR shows fluffy nodular shadows in upper zone, honeycomb lung, (ii) HRCT of chest, (iii) Lung function test (shows restrictive pattern with decrease CO transfer, (iv) CBC (No eosinophilia, may be leukocytosis), (v) Antibodies in the serum, (vi) Bronchoalveolar lavage shows high T lymphocyte and granulocyte.

Allergic bronchopulmonary aspergillosis is another possibility, which is characterized by wheeze, high eosinophil count, and proximal bronchiectasis in chest X-ray.

Diagnostic features of hypersensitivity pneumonitis (1) Evidence of exposure to a recognized antigen, (2) Clinical and radiographic features (cough, wheeze, fever, micronodular shadows in upper, mid or lower zones, restrictive lung defect), (3) Bronchoalveolar lavage with lymphocytosis (with low CD4 to CD8 ratio), (4) Positive inhalation challenge test, (5) Compatible histopathological changes. The diagnosis is possible without histological confirmation, if criteria 1 to 3 are present.

Treatment: Avoidance of allergen, prednisolone 30 to 40 mg daily for 1 to 2 weeks and then tapered over the next 2 to 4 weeks.

CASE NO. 233

a. Kallmann's syndrome.
b. Anosmia.
c. Measurement of gonadotropin releasing hormone (GnRH).

Note: Kallmann's syndrome results from disordered migration of gonadotropin releasing hormone (GnRH) producing neurons into the hypothalamus. This leads to failure of episodic GnRH secretion and subsequent failure of luteinizing hormone (LH), follicle stimulating hormone (FSH) and testosterone production. It is often familial, may be inherited as X-linked, autosomal dominant or autosomal recessive. 75% of sufferers have absent sense of smell (anosmia, which is due to hypoplasia of olfactory bulb). It is common in male, rare in female (male to female ratio 4:1). The syndrome is associated with cleft lip and palate, high arched palate, nystagmus and sensorineural deafness. In 55% cases, renal agenesis may occur. Also, there may be cryptorchidism, cerebellar dysfunction, cerebral abnormality (e.g. color blindness).

Treatment: GnRH hormone therapy restore pituitary function. In female, cyclic estrogen and progesterone therapy should be given. Fertility is possible.

CASE NO. 234

a. Osteomalacia.
b. X-ray of pelvis (to see looser's zone), serum 25-hydroxyproline (low or absent).

Note: Combination of bone fracture, hypocalcemia, hypophosphatemia, high alkaline phosphatase and high parathyroid hormone are highly suggestive of osteomalacia, due to vitamin D deficiency.

In vitamin D deficiency, there is increased parathyroid hormone, which maintains normal serum calcium concentration at the expense of the skeleton. Osteomalacia is a metabolic bone disease characterized by softening of the bone due to deficiency of vitamin D, resulting in inadequate mineralization of osteoid tissue. Ratio of osteoid tissue to calcium and phosphate is increased (low calcium, low phosphate and increased osteoid tissue. Alkaline phosphatase is also high).

CASE NO. 235

a. Pneumonia due to *Mycoplasma pneumoniae.*
b. Erythema multiforme.

c. Coomb's positive autoimmune hemolytic anemia.

d. Serum cold agglutinin estimation, serological test for *Mycoplasma*.

Note: Pneumonia associated with skin rash and hemolytic anemia is highly suggestive of *Mycoplasma pneumoniae* infection. Systemic upset, dry cough, fever, myalgia and arthralgia are common. WBC is usually normal. Extrapulmonary manifestations of *Mycoplasma* occur in up to 10% of cases, such as cold autoimmune hemolytic anemia, thrombocytopenia, renal failure, hepatitis, myocarditis, meningism and meningitis, transverse myelitis and cerebellar ataxia. Cutaneous manifestation includes erythema multiforme. Hemolysis is associated with the presence of cold agglutinins, found in up to 50% of cases of *Mycoplasma pneumoniae*. Low sodium is due to SIADH complicating pneumonia. Diagnosis is based on demonstration of anti-mycoplasma antibodies in paired sera.

Treatment: Macrolide antibiotic (clarithromycin 500 mg BD orally or IV or azithromycin 500 mg BD). Other drugs— erythromycin, tetracycline or doxycycline.

CASE NO. 236

a. Eaton-Lambert syndrome.

b. SIADH.

c. EMG, measurement of anti-VGCC (voltage-gated calcium channel) antibodies.

Note: The clinical picture is myasthenic myopathic syndrome (also called Eaton-Lambert syndrome). This is an autoimmune paraneoplastic phenomenon, most often associated with small cell lung cancer. It may present 2 years before primary malignancy is diagnosed. Clinical features are weakness and pain, especially in limb girdle muscle groups. Proximal myopathy of lower limb is more common. Ptosis and diplopia are present in 70% cases. Ocular-bulbar features are usually less severe than in myasthenia gravis. In contrast to myasthenia gravis, reflexes are diminished or absent, autonomic disturbance like dry mouth or impotence are common in myasthenic myopathic syndrome. EMG shows progressive incremental response (opposite to myasthenia gravis, where there is progressive decremental response). The underlying pathophysiology involves production of autoantibodies against P/Q type voltage-gated calcium channels (VGCC) at the neuromuscular junction, which impair release of acetylcholine from nerve terminals.

Treatment: 3, 4-diaminopyridine and pyridostigmine are effective. Immunosuppressive therapy may be given. Treatment of the primary cause.

CASE NO. 237

a. Subarachnoid hemorrhage.

b. CT scan of brain.

c. Lumbar puncture and CSF study.

d. Polycystic kidney disease.

Note: Subarachnoid hemorrhage is characterized by severe headache of sudden onset, as if being hit on the back of head, called hammer headache, followed by unconsciousness. It is due to rupture of berry aneurysm. Polycystic kidney disease is associated with berry aneurysm in 10% cases. CT scan should be done immediately. Fundoscopy may show subhyaloid hemorrhage.

Treatment: Control of blood pressure and administration of nimodipine. Surgical obliteration of aneurysm is the mainstay of treatment with an increasing tendency for early clipping of the aneurysm (within 3 days of initial bleeding).

CASE NO. 238

a. Cerebellar syndrome due to phenytoin toxicity.
b. Serum phenytoin and sodium valproate.

Note: The patient has signs of cerebellar lesion, which is more likely due to phenytoin toxicity. Nystagmus is present even in mild toxicity. Abnormal liver function is more likely due to sodium valproate, but may occur due to phenytoin. Hypotonia and reduced muscle power may be due to cerebellar syndrome. But in this case, it may be due to electrolyte imbalance. Though, CT scan is normal, MRI is the investigation of choice to detect lesion of cerebellum.

CASE NO. 239

a. Listeria meningoencephalitis.
b. MRI of brain.

Note: This patient has meningitis with brainstem involvement and CSF study shows high neutrophil, but no organism in gram staining. These features are consistent with *Listeria* meningitis. It should always be considered in patient with meningitis associated with brain-stem involvement. It is common in neonate, elderly, alcoholic, pregnant woman and in immunosuppressed patients. Focal neurological signs and cranial nerve palsy are recognized features. Viral, TB and fungal meningitis usually show a lymphocytic pleocytosis. Brainstem involvement with other bacterial meningitis is rare. Herpes simplex encephalitis involves the temporal lobes and therefore, presents with seizures, cognitive (memory) and behavior change. Brainstem involvement is absent.

Treatment: Gentamicin (5 mg/kg IV daily) and ampicillin (2 g IV 4 hourly daily). Alternative drugs — Imipenem and meropenem have excellent response in *Listeria*. Trimethoprim-sulfamethoxazole 50 mg/kg daily in 2 times daily plus ampicillin (2 g IV 4 hourly daily) is also effective.

CASE NO. 240

a. Allergic bronchopulmonary aspergillosis.
b. X-ray chest, serum IgE measurement, skin test to *Aspergillus fumigatus* (other—sputum for fungal hyphae of *A. fumigatus*).

Note: History of bronchial asthma, eosinophilia and perihilar infiltrates is consistent with allergic bronchopulmonary aspergillosis.

Diagnosis of allergic bronchopulmonary aspergillosis is made by (i) Bronchial asthma, (ii) Proximal bronchiectasis and parenchymal infiltrates in the perihilar area, (iii) High titers of IgE and IgG antibodies, (iv) Positive skin test to *Aspergillus fumigatus*, (v) Peripheral high eosinophil count, (vi) Fungal hyphae of *A. fumigatus* on sputum examination. X-ray chest shows pulmonary infiltrate, bronchiectasis (usually proximal).

Treatment: Prednisolone 40 to 60 mg daily and chest physiotherapy. Maintenance dose of steroid is 7.5 to 10 mg daily. Itraconazole 400 mg/day facilitated the reduction of steroid. If persistent collapse, bronchoscopy should be done in impacted mucous. For asthma, inhaled steroid should be given. Omalizumab (monoclonal antibody against Ig E) is in trial. Surgery may be done in some cases.

Differential diagnoses are—drug induced, tropical pulmonary eosinophilia or Churg-Strauss syndrome. In this case, no drug history to indicate an eosinophilic pneumonitis, nor a history of traveling to the tropics to suggest tropical pulmonary eosinophilia. Churg-Strauss syndrome is unlikely in the absence of vasculitis, neuropathy or renal involvement. Pure bronchial asthma does not cause pulmonary infiltrates.

Tropical pulmonary eosinophilia is an immune reaction to the infection with human filarial parasites *Wuchereria bancrofti* and *Brugia malayi*. It is characterized by non-productive cough, wheeze, fever, weight loss, lymphadenopathy, eosinophilia and patchy infiltrates in chest X-ray. The condition occurs in patient infected in the tropics. It is treated with diethylcarbamazine.

CASE NO. 241

a. Mixed obstructive and restrictive defect with a reduced KCO.
b. Diabetes insipidus.
c. Histiocytosis X (also called Langerhans cell histiocytosis).
d. Serum and urine osmolality, bone marrow study.

Note: In this patient, low FEV_1/FVC ratio is suggestive of obstructive airway defect and low residual volume suggests restrictive defect. Polydipsia, polyuria with respiratory involvement is suggestive of diabetes insipidus. Blood pictures show pancytopenia. In a boy with a mixed restrictive and obstructive defect, diabetes insipidus and pancytopenia are more likely due to histiocytosis X.

Transbronchial lung biopsy, liver biopsy or trephine aspirate may show histiocytes and small round cells.

Histiocytosis X is a syndrome of unknown etiology, characterized by formation of Langerhans cells from dendritic cells that involves the skin, bones, ears, lungs, eyes and reticuloendothelial and central nervous systems. Skin rash is common. Pathology—there is proliferation of Langerhans cells with collection of histiocyte, eosinophil and lymphocyte. Langerhans cells secrete prostaglandin E and IL-1, responsible for widespread osteolytic bony lesion.

Three types—(1) Letterer—Siwe disease—occurs in infant, fulminant visceral form of disease and confused with lymphoma. Involves liver, spleen, lymph node, skin, bone marrow. (2) Hand—Schuller—Christian disease posterior pituitary is commonly involved. Diabetes insipidus is common, multiple bone lesions, exophthalmos may occur. (3) Eosinophilic granuloma (adult type)—common in male and in smoker. Interstitial lung disease may occur. It may be focal, involve the bone (skull, jaw, spine).

Treatment:
1. Unifocal—no treatment needed, sometimes surgery or curettage may be needed.
2. Progressive disease—low dose radiation, chemotherapy (etoposide).
3. Systemic involvement
   - Stop smoking.
   - Drugs—steroid, vinblastin, methotrexate, etoposide.

- If interstitial lung disease- penicillamine may be given.
- Bone marrow transplantation in some cases.

CASE NO. 242
(See also case no. 161)

a. Leukemoid reaction.
b. PBF may show toxic granulations or Dohle bodies in the white cells, neutrophils show toxic shift to the left.
c. Bone marrow study.

Note: Leukemoid reaction may follow any sepsis or infection. In some cases of overwhelming infection, the 'sick' marrow releases immature cells into the bloodstream. Thus, there is plenty of myelocytes and normoblasts, confuses with leukemia, where the marrow is characteristically replaced by neoplastic cells. In leukemoid reaction, there is no lymphadenopathy or hepatosplenomegaly.

CASE NO. 243
(See also case no. 157)

a. Lupus anticoagulant syndrome.
b. ANA, anti-ds DNA, serum antiphospholipid or anticardiolipin.
c. Anti-phospholipid antibody.

Note: In any young patient especially female, it is important to exclude SLE or anti-phospholipid syndrome as a cause of CVD with hemiplegia. There is history of miscarriages, thrombocytopenia, high ESR, all of which are characteristic of lupus anticoagulant syndrome or anti-phospholipid syndrome. Echocardiography may show evidence of verrucous (Libmann-Sack) endocarditis. ASD is non-significant in this case.

CASE NO. 244

a. Pneumonia due to *Legionella pneumophila*.
b. Urinary *Legionella* antigen, direct immunofluorescent staining of sputum, anti-*Legionella* antibody.
c. Vomiting, SIADH, acute tubulointerstitial nephritis.
d. Oxygen therapy, antibiotic (erythromycin or azithromycin intravenously) plus rifampicin, correction of electrolytes.

Note: Pneumonia associated with confusion, hyponatremia, lymphopenia, hematuria and proteinuria are highly suggestive of *Legionella pneumophila* infection. Abnormal liver biochemistry (especially aminotransferases) and renal function occur in 50% of patients.

Outbreaks due to contaminated water-cooling systems, air-conditioning or showers. May be occupational history or recent hotel holiday. Usually, occurs in previously fit individuals. Males are affected more than female.

Incubation period is 2 to10 days and it typically presents with flu-like symptoms such as fever, malaise, myalgia and headache. The patient later develops cough, breathlessness and confusion, 50% develop gastrointestinal symptoms. Neurological features like confusion, hallucination, peripheral neuropathy, myelitis, rarely cerebellar syndrome may occur. Renal involvement like tubulointerstitial nephritis may occur.

Investigations: Hyponatremia, lymphopenia, hematuria, proteinuria and hypoxia. High SGPT, SGOT, alkaline phosphatase, CPK may occur.

Diagnosis: Quickest way is to detect urinary legionella antigen (90% positive in first week) and direct immunofluorescent staining of the organism in sputum (may be found in pleural fluid, or bronchial washings). Gram stain does not reveal organism. Fourfold rise in antibody titer to > 1:128 is helpful.

Treatment: Macrolide antibiotic (clarithromycin 500 mg BD orally or IV or azithromycin 500 mg BD for 10 to 14 days). Other drugs—erythromycin, tetracycline or doxycycline.

▋ CASE NO. 245

a. Brucellosis.
b. *Brucella* agglutination test or *Brucella* immunoglobulins (ELISA).
c. Tetracycline and rifampicin.

Note: Malaise, myalgia, headache and weight loss in association with neutropenia, hepatosplenomegaly, orchitis and erythema nodosum are highly suggestive of brucellosis.

Brucellosis is caused by *Brucella*, a gram-negative bacillus, contacted from cows, goats, pigs or sheep. Three species cause infection in man *B. abortus* (cattle), *B. melitensis* (goats/sheep) and *B. suis* (pigs). Infection occurs usually through gastrointestinal tract, due to consuming unpasteurized milk. From gastrointestinal tract, bacilli travel to the lymphatics and infect lymph nodes, and eventually there is hematogenous spread to other organs.

Onset is insidious. Malaise, headache, myalgia, weakness and night sweats are common. There is an undulant high fever. Lymphadenopathy is common. Hepatosplenomegaly may be present, splenomegaly usually indicates severe infection. Tenderness is relatively common. There may be arthritis, orchitis, endocarditis, osteomyelitis, and meningoencephalitis.

Brucellosis may be chronic, associated with fatigue, myalgia, depression, occasionally fever. Splenomegaly is characteristic. Infection may be localized to specific organs such as the bones, heart or central nervous system. In such cases, systemic features are absent in 60% cases and antibody titers are low.

Diagnosis is based on positive blood culture and rising anti-*Brucella* immunoglobulin titres. Blood cultures are positive in 50% cases. *Brucella* agglutination test is positive within 4 weeks of the onset of illness.

Treatment: As follows:
❖ Non-localized disease—Doxycycline 100 mg orally twice daily for 6 weeks plus gentamicin 5 mg/kg for 7 days **or** Doxycycline 100 mg orally twice daily plus rifampin 600 to 900 mg orally once daily for 6 weeks.
❖ Bone disease—Doxycycline 100 mg orally twice daily plus rifampin 600 to 900 mg orally once daily for 6 weeks plus gentamicin 5 mg/kg for 7 days. **Or** Ciprofloxacin 750 mg twice daily plus rifampin 600 to 900 mg orally once daily for 3 months.
❖ Neurobrucellosis—Doxycycline 100 mg orally twice daily plus rifampin 600 to 900 mg orally once daily for 6 weeks plus Injection ceftriaxone 2 g twice daily until CSF is clear.

❖ Endocarditis -Doxycycline 100 mg orally twice daily plus rifampin 600 to 900 mg orally once daily for six weeks plus trimethoprim 5 mg/kg for 6 month plus gentamicin 5 mg/kg IV for 2 to 4 weeks.

CASE NO. 246

a. Cervical myelopathy, cervical cord compression, motor neuron disease, multiple sclerosis.
b. Cervical myelopathy.
c. MRI of cervical spine.
d. C_5 and C_6 level.

Note: Progressive weakness of arms and hands with combination of lower motor neuron signs in upper limbs and upper motor neuron signs in lower limbs, more likely diagnosis is cervical myelopathy. Loss of vibration at ankles may be a normal finding in elderly, but may be due to dorsal column lesion.

Both cervical myelopathy and cervical cord tumor present with involvement of upper limb, which usually produces lower motor neuron disturbances at the level of the lesion and upper motor signs below it. MRI is the best investigation to differentiate between these two.

Absent supinator and biceps reflex, but exaggerated triceps reflex, indicates lesion at C_5 and C_6. Small muscle wasting in cervical myelopathy is due to reduced blood flow to the lower segments of the cord. Sensory disturbance in the upper limbs may be absent or very mild in cervical myelopathy.

Cervical myelopathy is due to bulging or extrusion of the disk into the cervical spinal canal, which results in pressure atrophy and ischemia. Common cause is osteoarthritis of cervical spine. Posterior columns (dorsal tracts carrying proprioception, vibration sense and light-touch fibers) and the lateral column (pyramidal tracts carrying upper motor neurons) are affected. C_5 to C_7 cervical segments are most commonly affected. Symptoms are those of lower motor neuron signs at these levels and upper motor neuron signs below. Neck stiffness and upper limb pain may be present. Spasticity of the lower limbs is common. Ataxia may occur owing to dorsal column involvement (sensory ataxia). Lhermitte's sign (electrical shock feeling down the spinal cord and into the legs) is recognized. This sign may also be found in cervical cord tumor, multiple sclerosis and subacute combined degeneration of spinal cord.

CASE NO. 247

a. Postpartum thyroiditis.
b. β-blocker.

Note: Postpartum thyroiditis occurs usually 2 to 6 months after delivery and is associated with transient hyperthyroidism, followed by hypothyroidism, which usually resolves but permanent hypothyroidism may occur. It occurs in 5% of females. Radioactive iodine test will show less uptake. Cause is unknown, but lymphocytic infiltration in thyroid is suggestive of autoimmunity. Symptoms usually resolve spontaneously, β-blocker may be given.

It may be confused with de Quervain's thyroiditis, which is associated with tender enlargement of thyroid gland, constitutional symptoms and high ESR.

Causes of high T_3 and T_4, but low radioiodine uptake are found in subacute thyroiditis, postpartum thyroiditis, iodine induced hyperthyroidism, factitious hyperthyroidism.

CASE NO. 248

a. Chronic lymphocytic leukemia.
b. Hemolytic anemia.
c. Autoimmune hemolytic anemia (warm type) and bone marrow infiltration.
d. May be due to high reticulocyte count secondary to hemolysis, megaloblastic anemia due to folate deficiency.
e. Direct Coomb's test.

Note: In elderly person with the above blood count, is highly suggestive of chronic lymphocytic leukemia.

This disease is common in elderly, 65 to 70 years. Male: Female = 2:1, involving B lymphocyte.

It may be asymptomatic, diagnosed incidentally in routine examination. General features like malaise, weakness, fatigue, weight loss, night sweating, and features of anemia. There may be recurrent infection, generalized lymphadenopathy, hepatosplenomegaly. Blood picture shows high lymphocyte count with smear or smudge cells. Bone marrow examination shows increased lymphocytes. Reticulocyte is high in autoimmune hemolytic anemia and Coomb's test is positive. Paraproteins may be increased and uric acid is also high, immunophenotyping-B cell antigen (CD19 and CD23) and T cell antigen (CD5). No treatment is necessary in asymptomatic case. If indicated, chlorambucil 5 mg daily, adjust the dose according to blood count. Fludarabine may be given. Prednisolone is given in marrow failure or autoimmune hemolytic anemia.

Local radiotherapy of lymph node causing discomfort or local obstruction and huge splenomegaly.

CASE NO. 249

a. Stevens Johnson's syndrome.
b. Toxic epidermal necrolysis.
c. Stop carbamazepine.

Note: Involvement of skin and mucous membrane of mouth is highly suggestive of Stevens Johnson's syndrome (or toxic epidermal necrolysis). In this patient, it is likely to be due to carbamazepine therapy. Stevens Johnson's syndrome is a severe form of erythema multiforme with widespread bullous lesion in skin and mucous membrane of mouth, eyes, genitalia associated with severe constitutional symptoms. In this case, <10% body surface area (BSA) is involved. When >30% BSA is involved, it is called TEN. Most commonly induced by same medications. Patient initially presents with SJS, may progress to TEN.

It is often idiopathic, but may be associated with viral infections, leukemia, lymphoma and drugs (sulfonamides and anticonvulsants).

Treatment: Carbamazepine is stopped. Symptomatic (IV fluid, antipyretic, antibiotic). Local care of eyes and mouth. In severe cases—IV immunoglobulin. Steroid- its use is controversial. Can be used and tapered rapidly. Because, once skin loss has occurred, it may aggravate morbidity and mortality, because of immunosuppression.

CASE NO. 250

a. Mixed restrictive and obstructive airway disease.

b. Pleural thickening, respiratory muscle weakness and chest wall disease (such as thoracoplasty or scoliosis).
c. Chest X-ray.

Note: In this case, FEV_1 and FVC are both reduced, producing a restrictive pattern. Also, there is low RV. DLCO is also reduced in restrictive defect. But high KCO is due to extrapulmonary restriction. This can be caused by pleural disease like thickened pleura, respiratory muscle weakness and chest wall disease like thoracoplasty or scoliosis.

Emphysema produces an obstructive airway defect on spirometry with increased RV, but decreased DLCO.

Cryptogenic fibrosing alveolitis produces a restrictive pattern, but KCO is reduced, although it can be normal but is never elevated.

CASE NO. 251

a. Cryptogenic fibrosing alveolitis (Idiopathic pulmonary fibrosis, IPF)
b. Restrictive airway disease.
c. Chest X-ray, CT scan of chest, lung biopsy.

Note: In restrictive lung disease, ratio of FEV_1/FVC is normal, or increased, but low TLC, low transfer factor for carbon monoxide. In this case, lung function demonstrates a restrictive defect with an increased ratio of FEV_1/FVC and decreased lung volumes. Both DLCO and KCO are reduced. DLCO is sensitive (but not specific), indicator of the integrity of alveolar capillary membrane and gas exchange function of the lung.

CASE NO. 252

a. Tumor lysis syndrome (TLS).
b. Serum phosphate (high), calcium (low).
c. Dialysis (mainly hemodialysis).
d. Serum uric acid (may be high) and LDH (high level is considered as a marker of bulky disease, with a risk of TLS).

Note: Tumor lysis syndrome (TLS) is characterized by hyperuricemia, hyperkalemia, hyperphosphatemia, and hypocalcemia and is caused by the destruction of a large number of rapidly proliferating neoplastic cells. Acidosis may also develop. Acute renal failure occurs frequently.

TLS is most often associated with the treatment of Burkitt's lymphoma, acute lymphoblastic leukemia and high-grade non-Hodgkin's lymphoma, but also seen in chronic leukemias and rarely, with solid tumors. This syndrome may be found in patients with chronic lymphocytic leukemia after treatment with nucleosides. TLS has been observed with administration of glucocorticoid, hormonal agents such as letrozole and tamoxifen, and monoclonal antibodies such as rituximab and gemtuzumab. TLS usually occurs during or shortly (1 to 5 days) after chemotherapy. Rarely, spontaneous necrosis of malignancy can cause TLS.

Effective treatment with chemotherapy kills malignant cells and leads to increased serum uric acid levels from the turnover of nucleic acids. Due to the acidic local environment, uric acid can be precipitated in the tubules, medulla, and collecting ducts of the kidney, leading to renal failure. The finding of uric acid crystals in the urine is a strong evidence for uric acid nephropathy.

Hyperphosphatemia, which can be caused by the release of intracellular phosphate pools by tumor lysis, produces a reciprocal depression in serum calcium, which causes severe neuromuscular irritability and tetany. Deposition of calcium phosphate in the kidney and hyperphosphatemia may cause renal failure. Potassium is the principal intracellular cation, and massive destruction of malignant cells may lead to hyperkalemia.

Treatment: Recognition of risk and prevention are the most important steps in the management of this syndrome. Preventive measures are allopurinol, urinary alkalinization, and aggressive hydration. Care should be taken to prevent worsening of symptomatic hypocalcemia by induction of alkalosis during bicarbonate infusion. Dialysis is often necessary and should be considered early in the course. Hemodialysis is preferred.

Prognosis is excellent and renal function recovers after the uric acid level is lowered to 10 mg/dL.

CASE NO. 253

a. Secondary polycythemia.
b. Doppler ultrasonography of left lower limb, venography of left lower limb.
c. Red cell mass estimation, arterial blood gases, erythropoietin level.

Note: This is likely to be a case of secondary polycythemia, as suggested by high hemoglobin and a raised PCV. Secondary polycythemia is due to raised levels of circulating erythropoietin (due to living at high altitude, chronic lung disease, or cyanotic heart disease) or due to inappropriate secretion of erythropoietin from various sources (such as renal cell carcinoma, polycystic kidney disease, hepatocellular carcinoma, cerebellar hemangioblastoma). In these cases, white cells and platelets are unaffected.

In pseudopolycythemia, both Hb and PCV are raised owing to hemoconcentration, resulting from any cause of reduced extracellular volume (dehydration, diuretics). Pseudopolycythemia can be differentiated from true polycythemia by red cell mass estimation, which is normal in former. In polycythemia rubra vera, in addition to raised Hb and red cell count, white cells are also increased in 70%, and platelets in 50% of cases. Physical examination may show palpable spleen.

Bone marrow examination will show erythroid hyperplasia and increased megakaryocytes, leukocyte alkaline phosphatase score is also high.

CASE NO. 254

a. Spontaneous pneumothorax.
b. Chest X-ray, ECG.
c. Marfan's syndrome.
d. Dissecting aneurysm.

Note: In any young patient presenting with severe central chest pain, one should consider spontaneous pneumothorax. Appearance of this patient is highly suggestive of Marfan's syndrome, in which pneumothorax may occur, also dissecting aneurysm may occur rarely.

Marfan's syndrome is characterized by triad of eye, skeletal and cardiac abnormalities. (1) Eye—blue sclera, sublaxation or dislocation of lens (ectopia lentis), iridodonesis (tremor of iris), heterochromia iris (various color of iris). Myopia, retinal detachment, glaucoma. (2) Skeletal- Tall, lean and thin, arachnodactyly. Hyperextensibility of joints, high arched palate, kyphosis or scoliosis. High pedal arch, pes planus, pectus excavatum or carinatum or asymmetry of chest. Arm span is greater than height and pubis-sole of foot is greater than pubis-vertex. (3) CVS-AR (due to aortic root dilatation, secondary to cystic medial necrosis), MR, mitral valve prolapse.

Aortic dissection or rupture are the commonest cause of death. Patient with Marfan's syndrome have a higher incidence of pneumothorax than the general population.

Marfan's syndrome may cause dissecting aneurysm, infective endocarditis and it may be associated with coarctation of aorta.

CASE NO. 255

a. Cystic fibrosis.
b. Meconium ileus equivalent.
c. Sweat test.
d. *Pseudomonas aeruginosa.*

Note: Diagnosis of cystic fibrosis should be suspected in any young patient who presents with chronic respiratory and chronic gastrointestinal problem. This girl is suffering from recurrent chest infections, bronchiectasis, malabsorption due to pancreatitis. She is also diabetic, secondary to pancreatic disease. Gastrointestinal problem in patient with cystic fibrosis is due to pancreatic insufficiency.

Diagnosis of cystic fibrosis is made by—1. Positive family history, 2. Sweat test—high sweat sodium concentration over 60 mmol/L 3. Blood DNA analysis of gene defect, 4. Blood immunoreactive trypsin (helpful for screening).

P. aeruginosa is the commonest organism, causing recurrent respiratory infection. Male with cystic fibrosis are infertile, due to failure of development of vas deferens and epididymis. About 20% of female with cystic fibrosis are infertile.

Cystic fibrosis is an autosomal recessive disease with a prevalence of 1/2,500, characterized by viscid respiratory and gastrointestinal secretions. Abnormality is in the gene encoding a chloride ion channel in the nasal epithelium, lungs, salivary glands, pancreas, intestine and bile ducts.

Clinical features are (i) Respiratory—recurrent infection, bronchiectasis, lung abscess, asthma, otitis media, nasal polyps, etc. (ii) Abdominal—meconium ileus (birth), rectal prolapse (neonate), steatorrhea (due to pancreatic insufficiency), malabsorption, gallstone, secondary biliary cirrhosis. There may be meconium ileus equivalent (infancy onwards), which is a bowel obstruction resulting from a combination of steatorrhea and viscid intestinal secretions, causing fecal impaction in ascending colon or in ileocecal junction.

Treatment: **Pancreatic** supplements, regular antibiotic, strict glucose control, mucolytic and regular physiotherapy with postural drainage.

If the patient presents with acute abdomen due to intestinal obstruction—nothing by mouth, intravenous fluid, and nasogastric suction should be given.

Other treatment: Acetylcysteine given intravenously or through the nasogastric tube has been shown to be very useful in resolving bowel obstruction.

Treatment of CF with lung disease—usually management of bronchiectasis is necessary. There is repeated chest infection with *Staph. aureus*, also *Pseudomonas* which should be treated with antibiotics.

Nebulized antibiotic either colistin or tobramycin is used between exacerbation to suppress chronic *Pseudomonas* infection.

Lung transplantation, if there is severe respiratory compromise.

CASE NO. 256

a. Achalasia of esophagus with aspiration pneumonia.
b. Barium swallows X-ray of the esophagus, endoscopy and biopsy, esophageal manometry.

Note: Achalasia of esophagus or cardia is a motility disorder, characterized by failure to dilate the lower esophageal sphincter due to absence or reduction of ganglion cells of Auerbach's plexus. Cause is unknown. There is failure of non-adrenergic non-cholinergic (NANC) innervation related to abnormal nitric oxide synthesis within the lower esophageal sphincter. Degeneration of ganglion cells within the sphincter and body of esophagus occurs. Common in middle age, but may occur at any age. Patients present with dysphagia, which is intermittent initially, worse for solid. Later, both solid and liquid. There is regurgitation of food, chest discomfort or pain (due to spasm). Sometimes, severe chest pain due to esophageal spasm (vigorous achalasia), repeated respiratory infection or aspiration pneumonia, loss of weight. Manometry is the confirmatory investigation in achalasia cardia.

Complications: Respiratory (recurrent aspiration pneumonia, bronchiectasis, collapse of lung), carcinoma of esophagus (squamous type in 5 to 10%), malnutrition (due to dysphagia).

Treatment: (i) Endoscopic dilatation by pneumatic bougie, may be repeated if necessary. Effective in 80% of cases, (ii) If repeated dilatation fails—surgery, open or laparoscopic. Heller's cardiomyotomy is done (circular muscle layer is cut). This may be complicated by perforation and reflux esophagitis. So, sometimes myotomy plus partial fundoplication may be done to prevent reflux esophagitis. Proton pump inhibitor (omeprazole) should be used, (iii) Endoscopic guidance of injection botulinum toxin in lower esophageal sphincter may be given. It helps in remission, but relapse may occur.

CASE NO. 257

a. Dementia of Lewy body type.
b. MRI of brain, thyroid function test, vitamin B_{12} assay.

Note: This patient has Parkinson's disease, hallucination and frequent falls (syncope), which is highly suggestive of dementia of Lewy body type. It is found in 10 to 20% of cases of dementia. Lewy bodies are intracytoplasmic inclusion bodies, composed of α-synuclein and ubiquitin, found in cerebral cortex and brainstem. Main clues to the diagnosis are severe neuroleptic sensitivity reactions, and presence of visual hallucinations for people and animal. Features of Parkinsonism are usually mild, memory impairment is also mild in early stage. Daytime drowsiness and sleepiness, falls, syncope and delusions may be present. There is overlap between Parkinsonism, Lewy body dementia and Alzheimer's disease. Day time sleepiness and drowsiness are more common in Lewy body dementia.

CASE NO. 258

a. Hypogonadotropic hypogonadism.
b. History of anosmia.
c. Kallmann's syndrome.

Note: Kallmann's syndrome is a rare disease, inherited as X-linked recessive trait, may be variable. It is characterized by deficient gonadotropin production by the pituitary, anosmia, cleft palate and color blindness. This patient has primary amenorrhea, with hypogonadotropic hypogonadism, but normal prolactin. Most likely diagnosis is Kallmann's syndrome.

CASE NO. 259

a. MRI of brain, lumbar puncture and CSF study.
b. Normal pressure hydrocephalus.
c. CSF drainage via repeated lumbar puncture.

Note: Triad of dementia, gait disturbance and incontinence is highly suggestive of normal pressure hydrocephalus. CT scan of brain shows enlarged ventricles with no obstruction to CSF. Lumbar puncture will show normal CSF pressure and normal composition. In this condition, dilatation of ventricular system is caused by intermittent rise of CSF pressure, related to impaired CSF absorption, occurs particularly at night and therefore may benefit from CSF shunting, but unpredictable. It occurs in old age.

CASE NO. 260

a. Iodine deficiency goiter with menopausal syndrome.
b. USG of thyroid gland, FNAC of thyroid, antithyroid antibody.
c. Thyroxine therapy.

Note: Normal FT_3, FT_4 and TSH with high radioiodine uptake is highly suggestive of iodine deficiency goiter. It may be confused with thyrotoxicosis, because of high radioiodine uptake. It is one of the commonest cause of diffuse goiter in endemic area. Intake of iodinated salt is the simplest way to prevent such goiter.

CASE NO. 261

a. Leptospirosis.
b. Dengue hemorrhagic fever, viral hepatitis due to E virus, falciparum malaria.
c. Blood culture, urine culture, anti-leptospira antibody (or microscopic agglutination test-MAT).
d. DIC.

Note: Evidence of hepatitis, renal failure and carditis is highly suggestive of leptospirosis. However, fulminant hepatic failure complicated by hepatorenal syndrome may follow viral hepatitis.

Leptospirosis is caused by the spirochete *Leptospira ictero-haemorrhagica*. Rodents, particularly rats, are the most important reservoir of infection. The organism is excreted in the urine and may survive in the soil for several weeks. Entry into the human host is through cuts and abrasions on the skin, or through intact mucous membranes. Occupations—most susceptible are sewerage workers, fishermen, vets and farmers. Replication occurs in the blood and tissue and multi-system involvement may occur, the kidneys and liver are commonly affected. Glomerular injury occurs, causing an acute interstitial nephritis and tubular necrosis. In liver, there is centrilobular necrosis in severe cases.

The incubation period is 1 to 2 weeks. Initial or septicemic phase is 4 to 7 days, characterized by fever, headache, myalgia, abdominal pain, vomiting, skin rash (macular, maculopapular or hemorrhagic) or conjunctival ingestion (blood shot eyes). Persistent headache may be due to meningitis. Proteinuria and hematuria may be present during this phase, and renal failure is evident in 50% of patients. Jaundice and impairment of liver function are present only in severe cases. 90% cases are anicteric. Hepatosplenomegaly is present in approximately 20%. Respiratory involvement is common, and manifests as dry cough, hemoptysis and confluent shadow in chest X-ray.

Second phase or immune phase last for 4 to 30 days. The patient is afebrile. Antibody titers to leptospira are rising. Deterioration in liver and renal function may continue. Meningism, uveitis and rash are common. Hematological manifestations include thrombocytopenia, hemolytic uremic syndrome characterized by fragmented red cells on the blood film and intravascular hemolysis. Endothelial injury may cause blood loss from the gastrointestinal tract and lungs. Pulmonary syndrome may occur during the outbreak of leptospirosis. It is characterized by hemoptysis, patchy lung infiltrate on CXR and respiratory failure. Bilateral lung consolidation and ARDS with multiorgan dysfunction may occur.

Blood culture in special media is positive in the first ten days. By the second week, urine culture is positive. IgM antibodies to leptospira are detectable in the first week. Microscopic agglutination test (MAT) is the investigation of choice. Leptospiral DNA by PCR is also helpful in blood and urine.

Treatment: Intravenous benzyl penicillin (1.5 mega unit 6 hourly) for one week. IV ceftriaxone 1 g daily equally effective. Doxycycline 100 mg 12 hourly for one week is also helpful. Renal failure may require dialysis. Doxycycline prophylaxis may be used in highly endemic area.

CASE NO. 262

a. Heart failure.
b. Cardiomyopathy, most likely hypertrophic cardiomyopathy.
c. Friedreich's ataxia.

Note: In young patient with pes cavus plus combination of cerebellar lesion (bilateral), UMN lesion (extensor plantar) and posterior column lesion (loss of vibration and position senses) is highly suggestive of Friedreich's ataxia. Differential diagnoses are multiple sclerosis, tabes dorsalis, spinocerebellar degeneration. Friedreich's ataxia is a type of hereditary ataxia, inherited as autosomal recessive (in some cases AD). Cause is unknown. Family history may be present. Features of Friedreich's ataxia are usual onset in young, <15 years (8 to 16 years). There is progressive difficulty in walking (truncal ataxia and ataxia of lower limbs), weakness of lower limbs, dysarthria. Diabetes mellitus is common. May be associated with kyphoscoliosis, pes cavus, cocking of toes, nystagmus, optic atrophy, hypertrophic cardiomyopathy. Normal mentation (may have mild dementia). Prognosis—usually progresses slowly, death occurs before 40 years of age (usually 20 years after the onset of symptoms).

CASE NO. 263

a. Infective endocarditis.
b. Serial blood culture, transesophageal echocardiogram (TOE).

Note: Any patient with fever, splenomegaly with cardiac murmur, infective endocarditis should be considered first. Blood culture is the single most important investigation, positive in 90% cases. Serial blood cultures should be performed; a single blood culture may be negative. Transesophageal echocardiography is useful to detect vegetation (>90%), more sensitive. Transthoracic echocardiography detect vegetation in 60 to 75% cases. Absence of vegetation does not exclude endocarditis, as vegetations <3 mm may not be seen. Routine blood culture may be negative, due to prior treatment with antibiotics before culturing the blood, or that the endocarditis is due to a fastidious organism. In immunosuppressed patient, endocarditis may be due to fungus that may be difficult to culture. Endocarditis may be a manifestation of SLE (Libmann Sacks endocarditis) or a manifestation of malignancy, called marantic endocarditis.

Features of endocarditis—fever, cardiac murmur, splinter hemorrhages, Osler's nodes (small, painful), Janeway lesions (macular, painless), Roth spots, splenomegaly, microscopic hematuria, nephritis.

Causes of culture negative endocarditis—Fungus, *Brucella, Coxiella burnetii, Chlamydia, Mycoplasma, Legionella, Haemophilus, Actinobacillus, Cardiobacterium, Eikenella* and *kingella* (HACEK) organisms.

Causes of non-infective endocarditis—Marantic endocarditis, SLE (Libman-Sacks).

CASE NO. 264

a. Magnesium toxicity.
b. Stop magnesium infusion, start IV fluid, diuretic, injection calcium gluconate.
c. Serum magnesium level and creatinine.

Note: Signs of hypermagnesemia include nausea, hypotension (due to myocardial depression and vasodilatation), bradycardia, drowsiness, respiratory depression. In severe cases, double vision, loss of deep tendon reflexes, coma and cardiac arrest may occur. Magnesium toxicity is more common when intravenous magnesium is given in the absence of hypomagnesemia such as preeclampsia and toxicity is exacerbated in presence of renal failure.

Treatment: Stop any drugs containing magnesium, promote urinary excretion of magnesium by loop diuretic, plenty of fluid, IV Ca-gluconate may be given to prevent cardiac arrest, dialysis may be needed in severe renal failure.

CASE NO. 265

a. Prolactinoma, drug induced hyperprolactinemia.
b. MRI of brain.
c. Drug induced hyperprolactinemia (due to metoclopramide or domperidone).
d. Stop antiemetic drug.

Note: In this young girl, after antiemetic drug, more likely domperidone or metoclopramide, she has developed galactorrhea and amenorrhea, with hyperprolactinemia. This is highly likely to be due to drug induced hyperprolactinemia. Pregnancy should be excluded, next possibility is prolactinoma. Prolactin above 5000 mU/L is suggestive of prolactinoma.

Features of hyperprolactinemia in female are galactorrhea, secondary amenorrhea, infertility, etc. In male, decreased libido, less secondary sexual character, lethargy.

CASE NO. 266

a. Primary hyperaldosteronism (or Conn's syndrome).
b. High resolution CT scan of suprarenal gland, lying and standing plasma renin and aldosterone.
c. Spironolactone.

Note: The patient has hypokalemic alkalosis with hypertension, highly suggestive of primary hyperaldosteronism. It is also called Conn's syndrome, caused by excess secretion of aldosterone by adrenal gland, which leads to salt and water retention, causing hypertension. Also, it causes hypokalemia resulting in muscular weakness, polyuria, polydipsia. Common causes is adrenal adenoma, sometimes may be due to hyperplasia of adrenal gland. High resolution CT scan of suprarenal gland is a very helpful investigation, >0.5 cm adenoma may be detected. Simultaneous measurement of serum renin and aldosterone in lying and standing position should be done. Renin is low, aldosterone is high in supine position. On standing suddenly, there is paradoxical drop of aldosterone level in adenoma, but exaggerated high aldosterone in patient with hyperplasia.

Treatment: If adenoma, surgery should be done. In hyperplasia, aldosterone antagonist like spironolactone should be given.

Causes of hypokalemic alkalosis with hypertension—primary hyperaldosteronism, Cushing's syndrome, Liddle's syndrome, hypertension treated with diuretic, renal artery stenosis, carbenoxolone therapy, congenital adrenal hyperplasia (11-β-hydroxylase deficiency).

CASE NO. 267

a. Kikuchi's disease.
b. Steroid should be given.

Note: Necrotizing lymphadenitis is suggestive of Kikuchi's disease. It is a rare, benign disorder of unknown etiology, characterized by enlargement of commonly cervical lymph nodes with or without systemic features. It is also known as histiocytic necrotizing lymphadenitis. Common in female.

Common manifestation of Kikuchi's disease is lymphadenopathy. It is usually localized, commonly affecting the cervical lymph nodes (80%), especially the posterior chain. Generalized involvement affecting axillary, inguinal and mesenteric nodes may occur. In 50% cases, lymphadenopathy is accompanied by fever and a flu-like prodrome. There may be headache, nausea, vomiting, malaise, arthralgia, myalgia, night sweat, rash, abdominal or thoracic pain and weight loss.

There may be maculopapular lesions, morbilliform rash, nodules, urticaria, and malar rash (resembling SLE), hepatosplenomegaly. Involvement of bone marrow, uvea, thyroid, parotid glands and myocardium is rare. Neurologic involvement include aseptic meningitis, acute cerebellar ataxia and encephalitis. Clinically, KD may be confused with lymphoma, tubercular lymphadenitis and SLE. Other differential diagnoses include viral or bacterial lymphadenitis, metastatic carcinoma, rheumatoid arthritis, infectious mononucleosis, sarcoidosis, cat scratch disease, Still's disease, tuberculosis.

CBC may show mild granulocytopenia or atypical lymphocytes. ESR and CRP may be elevated. LDH may be elevated, if liver is involved. Immunological studies for autoantibodies are generally negative. FNAC or biopsy of lymph nodes shows crescentic histiocytes, plasmacytoid monocytes and extracellular debris that suggest the diagnosis of Kikuchi disease.

Treatment is generally supportive. Reassurance is important. Fever and pain may be treated with NSAIDs. Corticosteroid is indicated in patient with severe extranodal disease, involvement of liver (elevated LDH) or nervous system, severe lupus-like syndrome (positive ANA) or generalized KD. Prednisolone 50 to 60 mg daily orally with tapering as symptoms resolve. Immunosuppressive drugs are used with steroid in severe, life-threatening cases.

Some patients respond to minocycline, ciprofloxacin, chloroquine and hydroxychloroquine. Kikuchi's disease is generally benign and self-limiting with a good prognosis. It usually resolves over several weeks to 6 months. Recurrence is unusual (3%) and fatalities are rare.

CASE NO. 268

a. Multiple myeloma.
b. Autonomic neuropathy.
c. Bone marrow study.

Note: Anemia, high ESR, hypercalcemia associated with severe bony pain are highly suggestive of multiple myeloma. The patient also has heart failure and nephrotic syndrome, which may occur in multiple myeloma with amyloidosis. Low sodium in this case is due to pseudohyponatremia, which occurs due to paraproteinemia in myeloma. Amyloidosis may cause autonomic neuropathy, which is responsible for dizziness or syncope.

CASE NO. 269

a. Sumatriptan subcutaneous or intranasal, high flow oxygen.
b. Cluster headache, migraine.
c. Verapamil.

Note: Most likely diagnosis is cluster headache. This is characterized by recurrent episodes of unilateral retro-orbital pain with associated autonomic features. Cluster headache can occur at any age, but common in 30 to 40 years, more in male, male: female is 9:1. Pain is severe, last for 15 minutes to 3 hours, radiates up over the frontotemporal region down to the jaw, neck or shoulder, associated with autonomic features like lacrimation, facial flushing, nasal or conjunctival congestion, meiosis. Ipsilateral eye is often red and watery, rhinorrhea or a blocked ipsilateral nostril.

Treatment in acute attack: Sumatriptan subcutaneous or intranasal and high flow oxygen 100% (10 to 12 L/min). Ergotamine, verapamil, lithium, sodium valproate and prednisolone have been used as prophylaxis, once the acute attack has resolved. Verapamil is the drug of choice for prophylaxis.

Differential diagnosis is migraine. Also, it may be confused with chronic paroxysmal hemicrania (CPH, which is treated with indomethacin). Features that distinguish CPH are: shorter duration of attacks (2 to 45 minutes), increased frequency of attacks, female preponderance and selective response to treatment with indomethacin.

CASE NO. 270

a. Another attack of myocardial infarction, acute pericarditis, rupture of chorda tendineae or papillary muscle causing mitral regurgitation, rupture of ventricular septum causing VSD, pulmonary embolism.
b. Pericardial rub to detect acute pericarditis, pansystolic murmur due to mitral regurgitation (or due to VSD).
c. ECG, transesophageal echocardiogram (TOE).

Note: In any patient with acute myocardial infarction, new onset of chest pain may be due to new myocardial infarction, acute pericarditis, rupture of the chorda tendineae or papillary muscle causing mitral regurgitation, pulmonary embolism. Presence of pansystolic murmur indicates mitral regurgitation due to papillary muscle rupture or ventricular septal defect (due to rupture of interventricular septum). Echocardiography, mainly transthoracic echocardiogram is preferable to transesophageal echocardiogram. Acute pericarditis is another complication, that occurs on 3rd or 4th day, a pericardial rub may be present. ECG will show elevation of ST, with upward concavity. Pulmonary embolism should also be considered in such case.

CASE NO. 271

a. T_3 thyrotoxicosis.
b. Serum FT_3 estimation.

Note: This patient's features are suggestive of thyrotoxicosis, TSH is very low, normal FT_4 but high radioiodine uptake. T_3 thyrotoxicosis is the likely diagnosis. The diagnosis of T_3 toxicosis should be suspected in patient presenting with symptoms of thyrotoxicosis, with or without goiter, in whom serum FT_4 is normal, low TSH with high radioiodine uptake.

CASE NO. 272

a. Superior vena caval obstruction.
b. Lymphoma.
c. Chest X-ray P/A view.
d. CT scan of chest, FNAC or biopsy of lymph node.

Note: The symptoms and signs in this patient are highly suggestive of superior vena caval obstruction, secondary to mediastinal lymphadenopathy. This is the common cause of SVC obstruction in early age. In elderly, commonest cause is bronchial carcinoma. First chest X-ray should be done, which will show mediastinal widening. CT scan of chest and also CT guided FNAC may be done. Blood count is done to exclude acute lymphoblastic leukemia. If lymphadenopathy is present, FNAC or biopsy of the lymph node should be done to confirm the diagnosis.

Treatment: High dose steroid, chemotherapy, radiotherapy to the mediastinum. To relieve SVC obstruction—IV furosemide, dexamethasone, expandable metallic stenting may be used.

CASE NO. 273

a. Pancytopenia due to azathioprine toxicity.
b. Septicemia with consolidation.

c. Broad spectrum antibiotic and azathioprine should be stopped temporarily.
d. Dose of azathioprine should be reduced.

Note: Allopurinol acts by inhibition of xanthine oxidase and thus inhibit the metabolism of 6-mercaptopurine, an active metabolite of azathioprine. Concomitant use of allopurinol with azathioprine is not recommended. If concomitant use is necessary, dose of azathioprine should be reduced along with regular blood count monitoring. Azathioprine toxicity—commonly bone marrow suppression, blood dyscrasias such as thrombocytopenia, leukopenia and agranulocytosis can also occur.

Cyclosporine levels can also rise with concomitant administration of allopurinol, but to lesser extent. Cyclosporine more commonly causes renal toxicity.

CASE NO. 274

a. Family history.
b. Huntington's disease.
c. MRI of brain, DNA analysis.

Note: Chorea may be due to many causes. In this case, there is no other history and taking any drugs. In Huntington's disease, chorea is associated with progressive dementia. It is inherited as autosomal dominant. Gene responsible is on short arm of chromosome 4.

Symptoms typically appear between 30 and 50 years of age. Genetic testing now provides an accurate method of establishing the diagnosis. Pathological changes—cerebral atrophy with neuronal loss in caudate nucleus and putamen. Changes of neurotransmitters—(i) Reduction of acetylcholine transferase and GAD (glutamic acid decarboxylase) in the corpus striatum. (ii) Depletion of gamma aminobutyric acid (GABA), substance P, angiotensin converting enzyme and metencephalin in substantia nigra. (iii) High somatostatin level in corpus striatum. CT scan or MRI shows atrophy of caudate nucleus and also cerebral atrophy.

Treatment: No curative treatment. Haloperidol or phenothiazine for dyskinesia. Tetrabenazine may be given. Psychological support. Institutional care for dementia. Genetic counseling is essential. Average lifespan after clinical onset is about 15 years.

CASE NO. 275

a. Amyloidosis.
b. Renal transplantation.
c. It can be reduced by using high flux dialysis membranes in patients who are likely to be on dialysis for a prolonged period.

Note: Amyloidosis is a common cause of neurological impairment in patient on longstanding dialysis. It is caused by beta 2 microglobulin accumulation. It causes joint pain and stiffness, usually upper limbs are involved more than lower limbs. The only treatment is renal transplantation. It can be reduced by using high flux dialysis membranes in patients who are likely to be on dialysis for a prolonged period.

Uremia may cause neurological symptoms. This is more common in men, and mostly affects the legs. Sensory symptoms (paresthesia, burning sensations and pain) occur before motor symptoms (muscle atrophy, myoclonus, and paralysis). Sensory symptoms may improve with starting or increasing the frequency of dialysis, but the motor symptoms are not reversible.

CASE NO. 276
(See also case no. 180)

a. Microangiopathic hemolytic anemia.
b. Reticulocyte count.
c. Metallic valve.
d. Anemic heart failure.

Note: In this patient, blood picture shows anemia, high bilirubin and LDH, but other normal enzymes, highly suggestive of hemolytic anemia. Blood film suggest microangiopathic hemolytic anemia. In any patient with replacement of metallic valve, mechanical hemolytic anemia may occur as a complication. In mild case, no interference is necessary. If severe anemia, metallic valve replacement may be necessary by tissue valve.

CASE NO. 277

a. Methanol poisoning.
b. CT scan of brain, serum methanol level.
c. Metabolic acidosis.

Note: As the patient is alcoholic and no history of other illness and there is severe metabolic acidosis, likely causes are methanol toxicity or ethylene glycol poisoning. Also, may be due to acute severe pancreatitis and acute hepatic failure. In this case, normal amylase excludes acute pancreatitis. Actual plasma osmolality is higher than the calculated plasma osmolality approximately 284 mOsm/L, suggesting the presence of an osmotically active substance, likely to be methanol or ethylene glycol. Methanol is metabolized to formic acid and ethylene glycol is metabolized to glycolic acid, which are relatively toxic.

Patient with methanol toxicity may complain of headache, nausea, vomiting, abdominal pain, dizziness, confusion, convulsion, stupor and coma. Formic acid can cause retinal injury. The patient suffers from reduced visual acuity, due to optic nerve damage by formic acid resulting from increased concentrations of formic acid. Mydriasis, reduced visual reflexes to light and hyperemia of optic disk are early features of methanol toxicity. If untreated, patient may develop blindness. Presence of visual abnormality in this patient indicates methanol poisoning (which is not a feature in ethanol poisoning).

Treatment: (i) Gastric lavage within 1st 4 hours, (ii) IV fluid, oxygen, (iii) Correction of acidosis—sodium bicarbonate in large dose (alkalinization enhances formic acid excretion), (iv) In early stage—ethanol is given (it inhibits methanol oxidation by competing the inhibition of enzyme). Ethanol is given 10 mL/kg of 10% ethanol IV or 1 mL/kg of 95% ethanol orally. (v), Thiamine (100 mg qid), pyridoxine (50 mg qid) and folate (50 mg qid), (vi) Folinic acid 30 mg IV every 6 hourly. It reduces ocular toxicity (accelerates metabolism of formic acid), (vii) Dialysis- indicated, if ingestion of methanol is >30 g or metabolic acidosis or blood methanol >500 mg/L.

Patient with ethylene glycol poisoning may present in the same way. However, reduced visual acuity is not a feature, whereas flank pain and renal failure due to crystallization of oxalic acid in the renal tubules is common. Urinalysis under Wood's light in patient with ethylene glycol poisoning may reveal oxalate crystals in the urine, but an absence does not exclude the diagnosis. Patient with ethylene glycol poisoning also develop severe cardiac failure if untreated. Presence of visual symptoms favor methanol intoxication (as in this case).

CASE NO. 278

a. Hypokalemic alkalosis.
b. Laxative abuse, self-induced vomiting.

Note: This patient has hypokalemic alkalosis and an appropriate hypokalemia. Urea is elevated, due to hypoperfusion of afferent glomerular vessels. This may occur in dehydration. Most probable cause of hypokalemia is loss of potassium from gastrointestinal tract. This is also causing dehydration and hence the elevated urea. There is no history of diarrhea or vomiting, but for her obesity, probably she is abusing laxatives or has self-induced vomiting in order to loss weight. Potassium may be lost via GI tract (diarrhea, vomiting, intestinal fistulae, villous adenoma, nasogastric aspiration) or the kidneys. Other causes of hypokalemia may occur in primary and secondary hyperaldosteronism, Cushing's syndrome, Liddle's syndrome or drugs.

Hypokalemia is generally associated with metabolic alkalosis, with the exception of RTA.

Many conditions associated with renal loss of potassium also cause hypertension. Most common cause of hypertension, hypokalemia and alkalosis are primary hyperaldosteronism (Conn's syndrome). However, other recognized causes include Cushing's, Liddle's syndrome accelerated hypertension, renal artery stenosis or hypertensive therapy with diuretics, Liddle's syndrome, carbenoxolone therapy, congenital adrenal hyperplasia (11-β-hydroxylase deficiency).

CASE NO. 279

a. Bronchial carcinoma with metastasis to the hilar lymph nodes, sarcoidosis, lymphoma.
b. CT scan of chest, FNAC of hilar lymph node (CT or USG guided).
c. Bronchial carcinoma with metastasis to the hilar lymph nodes.

Note: This patient has persistent dry cough, weight loss, hypercalcemia which are suggestive of squamous cell carcinoma of lung. Unilateral hilar lymphadenopathy may due to sarcoidosis, where hypercalcemia may occur. Other causes of unilateral hilar lymphadenopathy are lymphoma, tuberculosis. But in these cases, usually there is no hypercalcemia. Sometimes, in early case with small lung lesion, plain chest X-ray may not reveal the lung lesion. CT scan is more helpful. Sputum for malignant cells, bronchoscopy and biopsy should be done.

CASE NO. 280

a. Cerebral toxoplasmosis.
b. Tuberculous meningitis, cryptococcal meningitis, cerebral lymphoma, brain abscess, cerebral malaria.
c. CT scan of brain, anti-HIV, CSF study for tuberculosis, lymph node FNAC or biopsy.

Note: The patient was working abroad, may be associated with a high level of promiscuity and high risk for HIV infection. Confusion may be due to encephalitis, meningitis, cerebral abscess or cerebral malaria.

Toxoplasma encephalitis is the commonest cause of focal brain disease in HIV patient. This patient is confused, has focal neurological signs and chorioretinitis, which are suggestive of cerebral toxoplasmosis, TB or cryptococcal meningitis. Cerebral lymphoma does not cause chorioretinitis. Other recognized causes of chorioretinitis in patient with HIV include CMV and syphilitic infection.

Treatment: Many are self-limiting. In severe disease (eye or cerebral), 6-week regimen is as follows:

❖ Pyrimethamine (100 mg loading dose orally followed by 25 to 50 mg/day) plus sulfadiazine (2–4 g/day divided 4 times daily) OR

❖ Pyrimethamine (100 mg loading dose orally followed by 25 to 50 mg/day) plus clindamycin (300 mg orally 4 times daily)

❖ Folinic acid (leucovorin, 10 to 25 mg/day) should be given to prevent hematologic toxicity of pyrimethamine

❖ Trimethoprim (10 mg/kg/day) plus sulfamethoxazole (50 mg/kg/day) for 4 weeks.

Sulfadiazine or clindamycin can be substituted for azithromycin 500 mg daily or atovaquone 750 mg twice daily in immunocompetent patients or in patients with a history of allergy to the former drugs.

In pregnancy, spiramycin alone or sulfadiazine may be given.

Steroid may be given with radiologic midline shift, clinical deterioration after 48 hours, or raised ICP.

CASE NO. 281

a. Drug induced SLE.
b. Anti-histone antibody.

Note: History of this patient is suggestive of SLE. Her ANA is strongly positive and anti-ds DNA is negative. Also, history of taking minocycline. All the features are suggestive of drug induced SLE. CRP is usually normal in SLE. If it is high, indicates bacterial infection (or serositis). Minocycline may cause SLE, in which CRP, ESR are high, and ANA is strongly positive, but anti-ds DNA is negative.

Features of drug induced SLE: Sex ratio—equal, lung involvement is common, but renal and neurological involvement are rare. ANA is usually positive, anti ds DNA is negative, complements are normal. Antihistone antibody is positive in 95% of cases (characteristic, but not specific).

Drugs causing SLE like syndrome usually do not aggravate primary SLE.

Treatment: Withdrawal of drugs. Short course of steroid is necessary.

Drugs causing SLE—hydralazine is common (90%, slow acetylator), procainamide (rapid acetylator), anticonvulsant (carbamazepine, phenytoin), phenothiazine, INH, oral contraceptive pill, ACE inhibitor, penicillamine, methyldopa, minocycline.

CASE NO. 282

a. Behcet's syndrome.
b. Crohn's disease, herpes simplex, virus infection.

Note: This patient has oral and genital ulcer, iritis, arthritis, erythema nodosum. There is episode of bloody diarrhea and deep venous thrombosis, all are suggestive of Behcet's syndrome. Crohn's disease is another possibility, where genital ulcer and deep venous thrombosis are rare, which are common in Behcet's syndrome.

Behcet's syndrome is a vasculitis of unknown cause, characterized by recurrent oral, genital ulcer, ocular lesion and skin, joint and neurological lesion. Common in male. Oral and genital ulcers are present in most patients.

Ocular lesions are recurrent uveitis and iridocyclitis, retinal vascular lesions and optic atrophy, can lead to loss of vision in 50% of patients with ocular involvement. Erythema nodosum is a recognized feature. Other skin manifestations include diffuse pustular rash affecting the face, erythema multiforme. Pathergy test is a useful diagnostic sign. It is demonstrated by pricking the skin by needle, there is pustule formation at venipuncture site within 24 to 48 hours.

Seronegative arthritis occurs in about 40% patients, commonly involves knees, ankles and wrists. Recurrent thrombophlebitis is a significant feature of Behcet's syndrome, leading to venous thrombosis. Less often, superior or inferior vena caval thrombosis may occur. Abdominal pain and bloody diarrhea have also been documented. Asymptomatic proteinuria is a recognized feature, but rarely may cause renal amyloidosis. Neurological complications occur in 5% patients. Organic confusional states, meningoencephalitis, transient or persistent brainstem syndromes, multiple sclerosis and Parkinsonian type disorders are all recognized.

Behcet's syndrome is a clinical diagnosis. There is no specific diagnostic test. Criteria for diagnosis—Recurrent oral ulcer, at least three times in 12 months plus 2 of the—(a) Recurrent genital ulceration, (b) Eye lesion, (c) Skin lesion, (d) Positive Pathergy test.

Treatment: Oral ulcer can be treated by topical steroid. Also genital ulcers are treated with topical steroid. Thalidomide 100 to 300 mg/day for 28 days is effective in resistant oral and genital ulcer.

Systemic steroid, immunosuppressive agents and cyclosporine are used for uveitis and neurological disease. Colchicine is effective in erythema nodosum and arthralgia. Anti-TNF agent can be used in severe uveitis, neurological and gastrointestinal manifestations.

■ CASE NO. 283

a. Gastroesophageal reflux disease.
b. Endoscopy.

Note: Gastroesophageal reflux disease (GORD) is one of the commonest causes of chronic cough.

Her clinical presentation is typical of cough secondary to GORD; in which symptoms are worsen in talking and laughing. Lower esophageal sphincter closes at night leading to cessation of symptoms. Asthma is also a possibility. Cough secondary to ACE inhibitors may persist 3 months after the drug is stopped.

Gastroesophageal reflux disease usually causes heart burn. May also cause odynophagia, sometimes atypical chest pain which can mimic angina.

■ CASE NO. 284

a. Cardiac arrest.
b. ICD (implantable cardiac defibrillator).

Note: The patient is suffering from IHD, more likely ischemic cardiomyopathy. In such case, ICD implantation is the best treatment, as there is a clear morbidity and mortality benefit over the anti-arrhythmic drugs. β-blocker, ACE inhibitor, amiodarone, statin, etc. have benefit to reduce mortality, but use of ICD should be the first line. ICD resembles large cardiac pacemaker, consists of a generator device and lead or leads that are implanted into the heart via subclavian or cephalic vein. They can automatically sense and terminate life-threatening ventricular arrhythmia. ICD have all the functions of pacemaker. In addition, it can be used to treat ventricular tachyarrhythmias, using overdrive pacing synchronized cardioversion or defibrillator.

CASE NO. 285

a. Presence of anti-Ro/SSA antibody from maternal serum.
b. Pacemaker implantation.
c. To know whether the mother is suffering from SLE.

Note: If the mother is suffering from SLE having anti-Ro/SSA antibody in the serum, the baby may have congenital complete heart block, due to transplacental transfer of this antibody into the baby. Occurs in < 3% cases. Heart block is usually permanent; insertion of pacemaker may be needed. Though in many cases of congenital heart block, heart rate remains high and no treatment is necessary. In any mother suffering from SLE, screening for anti-Ro/SSA antibody must be done, if she wants to be pregnant.

CASE NO. 286

a. Strict glycemic control and control of hypertension.
b. ACE inhibitor, angiotensin receptor blocker.
c. Diabetic nephropathy.

Note: The patient has hypertension and probably microalbuminuria, that indicates nephropathy. Prevention of nephropathy is done by strict glycemic and blood pressure control. Good glycemic control delays the onset of diabetic nephropathy in patients who have no hypertension. In patient who has both diabetes and hypertension, diabetic nephropathy can be prevented by strict glycemic control and good control of blood pressure. Better glycemic control reduces glomerular basement membrane thickening and microalbuminuria.

If microalbuminuria has developed, there is little evidence that improving glycemic control alone delays progression of nephropathy. In such cases, control of blood pressure using ACE inhibitor or angiotensin II receptor blocker can retard the progression of nephropathy.

In young type I diabetic with microalbuminuria or proteinuria, ACE inhibitor should be given regardless of blood pressure. The target blood pressure in microalbuminuria is <120/70 mm Hg and with proteinuria is < 130/75 mm Hg.

In patient with type 2 diabetes mellitus, angiotensin II receptor blocker prevent development of proteinuria in patient with microalbuminuria. Target blood pressure is <130/75 mm Hg.

Smoking is a risk factor for the development of microalbuminuria. However, there are no prospective studies showing the benefit of cessation of smoking on renal function in type 1 diabetic.

CASE NO. 287

a. Q fever endocarditis.

b. Antibody against *Coxiella burnetii.*
c. Doxycycline and rifampicin.

Note: Q fever endocarditis is due to Coxiella burnetii, a rickettsial zoonotic disease. It is common in farmer, due to close contact with animal products of farm animals. Aortic valve is usually affected; chronic infection may cause hepatitis, osteomyelitis or endocarditis. Features include finger clubbing, hepatosplenomegaly and purpura or leukocytoclastic vasculitic rash. Laboratory tests often show features of hepatitis, anemia, high ESR, thrombocytopenia and hypergammaglobulinemia. Microscopic hematuria may be present. The disease may be complicated by immune complex-mediated glomerulonephritis and arterial emboli.\

Diagnosis is best made serologically and a Phase I antibody titer to *Coxiella burnetii* (IgG and/or IgA) greater than 1:200 is virtually diagnostic of Q fever endocarditis.

Treatment: Doxycycline and rifampicin or ciprofloxacin for long time. Combination of oral doxycycline (200 mg daily) and oral hydroxychloroquine (600 mg daily) for 2 years. Valve surgery may be required in refractory case.

CASE NO. 288

a. Chronic constrictive pericarditis.
b. Restrictive cardiomyopathy.
c. Echocardiography, cardiac MRI, cardiac catheterization.

Note: This patient has signs of severe right sided heart failure (raised JVP, enlarged tender liver and edema), but chest X-ray reveals a normal-sized heart. Also, dyspnea on exertion, atrial fibrillation, ascites, all are typical of chronic constrictive pericarditis. Differential diagnosis of severe heart failure in the absence of significant cardiac enlargement is chronic constrictive pericarditis and restrictive cardiomyopathy. Rarely, cardiac amyloidosis may occur, which is usually associated with multiple myeloma. In this case, patient is suffering from rheumatoid arthritis, also was suffering from tuberculosis; both may cause chronic constrictive pericarditis.

Causes of chronic constrictive pericarditis are infection (tuberculosis and coxsackie B infection), hemopericardium (due to trauma, myocardial rupture after infarction, dissecting aneurysm), collagen disease (rheumatoid arthritis), cardiac operation, mediastinal irradiation, fungal infection (histoplasmosis), rarely, after acute purulent pericarditis and also idiopathic.

Signs of chronic constrictive pericarditis—(1) Pulse—low volume, tachycardia. Pulsus paradoxus may be present. (2) JVP—raised. Kussmaul's sign positive (raised JVP on inspiration). Fall of Y descent (Friedrich's sign). (3) Precordium—no cardiomegaly. On auscultation-pericardial knock (a third heart sound), due to rapid ventricular filling. (4) Ascites—early feature, edema is a late feature (found in advanced stage). (5) Hepatomegaly.

Treatment: Surgery.

CASE NO. 289

a. Paradoxical cerebral embolus via patent foramen ovale.
b. Transesophageal echocardiography (TOE).

Note: This patient has long flight from Australia and therefore developed DVT, the thrombus passed through a patent foramen ovale, has caused left cerebral infarction. Other possibilities are ASD, VSD, etc. 2D echocardiography may be unable to detect foramen ovale. Transesophageal echocardiography is the investigation of choice to detect patent foramen ovale, although transthoracic echocardiography with contrast may be an alternative. A patent foramen ovale occurs when the primum and secundum septa fail to fuse completely, leaving a small flap-like communication, allowing the possibility of shunt. It may be present in 30% of general population, may be associated with right to left intracardiac shunt, responsible for systemic embolism (as in such case).

Treatment is closure using a mechanical device via right femoral vein.

CASE NO. 290

a. 24-hours ECG monitoring, blood pressure drops of 20 mm Hg during peak exercise tolerance testing.
b. Ventricular tachycardia (VT), ventricular fibrillation (VF).
c. Implantable automatic cardioverter defibrillator (ICD).
d. Hypertrophic cardiomyopathy (HCM).

Note: This patient is suffering from hypertrophic cardiomyopathy, presented with dizzy spells, is at increased risk of sudden cardiac death due to VF or VT. 24-hours ECG monitoring may demonstrate non-sustained ventricular tachycardia, presenting in 25% cases of HCM and it is a high-risk marker of sudden death. Five poor prognostic markers which are predictive of sudden cardiac death are (1) Syncope, (2) Family history of HCM and sudden cardiac death, (3) Maximum left ventricular wall thickness >3 cm, (4) BP drop during peak exercise stress testing, (5) Documented runs of non-sustained VT on 24 hours tape.

This patient is a high-risk group of sudden death, his father also died, more likely due to HCM. Ideal treatment is implantable automatic cardioverter defibrillator.

In HCM, 50% patients have chest pain and breathlessness, 20% present with dizziness or syncope. Sudden death is frequently the first presentation, particularly in adolescent, young adult and athlete. Mortality rate is 3%. Sudden death commonly occurs during or immediately after strenuous exertion. Diagnosis is made using echocardiography to demonstrate left ventricular hypertrophy, which is usually asymmetric, but can be concentric in up to 40% of cases. M-mode echocardiography shows systolic anterior motion of mitral valve, which is highly suggestive of HCM.

CASE NO. 291

a. Diabetes insipidus.
b. Urine osmolality.
c. Hypernatremia should be corrected slowly by giving 5% dextrose in aqua infusion.

Note: In this patient, there is severe hypernatremia with elevated chloride, but normal potassium and urea. There is history of severe head injury. The likely cause of this presentation is diabetes insipidus. Urine osmolality is therefore likely to be low.

Head injury is causing cranial diabetes insipidus. In such case, plasma osmolality is high (> 300 mOsm/L), urine osmolality will be low (<150 mOsm/L). Also, plasma sodium may be normal or high and urine sodium is usually low. To confirm the diagnosis, water deprivation test should done, which will show inability to concentrate urine, which response to administration of desmopressin.

Causes of cranial diabetes insipidus are familial, trauma, sarcoidosis, tuberculosis, histiocytosis X, cervical tumor, DIDMOAD syndrome, pituitary hemorrhage.

CASE NO. 292

a. Pancytopenia.
b. Felty's syndrome, folate deficiency causing megaloblastic anemia, methotrexate causing bone marrow depression.
c. Splenomegaly (in Felty's syndrome).
d. Bone marrow study.

Note: This patient has been suffering from rheumatoid arthritis and is on DMARD. So, there may be bone marrow depression by methotrexate. Also, prolonged intake of methotrexate may cause folate deficiency, responsible for pancytopenia. It may be also due to Felty's syndrome, which is characterized by triad of rheumatoid arthritis with splenomegaly with neutropenia. Her pancytopenia may be due to hypersplenism. Neutropenia is due to spleen produced antibody, which can shorten neutrophil lifespan, while large granular lymphocyte (LGL) can attack bone marrow neutrophil precursor. Felty's syndrome occurs in long-standing seropositive, deforming but inactive arthritis, in <1% of cases. It is more in female, may be associated with anemia, thrombocytopenia and abnormal liver functions.

CASE NO. 293

a. Serial blood cultures and transesophageal echocardiography.
b. Intravenous broad spectrum antibiotic, after sending blood culture.

Note: This is a clear case of infective endocarditis, which has developed after prosthetic valve replacement, indicating early prosthetic valve endocarditis. Commonest organism in early prosthetic valve endocarditis is coagulase negative *Staphylococcus epidermidis*, which is a normal commensal of skin. Others are *Staphylococcus aureus* and fungi. Organisms in late prosthetic valve endocarditis are similar to those causing infection on native valves.

Microorganisms usually reach the prosthesis by direct contamination during intraoperative period or via hematogenous spread several days or weeks after surgery. Patient commonly develops valve dehiscence and annular abscess. The risk of embolic phenomenon is also greater.

For diagnosis, three sets of blood culture should be taken at intervals of >1 hour within the first 24 hours.

Transesophageal echocardiography is more sensitive test (1 to 2 mm size vegetation can be detected), then transthoracic echocardiography to identify vegetation in prosthetic valve. Also, helpful to identify complications, like paravalvular abscess and fistula formation.

Treatment: High dose intravenous antibiotics (vancomycin and gentamicin) for 6 weeks. The need for surgical intervention is much higher than with native valve endocarditis. Indications for surgery in prosthetic valve endocarditis—(i) early endocarditis in first 2 months or less after surgery, (ii) murmur suggestive of valve dysfunction, (iii) moderate to severe heart failure, (iv) annular or aortic root abscess or new cardiac conduction abnormalities on ECG,

(v) persistent fever for 10 or more days despite appropriate antibiotic therapy, (vi) *Staphylococcus aureus* or fungi cultured from the blood.

CASE NO. 294

a. *Streptococcus bovis.*
b. Marantic endocarditis.
c. Colonoscopy and biopsy.

Note: This patient is suffering from endocarditis. In addition to the symptoms of endocarditis, he is also having altered bowel habit, which is highly suggestive of large bowel malignancy. *Streptococcus bovis* is a normal commensal of gastrointestinal tract. However, *S. bovis* bacteremia and endocarditis has a strong association with GI malignancy.

As the patient is probably suffering from carcinoma of large bowel, if blood culture is negative, there may be endocarditis associated with malignancy, called marantic endocarditis.

Treatment: IV benzyl penicillin, or flucloxacillin and gentamicin for 4 weeks.

CASE NO. 295

a. Cavernous sinus thrombosis.
b. CT scan of orbit, blood for C/S.
c. IV broad spectrum antibiotic, heparin, steroid IV.

Note: This patient has infection in upper lip followed by headache, fever and proptosis, all are highly suggestive cavernous sinus thrombosis.

Facial veins drain into the sinus and the most common source of infection is due to squeezing of nasal furuncle without antibiotic cover.

Other sources of infection include otitis media, sinusitis and dental infections. Commonest organism is *Staphylococcus aureus*. Patient with cavernous sinus thrombosis presents with severe periorbital headache, which also affects areas innervated by the ophthalmic and maxillary branches of trigeminal nerve. Fever and periorbital edema usually develop later. Ocular swelling, chemosis, ophthalmoplegia and drowsiness are recognized complications. Ophthalmoplegia is due to compression of the third, fourth and sixth cranial nerves. Headache with ophthalmoplegia are highly suggestive of cavernous sinus thrombosis.

The diagnosis of cavernous sinus thrombosis is either with high resolution CT scan of the orbit with contrast or a gadolinium-enhanced MRI scan of the orbit.

Treatment: Intravenous flucloxacillin and heparin. Corticosteroid may be used, which may improve inflammation around the cranial nerves.

Causes of cavernous sinus thrombosis—infections of the face, ear and sinuses, hereditary thrombophilic states, hyperviscosity states, oral contraceptive pill, Behcet's syndrome.

CASE NO. 296

a. Pregnancy.
b. Urine for pregnancy test.
c. Repeat FT_3 and FT_4.

Note: In case of recently married girl with weight gain, pregnancy must be excluded. In pregnancy, thyroxine binding globulin level is increased. So, her total T_4 and T_3 are elevated, but TSH level is normal. In pregnancy, FT_3 and FT_4 should be done, which are normal.

CASE NO. 297

a. Acute tubular necrosis (ATN).
b. Increased urinary sodium excretion, urine osmolality: plasma osmolality 1:1.1.

Note: In ATN, urine to plasma ratio osmolality should be <1.1, urinary sodium excretion is typically >60 mmol and urinary urea excretion is <160 mmol/L. If this patient had a physiological oliguria, there would still be preservation of urine concentration, with low urinary sodium. ATN is caused by renal ischemia, may be precipitated by hypovolemia, septicemia, drugs, rhabdomyolysis. It is usually characterized by oliguric renal failure, often reversible. Ischemia usually affects medullary area, therefore concentrating ability of the urine is diminished and sodium excretion is inappropriately increased.

CASE NO. 298

a. Organophosphorus poisoning.
b. Contaminated clothings should be removed, gastric lavage, airway should be cleared, high flow oxygen, injection atropine IV.
c. ECG, blood gas analysis, serum electrolytes, serum amylase and serum glucose.

Note: In this patient, it is likely to be a case of organophosphorus poisoning. Organophosphorus insecticides (e.g. malathion and parathion) are irreversible inhibitors of acetylcholinesterase, resulting in accumulation of acetylcholine at muscarinic and nicotinic synapses. Muscarinic effects include nausea, vomiting, abdominal pain, urinary and fecal incontinence, miosis. Increased pulmonary parasympathetic tone can result in wheezing due to bronchial hypersecretion and bronchospasm. In severe poisoning, bradycardia, hypotension, heart block and pulmonary edema may occur. Increased parasympathetic activity to salivary glands leads to hypersalivation. Nicotinic effects include twitching, fasciculations, muscle weakness, tachycardia, hypertension. CNS effects are headache, dizziness, confusion, drowsiness, fit and coma. Atropine 1.8 to 3 mg IV as a bolus dose, followed by double the dose every 5 minutes until atropinized (clear lung, dry tongue, normal heart rate, normal BP, pupil dilated). Antidote like pralidoxime or obidoxime may be given in selected case.

CASE NO. 299

a. Statin induced polymyositis.
b. Rhabdomyolysis.
c. Statin should be stopped.

Note: Myalgia, myositis and myopathy are all recognized effects of HMG-CoA reductase inhibitors (statins). There is an increased incidence, when statins are co-administered with a fibrate or when given to patients on immunosuppressants. Unless therapy is withdrawn, rhabdomyolysis may ensue, often associated with acute renal failure, secondary to myoglobinuria.

CASE NO. 300

a. Takayasu's arteritis.
b. Aortography.

Note: The history, high ESR, positive MT, may suggest tuberculosis. However, absent or feeble pulses, bruit in neck and femoral artery with high ESR in a young woman should raise the diagnosis of Takayasu's arteritis. Diagnosis is a clinical one and can be confirmed with aortography. Symptoms are systemic features (such as sweating, weight loss, anorexia and myalgia) and vascular insufficiency in the limbs affected. Physical signs include absence of pulse, usually in upper limb (also called reverse coarctation).

Takayasu's arteritis is a chronic inflammatory, granulomatous panarteritis of unknown cause, involving commonly the aorta and its major branches, carotid, ulnar, brachial, radial and axillary. Occasionally, may involve pulmonary artery, rarely abdominal aorta, renal artery resulting in obstruction. Female: Male = 8:1, more common in parts of Africa and Asia. Mean age of onset is 29 years, but it can occur from any age between infancy and middle age. It is very uncommon after middle age.

Takayasu's arteritis is of four types (i) Localized to aorta and its branches, (ii) Localized to the descending thoracic and abdominal aorta, (iii) Combined features of 1 and 2, (iv) Involve the pulmonary aorta.

Inflammation may be multi-segmental, interspersed with normal segments. Pathological changes are panarteritis, intimal hyperplasia, thickening of media, thickening of adventitia, and later on, fibrosis.

Hypertension is present in 50% cases. The causes of hypertension are renal artery stenosis, acquired coarctation and reduced distensibility of the aortic arch. Complications are those of long-standing hypertension, aortic regurgitation and congestive cardiac failure. Inflammatory markers are usually raised and there may be anemia of chronic disease.

Treatment: Prednisolone 40 to 60 mg daily or 1 to 2 mg/kg. If refractory to steroid or difficult to taper steroid, methotrexate up to 25 mg weekly. Reconstructive vascular surgery in selected cases.
Other drugs—Azathioprine, etanercept, cyclophosphamide, mycophenolate mofetil, leflunomide.

CASE NO. 301

a. Serum B_{12} estimation (also folic acid).
b. Bone marrow study.

Note: This patient has anemia with pancytopenia and raised MCV. With this picture, likely diagnosis is megaloblastic anemia due to B_{12} or folic acid deficiency.

CASE NO. 302

a. To take family history of hemochromatosis.
b. Liver biopsy for iron staining and quantitative measurement of iron.
c. DNA analysis to establish hereditary hemochromatosis.

Note: Hemochromatosis may present with generalized pigmentation only. Serum iron, ferritin all are very high in this case. TIBC also shows full saturation. Family history may be positive.

CASE NO. 303

a. Whipple's disease.
b. By demonstration of *Tropheryma whippelei* within the mucosa of a duodenal or jejunal biopsy by PAS staining.

Note: Whipple's disease is characterized by infiltration of small intestinal mucosa by 'foamy' macrophages, which stain positive with periodic acid-schiff (PAS) reagent. The disease is a multisystem one and almost any organ can be affected, sometimes long before gastrointestinal involvement becomes apparent. Middle-aged male are mostly affected.

Electron microscopy of small bowel biopsy reveals small Gram-positive bacilli (*Tropheryma whipplei*) within the macrophages. Villi are widened and flattened, densely packed macrophages occur in the lamina propria. These may obstruct lymphatic drainage, causing fat malabsorption.

Treatment: Injection ceftriaxone 2 g daily for 2 weeks, followed by oral cotrimoxazole for 1 year. Relapse may occur. In such case, same treatment should be given or doxycycline and hydroxychloroquine may be given.

CASE NO. 304

a. Celiac disease.
b. Endoscopy and jejunal biopsy.

Note: Celiac disease may be linked with type 1 DM. She has iron deficiency anemia, which supports the diagnosis. In some case of celiac disease, there may not be any GIT symptom.

CASE NO. 305

a. Megaloblastic anemia with cardiac failure.
b. Serum vitamin B_{12} and folate level.
c. Blood transfusion (this should be done very cautiously under diuretic cover).
d. Pulmonary edema.

Note: This patient is severely anemic, which is the cause of heart failure. Correction of anemia with blood transfusion, preferably packed cell volume should be the first measure.

CASE NO. 306

a. Methotrexate.
b. Folic acid deficiency.

Note: The patient is taking methotrexate which is the cause of macrocytosis due to folate deficiency. Folinic acid should be given.

CASE NO. 307

a. Amiodarone induced hypothyroidism.

Note: This is most likely a case of amiodarone induced hypothyroidism. Amiodarone which is used for atrial fibrillation inhibits the peripheral conversion of T_4 to T_3.

CASE NO. 308

a. Rhabdomyolysis due to trauma after fall.

Note: The patient has become unconscious in the street. He has renal impairment. There is high AST. These features are consistent with rhabdomyolysis due to trauma after fall.

CASE NO. 309

a. Neuroleptic malignant syndrome.

Note: For details, see Case No. 022.

CASE NO. 310

a. Hypercalcemia.
b. PTH assay.
c. Primary hyperparathyroidism.
d. Parathyroid adenoma.
e. Young patient <50 years with clear symptoms, complications such as peptic ulcer, renal stones, renal impairment or osteopenia.

Note: In primary hyperparathyroidism, there is autonomous secretion of PTH usually by a single parathyroid adenoma (90%), multiple adenoma (4%), nodular hyperplasia (5%), carcinoma (1%). Most of the patients remain asymptomatic or have vague symptoms. They should be reviewed every 6 to 12 months, with assessment of symptoms, renal function, serum calcium and bone mineral density.

CASE NO. 311

a. Bone marrow study.
b. Paraprotein deposition in renal tubule, hypercalcemia, infection, NSAIDs, amyloidosis, dehydration.

Note: Multiple myeloma is a malignant proliferation of plasma cells. In multiple myeloma, plasma cells produce immunoglobulin of a single heavy and light chain, a monoclonal protein called paraprotein. In some cases, only light chain is produced and this appears in urine as Bence-Jones proteinuria.

CASE NO. 312

a. Beta-thalassemia major.
b. Spinal cord compression.
c. X-ray of lumbodorsal spine.
d. Radiotherapy to vertebral body.

Note: In β-thalassemia major, there is extramedullary hemopoiesis, enlargement of the spines of vertebra, which may cause compression of spinal cord, leading to paraplegia. In such case, radiotherapy may help to reduce neurological symptoms.

CASE NO. 313

a. History of polyarthritis, skin rash, Raynaud's phenomenon, oral ulcer, drug history, occupation.
b. Butterfly rash, joint abnormality, alopecia, skin tightening.

Note: This history is suggestive of interstitial lung disease (DPLD). It may be cryptogenic or secondary to other diseases such as—collagen disease (rheumatoid arthritis, scleroderma, dermatomyositis), sarcoidosis, extrinsic allergic alveolitis, drugs (busulfan, bleomycin, methotrexate, amiodarone, nitrofurantoin), asbestosis, silicosis, pneumoconiosis, long-standing mitral valve disease, hemosiderosis.

High resolution CT scan is helpful in early diagnosis.

CASE NO. 314

a. Erythema induratum.
b. Biopsy and histopathology.

Note: Erythema induratum is a form of panniculitis, usually found in the calf of legs of young female, also called Bazin's disease. It is characterized by chronic, recurrent, tender, subcutaneous, ulcerated nodule.

CASE NO. 315

a. Methotrexate and PUVA.

Note: Methotrexate is indicated in severe progressive psoriasis or diffuse exfoliative psoriasis or progressive arthropathy (arthritis mutilans). It is helpful both in psoriasis and arthropathy.

CASE NO. 316

a. Eisenmenger's syndrome from reversal of patent ductus arteriosus (PDA).
b. Color Doppler echocardiography.

Note: The lady is most likely suffering from patent ductus arteriosus (PDA) with reversal of shunt. This is called differential cyanosis and clubbing.

CASE NO. 317

a. Pernicious anemia.

Note: She is suffering from pernicious anemia which is associated with other autoimmune disease like vitiligo in this case.

CASE NO. 318

a. Acrodermatitis from zinc deficiency.
b. Zinc therapy.

Note: Acrodermatitis enteropathica is a rare inherited disorder characterized by zinc deficiency. It presents 4–6 weeks after weaning or earlier in bottle-fed babies. Patients present with erythematous rashes or blisters around the perineum, mouth, hands and feet. It may be associated with photophobia, diarrhea and alopecia. Treatment is with lifelong oral zinc.

CASE NO. 319

a. Cutaneous leishmaniasis.
b. Biopsy of the skin lesion and staining for amastigotes.

Note: Cutaneous leishmaniasis is quite common in many Middle East countries. It is the most likely first diagnosis.

CASE NO. 320

a. Dermatitis herpetiformis.
b. Biopsy.

Note: Dermatitis herpetiformis presents with extremely itchy skin lesion and burning. Itching is paroxysmal and relapsing. Rarely oral mucosa may be involved. It may be associated with celiac disease, lymphoma and hypothyroidism. M:F is 2:1, 80% have HLA B8/DRw 3 and rare in childhood. It may be precipitated by taking iodide and gluten containing diet. Skin biopsy shows infiltration of neutrophils, eosinophils, fibrin at dermal papilla and subepidermal vesicle with neutrophil infiltration. Direct immunofluorescence in normal skin biopsy shows granular IgA deposition alone or with C3 at the dermo-epidermal junction with accentuation in dermal papillae (IgM and IgG are occasionally observed). Almost all patients have partial villous atrophy in jejunal biopsy, even without GIT symptoms.

Treatment: Gluten free diet, dapsone 50 to 200 mg daily.

CASE NO. 321

a. Middle cerebral artery territory.
b. Middle cerebral artery.

Note: Areas supplied by the middle cerebral artery include the most of the lateral surface of cerebral hemisphere (except for the superior part of the frontal and parietal lobes and the inferior part of the temporal lobe) and part of the internal capsule and basal ganglia. Its occlusion leads to paralysis and sensory loss of contralateral face and limbs and aphasia (when in dominant hemisphere). There may be homonymous hemianopia or quadrantanopia.

CASE NO. 322

a. IV magnesium.

Note: Acute severe asthma is managed at hospital with high flow oxygen (40–60%), nebulized salbutamol 5 mg (or terbutaline 10 mg) with ipratropium bromide 0.5 mg 4 hourly and IV hydrocortisone 200 mg 4 hourly for 24 hours followed by oral prednisolone 60 mg daily for 2 weeks. If there is no improvement, then magnesium sulfate 1.2–2 g IV over 20 minutes should be given. Other options are salbutamol 3–20 µg/min IV or terbutaline 1.5–5.0 µg/min IV. Ventilation should be considered, if $PaCO_2$ is more than 7 kPa.

CASE NO. 323

a. History of amenorrhea.
b. Ultrasonogram of whole abdomen.

Note: Ultrasonogram of whole abdomen will show whether the patient is pregnant or not. It will also reveal any ascites, hepatic or renal abnormality or any intra-abdominal mass lesion.

CASE NO. 324
(See also case no. 281)

a. Drug-induced SLE.
b. Antihistone Ab.

Note: Drugs causing SLE are hydralazine, procainamide, carbamazepine, phenytoin, phenothiazine, INH, OCP, ACE inhibitor, penicillamine, methyldopa, minocycline, etc. Sex ratio is equal in drug induced SLE. It commonly involves lung, but renal and neurological involvement are rare. ANA is usually positive, but anti-ds DNA is negative. Complements are normal. Antihistone antibody are positive in 95% of cases, this is characteristic but not specific. Drugs causing SLE like syndrome usually do not aggravate primary SLE. This is treated by withdrawal of drugs and short course of steroid, if necessary.

CASE NO. 325

a. SIADH.
b. Water restriction.

Note: Treatment of SIADH involves restriction of fluid intake to 500 to 1000 mL/day and correction of underlying cause, if possible. Plasma osmolarity, sodium and body weight should be measured frequently. If water restriction is not effective or poorly tolerated, then demeclocycline (600–1200 mg daily) may be given. In very severe cases, hypertonic saline and furosemide may be given.

CASE NO. 326

a. Bleomycin-induced pulmonary fibrosis.
b. HRCT of chest, lung function tests.

Note: In any patient who has received bleomycin, it can cause pulmonary fibrosis. Other drugs causing pulmonary fibrosis are busufan, amiodarone MTX, and nitrofurantoin. CXR may be normal in early stage. HRCT of chest is very helpful for early diagnosis.

CASE NO. 327

a. Refeeding syndrome.
b. Serum electrolytes, magnesium, calcium, phosphate.

Note: Refeeding syndrome may occur following nutritional support by artificial feeding, as in this case. It occurs as a result of shifts of fluid and electrolytes in malnourished patient receiving artificial nutrition (either enterally or parenterally). Typical findings are sodium—normal or lower normal, low potassium, magnesium and phosphate. Calcium is normal. Biochemical abnormality can lead to cardiac arrhythmias, pulmonary edema, seizures and death. The patient should be regularly monitored with regular blood tests to check for the characteristic picture of refeeding syndrome.

CASE NO. 328

a. Familial hypocalciuric hypercalcemia (FHH).
b. Follow-up the patient.

Note: This patient has mild hypercalcemia with normal phosphate and low urinary calcium concentration. He is asymptomatic. It may be confused with primary hyperparathyroidism, in which, urine calcium excretion will also be high. FHH is a benign cause of hypercalcemia that is characterized by autosomal dominant inheritance with high penetrance. Affected heterozygous patients typically present in childhood with the incidental discovery of: mild hypercalcemia, hypocalciuria, a normal PTH level and high-normal to frankly elevated serum magnesium levels.

CASE NO 329

a. Common variable immunodeficiency (CVID).
b. Regular intravenous immunoglobulin (IgG).

Note: Common variable immunodeficiency (CVID) is the common primary immunodeficiency diseases. The basic defect in CVID is failure of B lymphocyte differentiation into plasma cells that produce the various immunoglobulins . Patients with CVID have marked reduction of both IgG and IgA. About 50% of patients also have reduced IgM. The diagnosis is based on exclusion of known causes of defects of the humoral immune system. Most cases are sporadic, although familial cases exist that have various inheritance. Regular intravenous immunoglobulin infusions greatly reduce the frequency of recurrent respiratory tract infections.

Clinical manifestations of CVID include: (a) Recurrent infections: Mainly recurrent pyogenic infections of upper and lower respiratory tract. *Haemophilus influenzae*, *Moraxella catarrhalis*, *Streptococcus pneumoniae*, and *Staphylococcus aureus* are the organisms most commonly involved. Severe, recurrent infection with herpes simplex is also common (b) Autoimmune diseases: Rheumatoid arthritis, hemolytic anemia, thrombocytopenia, thyroid abnormalities, vitiligo may be present. (c) Lymphoid hyperplasia and granulomatous diseases, (d) Predisposition to malignancy—patients with CVID have a high risk of developing malignancy (commonly non-Hodgkin's lymphoma and gastrointestinal carcinoma). Other malignancies include—cancer of colon, breast, prostate, ovary, oral etc.

CASE NO. 330

a. Hypokalemia.
b. Diuretics mainly thiazide.

Note: Mild hypertensive cases are treated with diuretics like thiazide. Prolong use of this drug may cause hypokalemia. In this case, patient's weakness is likely due to thiazide induced hypokalemia. Her presentation may be confused with TIA or Mild CVD, but there is no focal neurological sign. Immediate serum electrolyte should be done.

CASE NO. 331

a. CXR.
b. Tension pneumothorax.
c. Pulmonary embolism, acute MI.

Note: Following FNAC, there may be complication like tension pneumothorax. In this elderly man, other possible causes of chest pain may be acute pulmonary embolism or acute MI, which should be excluded also.

CASE NO. 332

a. Metastatic carcinoma in the brain.
b. MRI of brain with contrast.

Note: There is history of carcinoma breast. Her headache is more likely due to metastasis in the brain, which may occur after many years. Plain CT scan or MRI of brain may be normal. Only contrast MRI may be diagnostic. History of trauma to head may indicate subdural hematoma, which is absent in this case.

CASE NO. 333

a. Wegener's granulomatosis (See also data 230).
b. Biopsy from nasal crusting, c ANCA.

Note: Combination of ear, nose, chest and renal involvement may be due to Wegener's granulomatosis. Frequently the patient use to consult ear or eye specialist. Chest X-ray shadow may be confused with pulmonary tuberculosis. There may be migrating or transient or recurrent shadow in the lung. High degree suspicion is essential for the diagnosis. Recently it is change to granulomatosis with polyangiitis.

Chapter

2

Answers

Data Interpreation of Cardiac Catheter

"The heart ... moves of itself and does not stop unless for ever."

— Leonardo da Vinci

CARDIAC CATHETER - 01

a. There is step-up in oxygen saturation between the right atrium and right ventricle with a further increase in right ventricular out-flow tract. This suggests a left-to-right shunt at ventricular level. Right ventricular systolic pressure is elevated (normally less than 30/8 mm Hg), which indicates left-to-right shunt at ventricular level.
b. Ventricle septal defect (VSD).
c. Perimembranous (at the junction of membranous and muscular part of septum).
d. Pansystolic murmur at the left 3rd or 4th intercostal space in lower sternal edge.

CARDIAC CATHETER - 02

a. Atrial septal defect (secundum type) and pulmonary stenosis.

Note: Peak systolic right ventricular out-flow tract gradient is 44 mm Hg, also pulmonary: systemic blood flow ratio is 3:1. Oximetry shows an abnormal step-up in saturation at the level of the mid right atrium, typical of secundum ASD. Right ventricular systolic pressure is high compared with the pulmonary artery pressure, suggestive of out-flow tract obstruction.

CARDIAC CATHETER - 03

a. Pulmonary stenosis, ventricular septal defect and dextroposition of aorta indicate Fallot's tetralogy.
b. Boot-shaped heart, pulmonary conus is concave (due to small pulmonary artery), right ventricle is enlarged (elevated apex), oligemic lung field.
c. Color Doppler echocardiography

CARDIAC CATHETER - 04

a. Patent ductus arteriosus with reversal of shunt.
b. Color Doppler echocardiography.

Note: If diastolic pressure in pulmonary artery and aorta is same, it indicates PDA. Oxygen saturation is reduced, which indicates reversal of shunt.

CARDIAC CATHETER - 05

a. Post infarction VSD.
b. Surgical correction after 6 months.

Note: There is step-up in oxygen saturation between the right atrium and right ventricle with a further increase in pulmonary artery. This suggests left-to-right shunt at ventricular level.

CARDIAC CATHETER - 06

a. Aortic stenosis, hypertrophic obstructive cardiomyopathy (HOCM).
b. Echocardiography.

Note: There is a gradient of 80 mm Hg across the region of the aortic valve. This could be due to stenosis of the valve or to hypertrophy of the outflow tract (HOCM). These conditions can be distinguished by measurement of subvalvular pressure, left ventricular angiography and echocardiography. Left ventricular end diastolic pressure is raised. This may be due to left ventricular hypertrophy (thick non-complaint muscle) or to left ventricular failure.

CARDIAC CATHETER - 07

a. Patent ductus arteriosus.
b. A continuous machinery murmur at the left upper sternal edge.
c. Step-up in oxygen saturation between the RV and PA and high pulmonary artery pressure.

Note: This data shows step-up in oxygen saturation between RV and PA, consistent with PDA (with left-to-right shunt).

CARDIAC CATHETER - 08

a. Three abnormalities are—(i) Right ventricular pressure and pulmonary artery pressure are high (>35 mm Hg), (ii) PCWP > LVEDP, (iii) There is pressure drop of 50 mm Hg across the aortic valve.
b. Above finding indicates mitral stenosis, with aortic stenosis and pulmonary hypertension.

CARDIAC CATHETER - 09

a. There is wide pulse pressure.
b. Aortic regurgitation.
c. Marfan's syndrome.

Note: The patient is tall, lean and thin, with aortic regurgitation, consistent with the diagnosis of Marfan's syndrome.

CARDIAC CATHETER - 10

a. There is increased systolic gradient between the left ventricle and femoral artery (195 - 155 = 40).
b. Coarctation of aorta.

CARDIAC CATHETER - 11

a. Pressure in right ventricle and pulmonary artery are grossly elevated, also exceeded than the left. Oxygen saturation is reduced in left ventricle.
b. Eisenmenger's syndrome.

Note: There is increased right ventricular pressure, also oxygen saturation in the left ventricle is low, which indicates right to left shunt.

CARDIAC CATHETER - 12

a. Oxygen saturation is more in right atrium than SVC. Normally, it should be same both in SVC and RA. Because of admixture of blood from LA to RA, there is increased oxygen saturation in RA.
b. Atrial septal defect.

Note: Normally, oxygen saturation should be same in SVC and RA. Because of admixture of blood from LA to RA, there is increased oxygen in RA.

CARDIAC CATHETER - 13

a. Possible diagnoses are—(i) Mitral stenosis, as the end diastolic pressure gradient is 30 mm Hg across the mitral valve. (ii) Pulmonary hypertension as the pulmonary artery systolic pressure is 70 mm Hg. (iii) Right ventricular overload, as normally right ventricular end diastolic pressure is less than 5 mm Hg (here it is 15 mm Hg). (iv) Tricuspid regurgitation, as right atrial pressure is very high, indicating TR.
b. Color Doppler echocardiography.

CARDIAC CATHETER - 14

a. Atrial septal defect with pulmonary hypertension with Down's syndrome.
b. Color Doppler echocardiogram.

CARDIAC CATHETER - 15

a. Chronic constrictive pericarditis.
b. Chest X-ray.

Note: The data shows elevated and equal right and left atrial pressure. Also elevated and equal left and right ventricular end diastolic pressure.

CARDIAC CATHETER - 16

a. Aortic regurgitation.
b. Early diastolic murmur in left lower parasternal area.

Note: The abnormality here is wide pulse pressure in aorta, indicating aortic regurgitation.

Chapter
3

Answers

Family Tree (Pedigree)

"The art of medicine consists of amusing the patient while nature cures the disease."

— Voltaire

FAMILY TREE - 01

a. X-linked dominant.
b. Vitamin D resistant ricket (other—pseudohypoparathyroidism).

Note: In this case, no male to male transmission is seen. As well as affected male transmits the disease to all of his daughters and affected female transmits the disease to 50% of her offsprings. Moreover, male and female both are affected by this disease.

Ricket, which is resistant to ordinary therapeutic dose of vitamin D is called vitamin D resistant ricket. Most common is hypophosphatemic vitamin D resistant ricket (VDRR), which is inherited as X-linked dominant. There is reduction of renal tubular reabsorption of phosphate and only biochemical abnormality is hypophosphatemia. The cause of renal abnormality is unknown. There is no overactivity of parathyroid or no deficiency or disturbance of vitamin D metabolism. Children with hypophosphatemic ricket presents with features of ordinary ricket, but deformity is more with dwarfism. In adult, calcification of ligamentum flava, which may lead to paraplegia.

Treatment: Very high dose of vitamin D, oral phosphate may be given.

FAMILY TREE - 02

a. X-linked recessive.
b. Hemophilia A and B, glucose-6-phosphate dehydrogenase deficiency, Lesch Nyhan syndrome, Fabry's disease, red-green color blindness (others—Hunter's syndrome, Duchenne and Becker's muscular dystrophy, congenital ichthyosis).

Note: In this case, only males are affected and here in second generation, the mother of the affected son is a carrier.

FAMILY TREE - 03

a. Autosomal recessive.
b. Cystic fibrosis, Wilson's diseases, Homocystinuria, α_1 antitrypsin deficiency, infantile polycystic kidney disease.

Note: Here neither parent is affected, which virtually excludes autosomal dominant diseases. Both males and females are affected. In second generation, the wife of the affected male is a carrier. So, 50% of the offsprings are affected.

FAMILY TREE - 04

a. Both autosomal recessive.
b. All affected.

Note: Here it is shown that neither parent is affected. So, it is not autosomal dominant. As both the couples are affected. So, chance of their children being affected is 100%.

FAMILY TREE - 05

a. Autosomal dominant with variable penetrance.
b. 1 in 2 (both 50% chance), son affected in 50% and daughter affected in 50%.

Note: Here, all the individuals inheriting the abnormal gene are affected. Also, there is male-to-male transmission (which excludes X-linked conditions).

FAMILY TREE - 06

a. Autosomal recessive.
b. If both parents are carrier, (i) 25% of their offspring are affected, (ii) 1/2 are carriers.

Note: In this case, male and female both are affected and male-to-male transmission is present. Also, it is seen that male and female both are carriers.

FAMILY TREE - 07

a. Non-germ line cytoplasmic inheritance.
b. None, no males transmit the disease.
c. Leber's optic atrophy.

Note: Here, it is obvious that both male and females are affected, but affected females transmit the disease to 100% offsprings and affected males cannot transmit the disease to offsprings.

FAMILY TREE - 08

a. Autosomal recessive.
b. Usually, only one generation is affected.

Note: In this case, both male and female are affected and in second generation, both parents are carrier and 25% of the offsprings are diseased, 50% of the offsprings are carrier and 25% have got no disease.

FAMILY TREE - 09

a. Translocation Down's syndrome, 46 xyt.
b. 100%.

Note: It is karyotype of Down's syndrome. Here, the mother has Robertsonian translocation 21q21q. This very rare carrier of 21q21q translocation, transmits the disease to all of the offsprings.

FAMILY TREE - 10

a. Autosomal recessive.
b. Autosomal recessive.
c. None, 100% will be affected.

Note: As first generation is not affected and both male and female are affected, this is autosomal recessive. If both parents are affected, 100% of their offsprings will be affected.

FAMILY TREE - 11

a. X-linked dominant.

b. 50%.
c. 50%.
d. Vitamin D-resistant rickets.

Note: See answer 01.

FAMILY TREE - 12

a. Like normal population.
b. Like normal population.

Note: Achondroplasia can occur as a result of new mutation or de novo mutation. There may be no family history of this disease. So, the chance of parents having another offspring with achondroplasia does not obey any Mandelian rule. It occurs like normal population.

FAMILY TREE - 13

a. Autosomal dominant.
b. 50%.
c. Huntington's chorea, neurofibromatosis, adult polycystic kidney disease, multiple polyposis coli, myotonic dystrophy (others—hereditary spherocytosis, tuberous sclerosis, acute intermittent porphyria, Marfan's syndrome, achondroplasia).

Note: This is autosomal dominant, as first generation is not affected and male and female are both affected. Male-to-male transmission is present. Also, 50% offsprings of the affected parents are suffering from the disease.

FAMILY TREE - 14

a. Klinefelter's syndrome.
b. Like normal population (1 in 500).
c. None, as the patient is sterile.

Note: This disease is due to chromosomal abnormality. It does not show any Mandelian inheritance. So, chance of parents to get another XXY child is like normal population (i.e. 1 in 500).

Notes on inheritance pattern

a. *Autosomal dominant:* It has the following characters:
  - Consecutive generations are affected.
  - Half of the offsprings are affected, both male and female are equally affected.
  - Unaffected individual cannot transmit the disease.
b. *Autosomal recessive inheritance:* It has the following characters:
  - Half the children of unaffected carriers will be carriers.
  - If both parents are carriers, then one-quarter of their offspring are affected, and one-half are carriers.
  - Usually only one generation is affected.
c. *X-linked recessive inheritance:* It has the following characters: (X chromosome gene)
  - Only males are affected, females are carrier.
  - Unaffected female carriers transmit the disease.

♦ Half of carrier female's offspring inherit mutation—males are affected and females are carriers.

♦ Affected males cannot transmit the disease to their sons, but all the daughters are carrier.

d. *X-linked dominant:* It has the following characters:

♦ X-linked diseases are rarely dominant.

♦ Females who are heterozygous for the mutant gene and males who have only one copy of the mutant gene on their single X chromosome will manifest the disease.

♦ Half of the male or female offspring of an affected mother will have the disease.

♦ All the female offspring of an affected man will have the disease.

♦ Affected man will always have affected daughter, never son.

♦ Women are more affected than men, M:F = 1:2.

♦ Affected males tend to have the disease more severely than the heterozygous female.

e. *Non-germ line cytoplasmic inheritance* (e.g. gene on mitochondrial DNA): It has the following characters:

♦ Males and females are affected.

♦ No males transmit the disease.

♦ Variable proportion of offspring from female are affected.

Chapter
4

Answers
Spirometry

"All these primary impulses, not easily described in words, are the springs of man's actions."

— *Albert Einstein*

SPIRO - 01

* ❖ FVC – 96%.
* ❖ FEV_1 – 83%.
* ❖ FEV_1/FVC – 86%.

This is a case of normal spirometry

Upper curve is called Flow Volume Curve (FVC). Only PEF is seen in this curve in liter per second.

Lower curve is called time volume curve. In this curve, FEV_1 is seen. The point in 1 second which cuts with the curve is taken as the result.

Normal value of FEV_1/FVC (in %) – >80%.

PEF: Vary according to age, sex, height, weight and race. PEF may be reduced in COPD, bronchial asthma, restrictive lung disease, extrathoracic compression.

FEV_1 may be reduced in obstructive and restrictive airway disease.

Three types of obstructive airway disease (on the basis of FEV_1):

Mild – 80 to 65%. Moderate – 65 to 50%. Severe – <50%.

SPIRO - 02

* ❖ FVC – 49%.
* ❖ FEV_1 – 33% (<50%).
* ❖ FEV_1/FVC – 69% (<75%).

This is a case of severe obstructive airway disease.

SPIRO - 03

* ❖ FVC – 86% (normal).
* ❖ FEV_1 – 79% (<80%).
* ❖ FEV_1/FVC – 92% (>75%).

This is a case of mild restrictive airway disease.

SPIRO - 04

* ❖ FVC – 36% (<50%).
* ❖ FEV_1 – 43% (<50%).
* ❖ FEV_1/FVC – 120% (>75%).

This is a case of severe restrictive airway disease.

SPIRO - 05

* ❖ FVC – 67%.
* ❖ FEV_1 – 45% (<50%).
* ❖ FEV_1/FVC – 67% (<75%).

This is a case of severe obstructive airway disease.

SPIRO - 06

* FVC – 45%.
* FEV$_1$ – 33%.
* FEV$_1$/FVC – 22%.

This is a case of severe obstructive airway disease.

SPIRO - 07

* FVC – 90%.
* FEV$_1$ – 72%.
* FEV$_1$/FVC – 80%.

This is a case of mild obstructive airway disease.

SPIRO - 08

* FVC – 69%.
* FEV$_1$ – 45%.
* FEV$_1$/FVC – 65%.

This is a case of severe obstructive airway disease.

SPIRO - 09

* FVC – 39%.
* FEV$_1$ – 25%.
* FEV$_1$/FVC – 64%.

This is a case of severe obstructive airway disease.

SPIRO - 10

* FVC – 52%.
* FEV$_1$ – 50%.
* FEV$_1$/FVC – 96%.

This is a case of mixed obstructive and restrictive airway disease.

Causes of mixed airway disease—(i) Ankylosing spondylitis, (ii) Kyphoscoliosis with bronchial asthma, (iii) Interstitial lung disease (commonly restrictive), (iv) Others—pneumothorax, pneumonectomy.

SPIRO - 11

* FVC – 88%.
* FEV$_1$ – 93%.
* FEV$_1$/FVC – 104%.

This is a case of normal spirometry.

SPIRO - 12

* FVC – 89.6%.
* FEV$_1$ – 104.5%.
* FEV$_1$/FVC – 97.18%.

This is a case of normal spirometry.

SPIRO - 13

- ❖ FVC – 76.1%.
- ❖ FEV_1 – 61.9%.
- ❖ FEV_1/FVC – 67.84%.

This is a case of moderate obstructive airway disease.

SPIRO - 14

- ❖ FVC – 91.7%
- ❖ FEV_1 – 71.2%.
- ❖ FEV_1/FVC – 67.70%.

This is a case of mild obstructive airway disease.

SPIRO - 15

- ❖ FVC – 75.6%.
- ❖ FEV_1 – 71.6%.
- ❖ FEV_1/FVC – 82.36%.

This is a case of mild restrictive airway disease.

SPIRO - 16

- ❖ FVC – 29.9%.
- ❖ FEV_1 – 23.4%.
- ❖ FEV_1/FVC – 62.94%.

This is a case of severe obstructive airway disease.

SPIRO - 17

- ❖ FVC – 74.8%.
- ❖ FEV_1 – 75.2%.
- ❖ FEV_1/FVC – 83.33%.

This is a case of mild restrictive airway disease.

SPIRO - 18

- ❖ FVC – 79.0%.
- ❖ FEV_1 – 89.5%.
- ❖ FEV_1/FVC – 98.44%.
- ❖ MMEF 75/25 – 65.9%

This is a case of small airways obstruction.

SPIRO - 19

- ❖ FVC – 49%.
- ❖ FEV_1 – 23.9%.
- ❖ FEV_1/FVC – 48.7%.

This is a case of severe obstructive airway disease.

SPIRO - 20

* FVC – 68.3%.
* FEV_1 – 81.8%.
* FEV_1/FVC – 117.7%.

This is a case of moderate restrictive airway disease.

SPIRO - 21

* FVC – 69.3%.
* FEV_1 – 25.5%.
* FEV_1/FVC – 36.6%.

This is a case of severe obstructive airway disease.

SPIRO - 22

* FVC – 65.0%.
* FEV_1 – 35.1%.
* FEV_1/FVC – 54.1%.

This is a case of severe obstructive airway disease.

SPIRO - 23(A)

* FVC – 99.8%.
* FEV_1 – 59.9%.
* FEV_1/FVC – 60.9%.

This is a case of moderate obstructive airway disease.

SPIRO - 23(B)

(Reversibility test of the previous).

FEV_1: Before salbutamol inhalation is 1.34 L (59.9% predicted), which is consistent with moderate obstructive airway disease.

After 20 minutes of 200 µg salbutamol inhalation shows, FEV_1 is 1.93 L (87.6% predicted).

So, there is 44% increased, which means positive reversibility (20% increase is needed to depict the reversibility as positive).

So, it is consistent with bronchial asthma.

SPIRO - 24(A)

* FVC – 93.8%.
* FEV_1 – 37.3%.
* FEV_1/FVC – 39.7%.

This is a case of severe obstructive airway disease.

SPIRO - 24(B)

(Reversibility test of the previous).

FEV$_1$: Before salbutamol inhalation is 1.32 L (37.3% predicted), which is consistent with severe obstructive airway disease.

After 20 minutes of 200 µg salbutamol inhalation, FEV$_1$ is 1.32 L (37.3% predicted).

So, FEV$_1$ is not increased, which means negative reversibility (20% increase is needed to depict the reversibility as positive).

So, it is consistent with COPD (also it may be found in severe persistent bronchial asthma).

SPIRO - 25

FEV$_1$: Before salbutamol inhalation is 1.01 L (32% predicted), which is consistent with severe obstructive airway disease.

After 20 minutes of 200 µg salbutamol inhalation, FEV$_1$ is 1.23 L (122% predicted).

So, FEV$_1$ is increased by 0.22 L and 90%, which means positive reversibility (20% increase is needed to depict the reversibility as positive).

So, it is consistent with bronchial asthma.

SPIRO - 26(A AND B)

FEV$_1$: Before salbutamol inhalation is 0.8 L (35.1% predicted), which is consistent with severe obstructive airway disease. After 20 minutes of 200 µg salbutamol inhalation, FEV$_1$ is 1.12 L.

So, FEV$_1$ is increased by 0.32 L and 75%, which means positive reversibility.

So, it is consistent with bronchial asthma.

Chapter
5

Answers

Pictures of Multiple Diseases

PICTURE 01

a. Left-sided Horner's syndrome.
b. Partial third nerve palsy.
c. To see the pupil, which is constricted, reacts to direct and consensual light.

PICTURE 02

a. Right-sided cervical lymphadenopathy.
b. Cold abscess.
c. FNAC or biopsy.

PICTURE 03

a. Palmar erythema, Dupuytren's contracture.
b. Chronic liver disease (Cirrhosis of liver).

PICTURE 04

a. Short 4th metacarpal bone in right hand.
b. Pseudohypoparathyroidism (Other causes of short 4th metacarpal bone are Turner's syndrome, Noonan's syndrome, sickle cell dactylitis, JIA, recurrent hand trauma).

PICTURE 05

a. Leonine face.
b. Lepromatous leprosy.
c. PKDL.

PICTURE 06

a. Multiple erythematous rash.
b. Dengue hemorrhagic fever.

PICTURE 07

a. Left-sided complete ptosis, right-sided partial ptosis.
b. Myasthenia gravis.

PICTURE 08

a. Osteosarcoma.
b. FNAC or biopsy for histopathology.

PICTURES 09 AND 10

a. Hyperextensibility of joint.
b. Steinburg sign.
c. Marfan's syndrome.

PICTURE 11

a. Turner's syndrome.
b. Buccal smear for karyotyping.
c. Primary amenorrhea.

PICTURE 12

a. Relapsing polychondritis.
b. Biopsy of the involved cartilage.

PICTURE 13

a. Periungual fibroma.
b. Tuberous sclerosis.
c. Epilepsy.

PICTURE 14

a. Rain drop pigmentation on back.
b. Source of drinking water.

PICTURE 15

a. SLE, MCTD, dermatomyositis.

PICTURE 16

a. Post kala-azar dermal leishmaniasis (PKDL).

PICTURE 17

a. Central retinal vein obstruction.
b. Diabetes mellitus, hypertension.

PICTURE 18

a. Clubbing with drum stick appearance.
b. Interstitial lung disease or Idiopathic pulmonary fibrosis (DPLD).

PICTURE 19

a. Wasting of muscles of both thighs.
b. Proximal myopathy.
c. Fascioscapulohumeral muscular dystrophy.

PICTURE 20

a. Pseudohypoparathyroidism.
b. Short stature, mental retardation.

PICTURE 21

a. Pyoderma gangrenosum.

PICTURE 22

a. Multiple hypopigmented patch over chest and both upper arms, multiple small nodular lesion over dorsum of hand and fingers in right side.
b. Lepromatous leprosy.
c. Sensory test on hypopigmented patches.

PICTURE 23

a. Erythema nodosum.
b. Sarcoidosis, primary pulmonary tuberculosis.

PICTURE 24

a. Abdominal striae, bilateral gynecomastia.
b. Prolonged use of steroid (causing Cushing's syndrome).

PICTURE 25

a. Diffuse goiter, bilateral exophthalmos.
b. Graves' disease.
c. Dermopathy.

PICTURE 26

a. Molluscum contagiosum.
b. AIDS.
c. Curettage of the lesion.

PICTURE 27

a. Huge ascites, engorged superficial vein on abdomen, bilateral gynecomastia and wasting.
b. Chronic liver disease (CLD).

PICTURE 28

a. Leukonychia.
b. Albumin deficiency (hypoalbuminemia).

PICTURE 29

a. Drug reaction (Stevens-Johnson syndrome).

PICTURE 30

a. Erythroderma.
b. Psoriasis.

PICTURE 31

a. Left-sided complete ptosis with a scar mark over left side of head.
b. Left-sided third cranial nerve palsy with possible intracranial surgery.
c. Intracranial space occupying lesion (ICSOL).

PICTURE 32

a. Chancre due to primary syphilis.
b. Chancroid.

PICTURE 33

a. Orf.
b. A pox virus.

PICTURE 34

a. Raw beefy tongue and angular stomatitis.
b. Deficiency of riboflavin, folic acid and iron.

PICTURES 35 AND 36

a. Myotonia.
b. Myotonic dystrophy.

PICTURE 37

a. Multiple nodules and cafe au lait spot.
b. Neurofibromatosis type 1.

PICTURE 38

a. Puffy face with baggy eyelids.
b. Hypothyroidism, superior vena caval obstruction.

PICTURE 39

a. Pes cavus.
b. Friedreich's ataxia.

PICTURE 40

a. Lupus pernio.
b. Sarcoidosis.

PICTURE 41

a. Adenoma sebaceum.
b. Tuberous sclerosis.
c. Periungual fibroma (around nail base), Shagreen patch (cobble stone-like plaque at the base of spine on back).

PICTURE 42

a. Cellulitis with foot ulcers.
b. Blood sugar.
c. Diabetic ulcer (Other causes are leprosy, syphilis, pyogenic infection).

PICTURE 43

a. Pectus carinatum.
b. Congenital, bronchial asthma from childhood, repeated respiratory tract infection, osteogenesis imperfecta, rickets, Marfan's syndrome.

PICTURE 44

a. Pectus excavatum.
b. Causes are:
   ♦ Congenital.
   ♦ Rickets.
   ♦ Marfan's syndrome.
   ♦ Homocystinuria.
   ♦ Osteogenesis imperfecta.
   ♦ Ehlar-Danlos syndrome.

PICTURE 45

a. To see the flow of engorged veins.
b. Superior vena caval obstruction, inferior vena caval obstruction.

PICTURE 46

a. Stevens-Johnson syndrome.
b. Carbamazepine, sulfonamide, thiacetazone.

PICTURE 47

a. Knuckle pads on the fingers.
b. Garrod's patch.

PICTURE 48

a. Psoriatic plaque with knee joint swelling.
b. Psoriatic arthritis.

PICTURE 49

a. Hyperkeratosis of palm, X-ray shows irregular narrowing of the lower end of esophagus suggestive of carcinoma esophagus.
b. Tylosis.

PICTURE 50

a. Angioid streaks in retina.
b. Pseudoxanthoma elasticum, Paget's disease, acromegaly, sickle cell disease, Ehlar-Danlos syndrome.
(**Note:** Angioid streaks underlie the retinal vessel and cross the fundus radially from the optic disk. They represent breaks/degeneration in the elastic tissue of Bruch's membrane with resultant fibrosis).

PICTURE 51

a. Pretibial myxedema.
b. Graves' disease.

PICTURE 52

a. Diabetic cheiroarthropathy.
b. Unknown.

PICTURE 53

a. Herpes zoster.
b. Complications are secondary infection, generalized zoster, purpura fulminants (local purpura with necrosis) and postherpetic neuralgia. Others are myelitis, meningoencephalitis, motor radiculopathy.

PICTURE 54

a. Guttate psoriasis.

PICTURE 55

a. Acute promyelocytic leukemia (with DIC).
b. Disseminated intravascular coagulation.

PICTURE 56

a. Behcet's disease.

PICTURES 57 AND 58

a. Budd-Chiari syndrome.
b. Ultrasonogram of hepatobiliary system, CT scan (or MRI) of upper abdomen).

PICTURE 59

a. Chronic tophaceous gout.
b. Aspiration from tophus to see MSUM crystal under polarized microscope (crystal is needle-shaped, negatively birefringent).

PICTURE 60

a. Pigmentation in surgical scar.
b. Addison's disease.

PICTURE 61

a. Deep jaundice, marked emaciation and pigmentation.
b. Carcinoma head of the pancreas.
c. CT-guided FNAC of pancreas.

PICTURE 62

a. Neurofibromatosis.
b. Sarcomatous change (<1% case).

PICTURES 63 AND 64

a. Stevens-Johnson syndrome.
b. Due to carbamazepine therapy.

PICTURE 65

a. Dengue hemorrhagic fever.
b. Total platelet count.

PICTURE 66

a. Left sixth cranial nerve palsy.
b. Causes are:
   ◆ Raised intracranial pressure (commonest cause).
   ◆ Idiopathic (common).
   ◆ Brainstem lesion (e.g. multiple sclerosis, neoplasia, vascular, etc.).
   ◆ Mononeuritis multiplex.
   ◆ Diabetes mellitus.
   ◆ Others are acoustic neuroma, nasopharyngeal carcinoma.

PICTURE 67

a. Basal cell carcinoma.

PICTURE 68

a. History of smoking.
b. Buerger's disease.

PICTURE 69

a. Polydactyly (6 toes in each foot).
b. Laurence-Moon-Biedl syndrome.

PICTURE 70

a. Pseudohypertrophy of calf muscles.
b. Gower sign.
c. Duchene muscular dystrophy.

PICTURE 71

a. Rheumatoid nodule, tophus, tendon xanthoma.

PICTURE 72

a. Hereditary hemorrhagic telangiectasia.
b. Epistaxis.

PICTURE 73

a. Carpo-pedal spasm.
b. Trousseau's sign.
c. Hypocalcemia.

PICTURE 74

a. Webbing of the neck.
b. Noonan's syndrome (male Turner).

PICTURE 75

a. Psoriatic plaque.

PICTURE 76

a. Chronic tophaceous gout.
b. Podagra.

PICTURE 77

a. Multiple bullous lesion.
b. Pemphigus vulgaris, bullous pemphigoid and toxic epidermal necrolysis.

PICTURE 78

a. Transformation into acute leukemia.

PICTURE 79

a. Skin lesion consists of small yellowish papules in confluent plaques (plucked chicken skin or cobble stone appearance).
b. Pseudoxanthoma elasticum.

PICTURE 80

a. Erythroderma.

PICTURE 81

a. Exfoliative dermatitis.
b. Lymphoma, leukemia, multiple myeloma, HIV infection, graft versus host disease (also in carcinoma of lung, rectum, other malignancy).

PICTURE 82

a. Spider angioma.
b. Chronic liver disease.

PICTURE 83

a. Nodular lesion on the ear lobule, prominent and thick great auricular nerve.
b. Lepromatous leprosy.

PICTURE 84

a. Tendon xanthoma.
b. Serum cholesterol.
c. Tophus of gout, rheumatoid nodule, neurofibroma, lipoma.

PICTURES 85 AND 86

a. Hyperuricemia (Picture- 85 indicates chronic tophous gout and Picture 86 indicate psoriasis which are associated hyperuricemia) .

PICTURE 87

a. Herpes zoster ophthalmicus.

PICTURE 88

a. Tendon xanthoma.
b. Serum lipid profile.

PICTURE 89

a. Bilateral gynecomastia.
b. The relevant causes for this young patient are.
   ♦ Puberty (normal physiological).
   ♦ Drugs (spironolactone, digoxin, cimetidine, INH).
   ♦ Testicular tumor (teratoma, Leydig cell tumor).
   ♦ Secondary testicular failure (trauma, orchidectomy, leprosy).
   ♦ CLD (due to Wilson's disease, alpha 1 antitrypsin deficiency).

PICTURE 90

a. Swan neck deformity of the thumb.
b. Rheumatoid arthritis.

PICTURE 91

a. Multiple erythematous rash in the chest and abdomen
b. Dermatomyositis

PICTURE 92

a. Osler's node.
b. Infective endocarditis.
c. Blood culture and sensitivity.

PICTURE 93

a. Xanthelasma.
b. Dyslipidemia.

PICTURE 94

a. Hirsutism with virilization.
b. Causes are:
   - Ovarian causes—
     - PCOS.
     - Androgen-secreting ovarian tumor.
     - Arrhenoblastoma.
   - Adrenal causes—
     - Late onset congenital adrenal hyperplasia.
     - Cushing's syndrome.
     - Adrenal carcinoma.
     - Androgen-secreting adrenal tumor.

PICTURE 95

a. Black tongue.
b. Causes may be:
   - Drugs (e.g. bismuth-containing drugs, tetracycline and chronic or extensive use of antibiotics).
   - Smoking.
   - Poor oral hygiene, tooth loss.
   - Bacterial or fungal infection of the tongue.
   - Sjogren's syndrome.
   - Radiation treatment to head or neck.

PICTURE 96

a. Multiple nodular lesions.
b. Lepromatous leprosy.

PICTURE 97

a. Hidradenitis suppurativa.
b. Treatment is mainly surgical which includes:
  ♦ Incision and drainage or lancing.
  ♦ Wide local excision (with or without skin grafting).
  ♦ Laser surgery.

PICTURE 98

a. To take history of repeated fracture of bone.
b. Osteogenesis imperfecta.

PICTURE 99

a. There is gap between first and second toes.
b. Down's syndrome.

PICTURE 100

a. Perforation of hard palate.
b. Fungal infection (invasive aspergillosis, mucormycosis), Wegener's granulomatosis, syphilis, acute lymphoblastic leukemia.

PICTURE 101

a. Target lesion.
b. Erythema multiforme.

PICTURE 102

a. Pustular psoriasis.
b. Steven Jonson's syndrome.

PICTURE 103

a. Butterfly rash.
b. SLE
c. ANA and Anti-ds-DNA

PICTURE 104

a. Vesiculopapular rash.
b. Herpes genitalis.

PICTURE 105

a. Multiple hemorrhage (blot and flame shape), soft and hard exudates.
b. Proliferative diabetic retinopathy.

PICTURE 106

a. Gangrene in great toe and ulcer in second toe with pigmentation over the ankle joint.
b. Diabetic foot.

PICTURE 107

a. Genital warts.

PICTURE 108

a. Gibbous.
b. Spinal tuberculosis (Pott's disease).

PICTURE 109

a. Generalized edema with swelling of face.
b. Nephrotic syndrome.

PICTURE 110

a. Redness with puckering of the skin.
b. Erythroderma.

PICTURE 111

a. Gangrene with pigmentation at the front of the leg.
b. Pyoderma gangrenosum.

PICTURE 112

a. Knock knee.
b. Rickets.

PICTURE 113

a. Pseudohypertrophy of calf muscles of both legs, more in right side.
b. Duchene muscular dystrophy.

PICTURE 114

a. Multiple nodular skin lesion.
b. Neurofibromatosis.

PICTURE 115

a. Hypopigmented and some pigmented skin over the face and whole body with contracture of finger joints.
b. Systemic sclerosis.

PICTURE 116

a. Erythematosus maculopapular rash in the forehead and the butterfly distribution of the face.
b. Dermatomyositis.

PICTURE 117

a. Port wine stain along the maxillary division of the trigeminal nerve.
b. Sturge–Weber syndrome.

PICTURE 118

a. Rose spot.
b. Enteric fever.

PICTURE 119

a. Engorged and tortuous vein in abdomen and chest wall.
b. SVC, IVC, and portal venous obstruction.

PICTURE 120

a. Prominent temporal artery.
b. Temporal arteritis.

PICTURE 121

a. Erythematous elevated skin lesion in the right side of the cheek.
b. Lupus vulgaris.

PICTURE 122

a. Beau's line.
b. Prolong fever, pneumonia, any malignancy.

PICTURE 123

a. Healing Stevens-Johnson syndrome.

PICTURE 124

a. Six toes (polydactyly) in both feet.
b. Laurence Moon Biedel syndrome.

PICTURE 125

a. Multiple gangrene and amputation right second toe.
b. Peripheral vascular disease (Buerger's disease).

PICTURE 126

a. Erythematous swelling at the left great toe.
b. Acute gouty arthritis (this sign is called podagra).

PICTURE 127

a. Pigmentation in scar.
b. Addison's disease.

PICTURE 128

a. Right sided 7th nerve palsy.
b. Ramsay Hunt's syndrome.

PICTURE 129

a. Multiple vesicular lesion with some rupture vesicle.
b. Pemphigus vulgaris.

PICTURE 130

a. Hyperpigmentation and hypopigmentation in the forearm and dorsum of the hand.
b. Dermatomyositis.

PICTURE 131

a. Hypothyroidism.

PICTURE 132

a. Pectus carinatum.
b. Congenital, Rickets.

PICTURE 133

a. Multiple ulcer with irregular margin.
b. Pyoderma gangrenosum.

PICTURE 134

a. Bilateral parotid swelling.
b. Mumps, sarcoidosis.

PICTURE 135

a. Heberden's nodes in DIP.
b. Osteoarthritis.

PICTURE 136

a. Multiple telangiectasia in upper and lower lip.
b. Hereditary hemorrhagic telangiectasia.

PICTURE 137

a. Scar with pigmented lesion.
b. Healed herpes zoster.

PICTURE 138

a. Molluscum contagiosum.

PICTURE 139

a. Multiple ulcer in the inner side lower lip.
b. Aphthous ulcer.

PICTURE 140

a. Erythematous rash in the left side of face, upper lip and eye lids.
b. SLE, dermatomyositis.

PICTURE 141

a. Multiple ulceration with some crust along the ophthalmic division of trigeminal nerve.
b. Herpes zoster ophthalmicus.

PICTURE 142

a. Multiple sinuses with cervical lymphadenitis.
b. Tuberculous lymphadenitis (scrofula).

PICTURE 143

a. Onycholysis with nail pitting with redness of the skin of finger.
b. Psoriasis.

PICTURE 144

a. Molluscum contagiosum.

PICTURE 145

a. Multiple ulceration with peeling of skin.
b. Stevens-Johnson syndrome.

PICTURE 146

a. Erythematous nodular lesion at the root of the left side of neck.
b. Cold abscess.

PICTURE 147

a. Rain drop pigmentation in the back.
b. Arsenicosis.

PICTURE 148

a   Dupuytren's contracture with palmar erythema.
b. Cirrhosis of the liver.

PICTURE 149

a. Whitish patch on the dorsum of the tongue with gum hypertrophy.
b. Oral candidiasis with gingivitis.

PICTURE 150

a. Syndactyly.
b. Congenital anomaly.

PICTURE 151

a. Swelling of the lips.
b. Angioedema.

PICTURE 152

a. Bilateral parotid swelling
b. Sarcoidosis, mumps

PICTURE 153

a. Buffalo hump, striae, hirsutism and puffy face.
b. Cushing's syndrome.

PICTURE 154

a. Scar of venous resection site (left leg), pigmentation on the shin of right leg.
b. CABG with diabetic dermopathy.

PICTURE 155

a. Prominent artery in the temporal region.
b. Temporal arteritis.

PICTURE 156

a. Multiple nodular lesion.
b. PKDL, cutaneous sarcoidosis, lepromatous leprosy.

PICTURE 157

a. Fixed drug eruption.
b. History of drug intake.

PICTURE 158

a. Gibbus.
b. Pott's disease.

PICTURE 159

a. Multiple erythematous rash along the butterfly distribution and forehead with baggy eyelids.
b. Lupus nephritis.

PICTURE 160

a. Eruptive vesicular lesion in the scrotum and penis.
b. Herpes genitalis.

PICTURE 161

a. Hidradenitis suppurativa.

PICTURE 162

a. Pigmentation involving the whole of the back with a Nodular swelling.
b. Malignant melanoma.

PICTURE 163

a. Multiple black pigmented rash with variable size involving whole of the body.
b. Malignant melanoma.

PICTURE 164

a. Generalized hypopigmentation with extreme cachexia.
b. Albinism.

PICTURE 165

a. Polydactyly (fingers and toes).
b. Congenital, Laurence-Moon-Bardet-Biedl syndrome.

PICTURE 166

a. Progeria.

PICTURE 167

a. Pigmented gangrenous area.
b. Pyoderma gangrenosum.
c. IBD, multiple myeloma.

PICTURE 168

a. Multiple skin rash.
b. Xeroderma pigmentosum.

PICTURE 169

a. Multiple nodular lesion on the dorsum of the both feet.
b. Chronic tophaceous gout.

PICTURE 170

a. Koilonychia and leukonychia.
b. Iron deficiency anemia with hypoprotenemia.

PICTURE 171

a. Spindle shape swelling of all PIP joints.
b. JIA.

Bibliography

1. Beynon HLC, van den Bogaerde JB, Davies KA. Data Interpretation Questions and Case Histories, 2nd Edn. Churchill Livingstone. 2000.
2. Longo DL, Fauci AS, Kasper DL, Hauser SL, Jameson JL, Loscalzo J, Harrison's Principles of Internal Medicine, 18th Edn. McGraw Hill. 2012.
3. Kumar P, Clark M. Kumar and Clark's Clinical Medicine, 8th Edn. Saunders Elsevier. 2012.
4. Walker BR, Colledge NR, Ralston SH, Penman ID. Davidson's Principles and Practice of Medicine, 22th Edn. Elsevier Science Ltd. Churchill Livingstone. 2014.
5. Sawyer N, Gabriel R, Gabriel CM. 300 Medical Data Interpretation Questions for MRCP, 3rd Edn. Butterworths. 1989.

Bibliography

Index